Health Planning
for
Effective Management

Health Planning
for
Effective Management

Edited by
WILLIAM A. REINKE

New York   Oxford
OXFORD UNIVERSITY PRESS
1988

Oxford University Press

Oxford   New York   Toronto
Delhi   Bombay   Calcutta   Madras   Karachi
Petaling Jaya   Singapore   Hong Kong   Tokyo
Nairobi   Dar es Salaam   Cape Town
Melbourne   Auckland

and associated companies in
Beirut   Berlin   Ibadan   Nicosia

Library of Congress Cataloging-in-Publication Data

Health planning for effective management.

Includes bibliographies and index.
1. Health planning.   2. Rural health services—
Developing countries—Planning.   3. Public health
administration.   I. Reinke, William A.   [DNLM:
1. Health Planning.   2. Public Health Administration.
WA 525 H4345]
RA393.H415   1988   362.1'068   87-15386
ISBN 0-19-505337-0

Preface

To be facile in applying planning techniques, health planners must be quite knowledgeable in a number of disciplines. The assessment of health needs requires basic literacy in the terms and techniques of epidemiology. Relating those needs to particular population groups of specified size requires some understanding of the methods of demography. Program planning without careful analysis of the economics involved would be foolhardy. The list could be extended, but the wide range of considerations brought to bear on health planning should be apparent.

Two decades ago, when we were about to introduce an international program in health planning into the curriculum of the Johns Hopkins School of Public Health, we were reluctant to compel students to fully absorb the vast literature in each of the relevant disciplines merely to extract key features for planning. Instead, we prepared a set of course notes that contained a digest of planning principles and methods adapted from various disciplines, as well as a presentation of planning techniques. Finding that the notes facilitated learning, we edited and published them in a volume entitled *Health Planning—Qualitative Aspects and Quantitative Techniques*. The volume, adopted as a textbook in a number of other courses in health planning and as a reference work by health planning practitioners, is now in its seventh printing. Because of their proven value, many of the sections of that volume have been incorporated into the present one, and have been updated when necessary.

This is not simply a second edition of the earlier book, however, for experience has indicated the importance of three additional emphases. The first arises from recognition that impressive *plan* documents are far more numerous than examples of successfully executed *planning*. The latter requires vigorous attention to a continuous process that integrates planning with sound management, evaluation, and problem-solving research. The present volume therefore focuses on the practical aspects of planning for implementation. This is especially stressed in the first four chapters that Part I comprises.

The concern for planning practice leads to the second new feature. Whereas much of the material from the earlier volume relating to planning principles and methods has been transferred to Part II of the present work, as we have said, Part III has been organized to provide "how to" information for the practitioner. To illustrate, discussion of manpower planning in Part II considers the interrelationship among the supply of manpower, worker productivity, and demand for services. Presentation of the same topic in Part III includes a description of the calculations necessary for deriving annual training requirements to bring supply and demand into dynamic equilibrium.

The third noteworthy point of emphasis is on development. Though many of the methods and techniques described are widely applicable, special attention has been given to the difficult task of providing essential health services to relatively scattered rural populations in developing countries with severely limited resources. In short, primary health care is the underlying theme of much of the discussion.

Since the material in this volume reflects many years of experience in teaching and working with planners, a special word of gratitude is due our students, who have been such willing learners, and to our colleagues in health care agencies around the world, who in many respects have been our most able teachers. As the editor of this volume, I wish to acknowledge with both gratitude and thanks the contributors' investment of time and knowledge in the face of numerous competing demands for their attention. Their contributions would have been for nought, of course, had it not been for the dedicated efforts of Carol Buckley, who typed numerous drafts of the manuscript and took responsibility for so many of those thankless but essential administrative tasks that are linked to manuscript preparation.

Baltimore, Md.   W.A.R.
June 1987

Contents

Contributors

Unless otherwise noted, the contributors to this volume are members of the faculty of The Johns Hopkins University School of Hygiene and Public Health.

Timothy D. Baker, M.D., M.P.H., Professor of International Health, Health Policy and Management, and Environmental Health Sciences

Margaret Bright, Ph.D., Professor Emerita, Behavioral Sciences and Health Education

Thomas L. Hall, M.D., Dr.P.H., Policy Scholar, Institute for Health Policy Studies, Adjunct Professor of Medicine, University of California, San Francisco

William A. Reinke, Ph.D., Professor of International Health, Health Policy and Management, and Biostatistics

Alan L. Sorkin, Ph.D., Adjunct Professor of International Health

Carl E. Taylor, M.D., Dr.P.H., Professor Emeritus of International Health

Health Planning
for
Effective Management

1

The Integration of Planning with Action

Planning has moved from an intuitive, spontaneous, and subjective projection of activity based on past experience to a much more deliberate, systematic, and objective process of mobilizing information and organizing resources. Carefully considered plans frequently remain unfulfilled, however, because of inadequate attention to implementation. All too often health planners have felt that their responsibility ended when they produced a plan document, thinking they could then turn over the actual work to health administrators. This tendency to remain shielded from the facts of daily life and the process of implementation is responsible for the frequently heard criticism that health planners tend to be impractical and their plans irrelevant. While some administrative separation is necessary for the objectivity required for good evaluation, continuing involvement at the peripheral field level is absolutely essential for practical planning. In the perspective of cyclic planning, implementation must be viewed as the crucial activity toward which all prior steps of planning build.

Two principles emerge from these considerations. First, planning must be recognized as part of a total process that includes policy analysis, plan preparation, management of implementation, evaluation, and research. Second, responsibility for the planning function rests in delicate balance between groups of professional planners organized into well-structured, viable units and a wide array of providers and consumers who have an identifiable stake in the outcome of planning.

With respect to the first principle, planning takes place along lines established through policy decisions. Is health in the workplace a greater political concern than health in the classroom? What are the preferred options in paying for services? Are there feasible ways of attracting physicians to underserved areas? These are questions that require systematic appraisal and resolution, often in the form of legislative mandates or executive directives. The planner can contribute to the appraisals and must be guided by the results. Policy decisions impose constraints upon the planner, but these cannot be treated as insurmountable obstacles. A key element in the art of planning is sensitivity to the necessity and feasibility of policy change in some circumstances and the need to work creatively under existing policy in other cases. In short, a two-way flow of communication between the policymaker and the planner is essential.

Policy analysis determines the routes to be traveled and the destinations, while planning establishes the means whereby the terrain is to be traversed. In carrying out this task, the planner must not only consider the feasibility of implementation, but also facilitate the implementation of what is feasible and desired. If the destination is more efficiently reached by truck than by oxcart, the road must be paved and signposts erected along the way. More directly, a plan to immunize preschool children can only succeed if careful attention is paid to worker training and motivation, adequacy of supervision and logistical support, a means of ensuring the availability of effective vaccines, and other considerations of sound management. Throughout the planning process the planner needs to work closely with the would-be program managers and service recipients to gain dedicated support resulting in realistic solutions to the problems at hand.

The need for monitoring and evaluation of planned performance is evident. Objective mechanisms for forward-looking evaluation can signal problems requiring management attention, replanning, or even policy changes. Evaluation is therefore an ongoing part of an integrated effort, not simply a police action tagged on to the end of the planning process. The consequent need to include an evaluation plan within the overall process, however, is often given inadequate attention.

Planning presupposes innovation, often with uncertain and untested results. This indicates the critical importance of small-scale pilot projects in planning. Moreover, the evaluative process is expected to uncover field problems in need of operations research. Action-oriented health services research is thus another integral component of effective planning that has generally received inadequate attention.

The broad view of the planning process espoused herein should be apparent from the foregoing remarks. In Chapter 1 we focus in more detail on the structure and functions of planning units themselves. Subsequent chapters detail implementation and management, health services research, and evaluation as they relate to the overall planning process. While the topics are most conveniently discussed separately, we must not lose sight of their interrelatedness in successful planning.

The Process, Structure, and Functions of Planning

CARL E. TAYLOR AND WILLIAM A. REINKE

Effective planning requires stepwise application of selected multidisciplinary methods and procedures to designated programs and projects within specified timeframes. Planning is not simply a technical exercise, however. It is an ongoing process of learning, adapting to change, and educating. Both features should be kept in balance in the discussion that follows.

PLANNING SCOPE AND STRUCTURE

On the basis of the scope of subject matter covered, planning can be separated into comprehensive planning, program planning, and project planning. Comprehensive planning normally provides a framework for the other types and is more closely associated with policy analysis than with details of implementation. Although concerned with practicability and feasibility, attention is on general considerations such as priorities and the relative contributions to be achieved by various types of health investment. A major interest is the balance between health services and the other important facets of socioeconomic development. With the increased specificity associated with program and project planning, greater attention to implementation, especially in relation to time scale and target setting, is obviously needed.

Plans are also distinguished according to the planning horizon encompassed. Long-term perspective plans typically cover twenty years. Intermediate-term plans most often look five years forward. Finally, there are annual plans closely tied to the yearly budgeting cycle. As in the case of comprehensiveness, the time dimension of planning bears on proximity to implementation. Perspective plans establish long-term policy directions. At the other extreme, annual plans are closely targeted plans of work for direct administrative action.

In practice, intermediate-term plans have been the most common. Often these have borne little resemblance to annual budgetary allocations which serve as the basis for action. Plan implementation has suffered as a consequence. Intermediate-term plans have also been constrained in their ability to innovate. Development of health personnel and facilities is a time-consuming endeavor that requires a prospective view extending beyond five years. More broadly, basic changes in the balance between sophisticated hospital care and community-based primary health care are not accomplished quickly or easily.[1] Increasingly, therefore, long-term perspective planning is employed to provide the basic framework within which rolling intermediate-term planning and annual plan implementation take place. The structural framework for planning must be adjusted to reflect this orientation.

Full-Time/Part-Time Dilemma

In the interest of providing continuity between planning and implementation, an early decision must be made about the relative balance of planning responsibilities to be given to representative consultant groups and to a planning unit composed of full-time staff professionals. A spectrum of different arrangements may be necessary at various levels in the planning hierarchy. These range between two polar types which will be briefly discussed.

The process of bringing together appropriate groups of health officials, members of professional societies, interested voluntary agencies, and general consumer representatives under whatever title or terminology will be called for present purposes the *part-time committee approach*. This approach is exemplified by the pattern of health planning developed in India in the preparation of the health components of the successive five-year plans.[2] The National Planning Commission was composed of cabinet members and distinguished leaders representing many disciplines. The Health Panel of the Planning Commission similarly was composed of distinguished leaders interested in health services. Under this Health Panel there were numerous committees which had the primary responsibility for decisions required in formulating the plan. Staff support for all of this intensive committee work was provided mainly by officials from the Health Ministries, both Central and State.

In the other polar type of organization, planning has revolved around an elite full-time professional group of planners. The classic example is the Soviet system of planning.[3,4] As in India, a major burst of activity tends to occur during the preparation of a five-year plan; with a full-time professional group, however, planning tends to be done more on a continuing basis. The professional planners tend to work through their own hierarchy, which reaches out from the center.

Evidence is increasing that the best planning requires an appropriate mixture of the committee approach and a full-time professional planning unit. In an analogy with political organization, the planning unit can be compared with the executive branch, while the various commissions, councils, and committees have functions which more nearly resemble legislative responsibilities. In general, an approximately equal balance of the two components is probably desirable in the central organization of planning. At the middle level effective professional units are probably more important. At the local level the committee approach becomes particularly important.

The balance of the two organizational components also varies according to the type of planning activity. The committee approach is particularly necessary in comprehensive and perspective planning, while professional expertise is most needed in program and project planning and in preparation of annual plans of work. Perhaps this is one of the reasons why thus far project and program planning have been more effectively carried out than comprehensive planning.

The professional composition of the planning unit staff is determined by the local situation and traditions. Certainly, nothing causes planning to fall into disrepute among health personnel as quickly as a lack of health professionals in the planning groups. These health professionals should be respected for their practical experience and technical competence.[5] Although a new specialty of health planning seems to be developing, it seems desirable that professionals who take this special training should first have practical experience in general health programs. Of great importance in organizing the information system and undertaking the necessary analyses is strong representation of statistical skills. In view of the mounting evidence that the new techniques of systems analysis and operations research have much to contribute to health planning, some representation from this area should be incorporated, especially at the higher levels in the planning hierarchy. The planning team should also include a member with competence in health economics. Additional specialties which can profitably be included, perhaps through consultant arrangements, are public administration and the social sciences. Because of the tremendous importance of budgeting procedures in ensuring implementation, special expertise in budgeting and accounting is valuable. Finally, as planning focuses on particular substantive areas, such as the control of particular diseases or special subjects such as sanitation, the best technical experts in these areas must be available.

In setting up a smoothly functioning planning machinery, it is vital to define clearly the role of each member of the planning team.[6,7] Assigning technical responsibilities usually appears fairly obvious. Clear statements of responsibility are needed, however, to define the relationships among the professional planners and the innumerable other groups and individuals who should be involved in the planning process. Such liaison relationships may sometimes be shared among members of the planning team. Some of these, such as associations with special consumer groups and professional societies, require the careful choice of appropriate individuals and delicate handling. For optimum implementation a direct linkage with all levels of the administrative hierarchy and with the institutions where health activities are carried out is also necessary. Some planners feel that they must have their offices located in direct proximity to the highest executive authority, even in the office of the president. Just as important in the long run, however, are good channels of access to all levels of the official hierarchy.

Centralization/Decentralization Dilemma

No unresolved problem in the planning process recurs as continually as the question of the appropriate balance between centrally directed and peripherally initiated activities. One reason that this issue continues to be so pervasive is that generalizations are difficult. On the spectrum ranging between complete centralization and decentralization, the appropriate balance point in any planning situation must be determined by complex local considerations. In general, the most important determinants are intangibles in the local political and social milieu. Popular participation is largely conditioned by tradition and culture. In those health programs whose success is determined primarily by the extent to which individuals cooperate, it may be important for participants to feel that the whole plan was their own idea in the first place. The extent to which people are willing to take direction from outside may also show great local variations. Judgment about such matters requires the experience that comes from practical involvement with particular groups of people.

A generalization derived from experience is that the usual tendency is to have too much centralization initially.[8] This may be partly because most early efforts in planning were in situations which provided maximum centralized control, such as the typical United States corporation or the Soviet political system. This is certainly the most comfortable situation in which to plan. The planner works in a clear hierarchy. Assuming that it is possible to convince the decision makers at the top about the appropriateness of the plan, the planner has the feeling that implementation will naturally follow. Reasonable as this may appear, the clearest evidence from past experience is that such reliance on central control does not work. Even the Soviets are finding that they have to move increasingly toward decentralization of their elaborate planning machinery.

Some mass health programs do tend to have highly centralized planning and implementation. This is usually most successful when activities are directed primarily toward changing the environment, with minimum need for modifying the habits of people. Sanitation and malaria eradication are examples that come to mind. Even in such programs, however, planners have found it wise to work hard at gaining local participation and interest. Health activities more closely related to personal living require progressively greater decentralized involvement.

Enthusiasm in implementation is directly correlated with the extent of local involvement in planning. On the other hand, planning just does not happen spontaneously, and the move to decentralization can be carried too far. Certain responsibilities can be handled best from the center and others better at the periphery. An attempt will now be made to distinguish among some of the elements that need to be considered in this balance of functions.

Centralized Responsibilities

Early in the planning process aims must be defined, and this requires a large measure of central direction. Local units, of course, should have some opportunity to contribute ideas and suggestions. The real work of defining plan goals and balancing their importance, however, requires the highest level of responsible policy-making representation. A broad range of understanding is necessary, especially in relation to other aspects of development such as roads, communications, education, and economic growth.

Another major responsibility which must be primarily central is the specification of resource constraints. Planners must be told what the health services will have to work with, and then judgments must be made at the central level concerning limitations to be placed upon the funds and personnel which are centrally controlled. The central unit must also make overall estimates of contributions expected from local participation, allowing for variation in what individual peripheral units actually decide to contribute to particular health activities; such local decisions are, however, usually in the direction of expanding a particular project or program above the average for other local units.

A third responsibility which is primarily centrally controlled is adherence to basic plan priorities. This means that in the implementation process special central effort will have to be directed toward stimulating action in areas of deficiency.

Similarly, the establishment of the total organization and machinery of planning is primarily a central responsibility. The objective should be to have the planning machinery reach out as far as possible through the total range of public and private health services. The participation of private agencies is often one way to obtain the particularly important general objective of including representatives of all consumer groups. The significant organizational effort which is required to ensure this range of involvement must be initiated by the central planning unit. Efficiency demands a certain degree of standardization in relationships.

Another central responsibility must be the review of project plans and area plans prepared by peripheral groups. Local judgments based on knowledge of specific situations must be transmitted through a progressive screening process. Final approval, then, must be at some appropriate regional or central level where a sufficient range of proposals can be studied to give a balanced overall view of priorities.

A final planning activity that is primarily a central responsibility is evaluation. Some continuing evaluation, of course, has to be built into the routine of any good local administration; the principal responsibility for evaluation as part of the planning process should, however, provide a considerable degree of external objectivity. An important part of such overall evaluation is comparison with other areas and projects, and this can clearly be done best at the central level.

Decentralized Responsibilities

Simply stated, the components of decentralized responsibility in planning are those residual functions not assumed by central authorities. However, the appropriate locus for the initiation of action in specified circumstances must be defined explicitly.

Effective data gathering is organized centrally, but the quality obviously depends on local involvement. If personnel at the periphery where the data originate know the purpose for which the data will be used, then there will be much more interest and precision in obtaining valid information. Any sort of feedback by which peripheral units can see the tangible contributions of their data will lead to an automatic improvement in validity.

Although general priorities usually originate in central planning groups, permitting considerable flexibility to local units in final determination of priorities has great advantage. Great effort can go into educating local groups to accept centrally chosen priorities. On the other hand, by taking care of problems which are already of local concern, it is frequently possible to induce communities to move on to other priorities of which they were at first not aware.

Particularly important is that planning detailed programs be done by peripheral units.[9,10] Nothing promotes successful implementation as much as having communities feel that the planning hierarchy has been set up mainly to help them with their own planning. The most successful planners create a feeling of participation at peripheral levels so that credit for achievement is also decentralized.

Even more than other parts of the planning process, final implementation should be worked out at the local level. One of the more important considerations in implementation is allocation of responsibility for particular functions; this obviously requires knowledge of and accommodation to local organizational pressures and personal claims. More positively, implementation is mainly a process of finding the right persons to do particular jobs, and this can be best achieved locally with appropriate opportunity for self-selection.

At the local level, success in plan implementation depends on the participation of several diverse groups.[11,12] Perhaps most important are the local professionals who are directly responsible for health services. No other group can so completely block the implementation of a plan. This may happen even when they agree with the concepts and practical decisions proposed. If they were left out of earlier stages of the planning process and feel that something is being imposed on them, they can obstruct implementation just by withholding support. Obtaining effective participation of professionals is usually not difficult if it becomes evident to them that this is the best way of protecting their own interests and status. The proliferation of professional associations of doctors, nurses, midwives, all ranges of specialists, and numerous paramedical groups may seem too complex to make it worth the trouble of maintaining liaison. One advantage of keeping in touch with all groups, however, is that those who are most cooperative can influence the others. It should even be possible to develop a desirable spirit of competition among professional groups who realize that they might be left behind.

Efforts to include lay and consumer groups in the planning process also facilitate effective implementation. A major benefit is that such involvement can provide direct access to major gaps and areas of deficiency in services. Consumer participation is most essential in programs which have a large component of personal services. Since identifying appropriate community leaders is usually difficult, simply including representatives of interested agencies, especially those that are voluntary, is tempting. This does not necessarily ensure representativeness of consumer groups, however, and it is usually necessary deliberately to reach out to include those most in need.

As a local planning unit undertakes implementation of plans, it is important to recognize that a major ingredient of success is the art of capturing the right moment. Since implementation requires the simultaneous interaction of multiple forces, a high degree of opportunism is needed. Transitory shifts in opinion or personnel and temporary availability of funds may produce openings that require alert implementation even if all planning details have not been worked out.

PLANNING AS AN EDUCATIONAL PROCESS

Important as organizational relationships and responsibilities are in planning, success depends ultimately on individual attitudes, motivations, and competencies. Planning is largely an educational process. Planners' efforts will be proved effective not so much by what they do themselves as by what they persuade others to do. In spite of all that is said about the difficulty of educating the public, planners often need to concentrate even more educational effort on administrators and health personnel. The opinions of health workers are often harder to modify than public attitudes because of their greater personal investment in traditional ways of doing things.

A simple definition of *organized planning* is the use of systematic approaches to enable diverse individuals to agree on mutually satisfactory ways of carrying out complicated activities. Left to themselves, individuals naturally do things in their own way. They feel that methods they have learned or worked out are inherently best. Much mutual education, along with friction, occurs when individuals from different backgrounds work together. With the increasing complexity of health services such friction can be more disruptive than educational, however. Good planning should facilitate smoother mutual learning. Like most educational efforts, this should be realistically recognized to be a slow process.

Developmental change is primarily dependent on improved motivation. Public motivation starts with an interest in the immediate benefits of medical care. Professional guidance is needed in adjusting to a time scale of expected health improvements in which the public learns to think beyond immediate needs for curative services to the greater, though delayed, benefits of preventive and promotive activities.

Health personnel and administrators tend to be somewhat ambivalent in their approach to planning activities. Their investment in traditional activities and personal career goals makes them suspicious of planned change. A favorable motivation to change can be induced most readily by deliberate manipulation of incentives. Career and monetary rewards can be related directly to demonstrable improvements in services offered. An educational approach to plan implementation should be characterized by efforts to promote cooperation rather than to impose coordination.

STAGES OF THE PLANNING PROCESS

Experience in health planning has led to the identification of a series of systematic stages in the planning process.[13] To a considerable extent these stages parallel the commonly accepted steps of the scientific method as applied to research. Planning explores the uncertainties of how the best use can be made of limited resources to meet priority needs. It has, therefore, much of the intellectual challenge of research.

Planning is a dynamic process; hence it is not in practice a single movement up a rigidly structured static stairway of steps. Rather it is an unending upward spiral of incremental efforts toward improvement. The purpose of the present categorization of the elements of the planning process is to provide a general framework or outline of functions to be performed to ensure a systematic approach.

In reality, many activities should be carried out concurrently, providing a mutually supportive flow back and forth among various stages of the process, depending on local conditions and requirements. Such variations lead at different times and places to great differences in the balance among the amounts of planning input required for various steps of the process. Important determinants are the level of development of the country and such mundane questions as whether data are already available or must be laboriously gathered. The structure and function of the planning machinery must also be adjusted to local conditions. Flexibility is desirable, especially at the start, when adaptations are more necessary and frequent.

Developing Planning Competence

In any planning structure the policy-making body must represent the political power structure, the general public, and health professionals.[2,9,11,12,14] The balance among these three groups is determined largely by the type of planning to be undertaken. In broad-gauge comprehensive planning it is particularly important to ensure that the health activities fit general public desires; hence the proportionate representation of consumers should be great. In many types of program planning and project planning, which should themselves fit in with a general comprehensive plan, the particular competence required is more technical in nature; thus, representation on the policy-making group can be weighted more toward the health professional.

In general, the planning unit should be closely associated with the administrative structure but not directly involved in administration. Its success is often determined by its ability to make itself useful to administrators. This may involve undertaking a variety of service tasks for the administrative or institutional units with which the planners work. Effective planning, however, requires the ability to move easily at all administrative and organizational levels and lines of communication. It is, therefore, important to avoid being tied down with routine chores. While it is desirable to be as high as possible in the administrative hierarchy in order to gain as much authority as possible, it is also important to refrain from dissipating too much technical energy around conference tables of policymakers and committees which talk rather than act. Moreover, access to the most peripheral units in fieldwork brings an important realism into planning.

Since planning is largely an educational enterprise, substantial effort must be devoted to teaching the planning methods to be used throughout the administrative structure. Once the members of the planning unit have themselves received the best training available, they should organize special training programs for those with whom they work. Some of the most effective planning organizations have devoted a great deal of energy to organizing short courses in planning which are attended by all levels of health personnel.[15] In addition to teaching technical planning, data gathering skills, economic theory, and analytic methodology, such a systematic educational program can have a unique impact by developing enthusiasm and an esprit of cooperative action.

Statements of Policy and Broad Goals

Planning policies and goals must be politically determined.[11,14] The first lesson for the health planner to learn is to avoid imposing personal predilections on the planning process. Instead, skill must be developed in gauging and mobilizing political opinions. In order to set the stage for effective implementation of the plan it is essential to make sure at the start that planning goals fit the policies of the political group responsible for implementation.[16,17]

One of the best educational maneuvers that a planning group can use in conditioning the political structure to which it is responsible is to require the policy-making group to go through the difficult exercise of explicitly stating plan aims. Too often goals are left so vague and general that they are little more than platitudes. By taking the time at the beginning to induce policymakers to arrive at explicit statements, much time is saved later when the details of planning and implementation are being worked out. An important step at this stage is to distinguish clearly between long-term goals and short-range objectives. Both should be stated with clear recognition of time and priority implications.

Planners can profitably promote the idea among policymakers that planning is their best way of being leaders rather than followers of public opinion. To ensure that planning is dynamic rather than static, they must recognize its cyclic nature. After following the steps of the planning process through a plan period, the time comes when policymakers are back to the first step again and must revise the plan objectives on the basis of experience gained. Continuity must be maintained by constantly looking ahead to the next plan period.

Information for Planning

If planning had no other reason to exist, it would not be hard to justify it on the basis of improvements made in the information systems within the health services. [15,18] Some planning groups serve primarily as statistical units, and just by making information available to appropriate decision makers they have a major planning impact. For instance, the National Health Council has for many years fulfilled a useful voluntary role in the United States by collecting and analyzing information. [12,19] The relative amount of time which a planning unit must devote to data gathering depends, of course, on the existing statistical organization. Where the sources of information are good, the planning unit needs only to adjust the data to particular planning objectives. Where data are deficient, the planning unit may have to design its own surveys or establish other data gathering systems.

A particular benefit of good planning is that it provides a basis for judgment in sharpening the selection of truly useful data. A well-known weakness of statistical organizations is that they collect so much junk. Tradition and habit, along with outmoded reporting formats, maintain a flow of irrelevant and redundant numbers which make it difficult to sort out truly meaningful data. To start with, the burden of excessive form filling may cause outright fabrication or at the best rushed estimation at the peripheral unit where the data start. Excessive flow through the information system means that not only are the data not trusted but they are not even looked at. Good planning requires early attention to eliminating from the information system all items not related to clear plan objectives and functional use.

In health planning, data customarily start with demographic information. The basic unit of health care is obviously the number of people to be served and their distribution. Because of the rapid rate of population growth in most developing countries, it is particularly essential to have the most accurate population projections possible.

The second category of information is epidemiologic, specifically information on the frequency and distribution of major health problems. In developing countries this is often very spotty. Because of the chronic difficulty of collecting accurate mortality and morbidity information, an immediate need is oftentimes to organize some sort of sample survey. Certainly the patient selectivity factor makes hospital and other institutional reports of disease only minimally useful.

In many places the most serious deficiencies of planning information are in economic data. Most health people have little idea of what sort of information might be useful for economic analyses. The simplest type of information is usually accurate cost accounting of specific health activities, although the calculations become more complicated with the inclusion of indirect costs. Many of the more sophisticated measurements of items which would be useful in economic analysis, especially of the cost-benefit type, are still to be developed.

Another category of information which usually must be specially developed for planning purposes concerns the utilization of facilities and the functional patterns of work of various types of personnel.[20] Planning can make its most dramatic contributions in short time periods by increasing efficiency of utilization. This requires careful attention to the process of setting work standards and performance budgeting. Without an adequate data system, such rationalization of the services is obviously impossible. A related type of information is basic administrative data on the availability and projection of both personnel and facilities resources. Finally, more sophisticated research is necessary to develop ways of measuring demand for various categories of services.

Priority Statement of Health Problems

Setting priorities is considered by most health administrators to be the heart of the planning process. The steps leading up to this point can in a way be considered preparation for the crucial decisions involved in priority setting. Once priorities have been set, the subsequent steps can be considered progressive moves toward implementation. In priority setting judgment and wisdom are most needed, together with a unique ability to synthesize the numerous relevant details. It is the part of the planning process which is usually considered most intuitive. Priority setting, however, can perhaps benefit more than any of the other steps from being made an explicit and clearly defined exercise.

The greatest skill required in priority setting is to balance variables which have very different quantitative relationships and in fact lie in different dimensional scales. Too often mistakes arise from giving undue stress to one dimension. The epidemiologist tends to view priority setting as primarily a matter of defining relative mortality and morbidity from specific health problems. This approach was overdone in the first versions of the "Latin American method" of health planning.[21] Social scientists, politicians, and the public tend to view priority setting as mainly a response to popular feelings about what is important. To them the important considerations are what the public wants done and what health programs will be acceptable. Administrators tend to view priorities mainly in terms of what the Latin American health planning method has called the "vulnerability" of particular health problems. The concern is with the availability of technical methods for controlling the diseases or conditions requiring attention. Perhaps the most serious limitation in developing countries, often even more restrictive than lack of money, is the question of whether there is an administrative framework to provide services and necessary personnel.

Economists lay particular stress on cost. This is usually the final constraint which determines what will be done, and the relative costs of various control programs must be balanced. The underlying policy in balancing costs in health planning generally is to put more stress on providing adequate care for the maximum number of people, rather than the highest-quality care for a selected few.

The health planner must develop skills in all of the preceding disciplines sufficient to provide a balanced approach to each. Particularly needed are valid specific indices for both the quantitative and qualitative types of information implied in these judgments. Despite all attempts at measurement and specific categorization, the planner will in the end have to rely on the indefinable elements of wisdom from experience or from evaluation of previous plans in making the final decisions.

Plan Outline with Statement of Major Alternative Proposals

With the priority decisions in hand, it is necessary to begin to work out the alternative proposals which represent possible ways of coping with the health problems defined. A clear statement of alternative approaches provides a basis for deciding what should in fact be done. This involves actually specifying many of the underlying considerations which were gathered and balanced in the course of priority setting. The advantages at this stage of a clear outline for each alternative approach is that it provides a ready basis for comparison. Of the four approaches to analysis listed in the discussion of priority setting, the attention now shifts largely to the latter two: administrative and economic. Particular points to be included in the outline include (1) a clear definition of the technical aspects of the program, (2) the organization framework required, (3) the personnel and facilities needed, (4) costs in comparable financial terms, and (5) approximate benefits to be expected in relation to priority of concern.

One of the more complicated issues at this stage is the problem of deciding whether to undertake health activities that have multiple impacts on several health problems or those that have only a single impact. Since decisions between alternatives must be based largely on a cost-benefit type of judgment, it seems that benefits should be greater in programs that have multiple health contributions. At this stage in planning methodology, however, these essentially intuitive and approximate cost-benefit judgments usually cannot be put into the economic formulations normally associated with cost-benefit analysis.

At this point, the distinctions among comprehensive planning, program planning, and project planning should be recalled. Comprehensive planning provides the general framework for development; it is particularly concerned with the problem of priorities and the relative stress to be given to various programs and projects. It provides the overall conceptual structure within which program and project planning can be done. The most effective detailed planning, then, is at the program and project level. Program planning is directed toward broad-impact activities that affect a number of health problems. Project planning is the most focused and limited; it tends to be concerned with high-impact health activities directed against single health problems. It also tends to be more clearly limited in its time perspective.

Development of Detailed Plan with Targets and Standards

Construction of a detailed plan document is usually worked out in phases. Long-term goals are specifically stated, along with the proposed steps necessary to carry them out. Any programs requiring several years must be stated in flexible terms. Increasing detail and specificity can be introduced for more immediate periods, such as the next year.

As already noted, one difficult issue to be decided is the balance between centralization and decentralization in the planning process. The probability of achieving successful implementation of a detailed plan is proportionately increased with greater local involvement in the programming. If local units can be assigned responsibility for developing detailed programs on the basis of general procedures set up by the central unit, more spontaneous enthusiasm and active participation will be brought to the task.

In shifting the planning balance toward decentralization and local involvement, two major controls should be built in by central planning units. The first is the development of appropriate standards for performance. Since a good set of realistic standards can evolve only through experience, the initial set will necessarily have to be arbitrary and approximate. A major advance can be expected in subsequent cycles, however, if deliberate effort has been devoted to gathering the necessary information to permit more precise standard-setting as the plan is implemented.

Similarly, target-setting is an appropriate part of the central unit's responsibility. Targets should be specified according to quantitative indices of performance and within a clearly stated time framework. As with standard-setting, establishment of precise targets can be expected to improve with progressive implementation in successive plan periods. Both standard-setting and target-setting should be attempted from the beginning, however, in order to provide a rational basis for evaluation. Above all they should be realistic and based on the general human response that work effectiveness improves most if built on a reasonable experience of success. They should never be so likely to produce failure as to be punitive devices.

Implementation as Part of the Planning Process

The concept of planning as a dynamic and continuing activity requires that implementation be an integral part of health planning.[8] Early experiences in planning concentrated merely on the development of the plan as a document. Implementation was considered the responsibility of the service organizations assigned particular activities. No error in planning is more common or more serious than such a narrow perspective on the planning process.

Implementation can be considered an important part of the planning process from two quite distinct points of view. Traditionally, comprehensive planning has been considered a process in which the entire health service should be involved; planning has been viewed as only a normal step in good administration. In this inclusive view implementation is intimately associated with both planning and administration, so that the three aspects are not easily separated.

More recently health planning has gained recognition, at least potentially, as a discipline in its own right. Such a view clearly distinguishes the planner from those responsible for ongoing activities. If the planner is thus to be placed in an atmosphere of objective detachment, important questions arise concerning the planner's role in the process of implementation. Clearly, the plan itself must incorporate detailed planning for implementation, but the health planner must set up the conditions which give the plan the greatest likelihood of being successfully carried out.

The first tactical step in plan implementation is to gain acceptance of the plan. A completely innocuous plan which merely confirms existing conditions, of course, has the best chance for acceptance. The more innovative the plan proposal, the more difficulty there will be in inducing political leaders, health personnel, and the public to agree. If a plan is to do some good, it should contain the seeds of progressive change.

The probability of acceptance of plan proposals increases proportionately with the extent to which health personnel, political leaders, and the consumer public participate in the planning process. The document produced will probably be less coherent and polished than one produced by planning technicians alone. Still, it seems wise to keep the balance as much toward decentralization as possible. Each particular situation requires an individualized determination of what this balance should be.

Evaluation and Replanning

Evaluation is such an important part of the total dynamic process of planning that many functioning units are called *planning and evaluation units*. At one time there was a conceptual problem growing out of the notion that we were dealing with three separate activities: planning, implementation, and evaluation. The modern view, however, is that it is all one process of a cyclic nature, with the evaluation step leading directly into the initiation of a new planning cycle.[22]

Two fundamentally different types of evaluation must be distinguished: continuing evaluation for administrative purposes and periodic, more focused evaluation specifically for plan revision. Particularly important to the administrator is continuing self-evaluation by local administrative health units. If the planning process can encourage local units to undertake systematic self-evaluation and provide them with appropriate know-how and mechanisms, this will be perhaps the best possible means of building in continuous improvement. In addition, a major role of the planning organization is to undertake continuing administrative evaluation to see that standards and targets are being met. One of the best ways for planners to establish their usefulness is to show that they can fulfill an important service role to the administrators. A natural service activity with great practical value to most senior administrators is a tough, frank approach to evaluation. In any centralized/decentralized balance, this naturally tends to continue as an important role of the central units.

The second major type of evaluation is more definitely related to the planning process. A centrally directed activity has to be set up with the primary purpose of quantifying achievement in particular planning periods. Such activity tends to be timed to precede the evolution of a new major plan or the modification of an existing one. This kind of exercise should extend considerably beyond mere measurement of achievement in terms of previous standards and targets. It should concentrate on assessment of such basic issues as whether the original goals and objectives were in fact appropriate; whether resource development is actually moving in the direction most suited to local conditions, in terms of both facilities and personnel; whether the priority setting was, in fact, justified by further experience; and especially whether the data gathering system is producing useful information. Such an evaluation does not happen spontaneously. It has to be worked out with as much ingenuity and innovative precision as any other part of the planning sequence.

A final comment must be made about the need for objectivity in evaluation. One of the more intractable obstacles to change is the innate human conviction that whatever one is used to doing must be right. Normal human pride of involvement leads to an almost uncontrollable subjective bias. Innovation requires both a willingness to give up even the most sacrosanct culturally accepted ways of doing things and an openness to the new.

REFERENCES

1. Djuikanovic, V., and E. P. Mach, *Alternative Approaches to Meeting Basic Health Needs in Developing Countries*, Geneva: World Health Organization, 1975.

2. Government of India, Administrative Reforms Commission, *Study Team on the Machinery for Planning: Final Report*, New Delhi: Government of India Press, 1968.

3. Field, Mark G., *Soviet Socialized Medicine*, New York: The Free Press, 1967.

4. Zhuk, A. P., *Public Health Planning in the USSR*, Bethesda, MD: Fogarty International Center, 1976.

5. *Training in National Health Planning*, WHO Technical Report Series No. 456, Geneva: World Health Organization, 1970.

6. Takulia, Harbans S., et al., *The Health Center Doctor in India*, Baltimore: The Johns Hopkins University Press, 1967.

7. Department of International Health, Johns Hopkins University, *The Functional Analysis of Health Needs and Services*, New Delhi: Asia Publishing House, 1976.

8. Waterston, A., "An Operational Approach to Development Planning," *International Journal of Health Services*, 1:223–252, 1971.

9. Hochbaum, G. M., "Consumer Participation in Health Planning: Toward Conceptual Clarification," *American Journal of Public Health*, 59:1698–1705, 1969.

10. Blendon, R. J., and C. R. Gaus, "Problems in Developing Health Services in Poverty Areas: The Johns Hopkins Experience," *Journal of Medical Education*, 46:477–484, 1971.

11. Conant, Ralph W., *The Politics of Community Health*, Washington: Public Affairs Press, 1968.

12. National Health Forum, *Planning for Health*, New York: National Health Council, 1967.

13. *National Health Planning in Developing Countries*, WHO Technical Report Series No. 350, Geneva: World Health Organization, 1967.

14. Arnold, M. F., "Basic Concepts and Crucial Issues in Health Planning," *American Journal of Public Health*, 59:1686–1697, 1969.

15. Hall, T. L., "Planning for Health in Peru–New Approaches to an Old Problem," *American Journal of Public Health*, 56:1296–1307, 1966.

16. Kissick, W. L. (ed.), "Dimensions and Determinants of Health Policy," *Milbank Memorial Fund Quarterly*, 46, No. 1, Part 2, January 1968.

17. Kissick, W. L., "Health Policy Reflections for the 1970's," *New England Journal of Medicine*, 282:1343–1354, 1970.

18. Kennedy, F. D., *Basic Concepts Required in the Development of a Planning Information System*, RM-OH-387-1, Research Triangle Park, NC: Research Triangle Institute, November 1968.

19. National Commission on Community Health Services, *Comprehensive Health Care: A Challenge to American Communities*, Washington: Public Affairs Press, 1967.

20. Bice, W., and K. L. White, "Cross-National Comparative Research on the Utilization

of Medical Services," *Medical Care*, 9:253–271, 1971.

21. Ahumada, J., et al., *Health Planning: Problems of Concept and Method*, Scientific Publication No. 111, Washington: Pan American Health Organization, 1965.

22. *Methods of Evaluating Public Health Programmes*, Copenhagen: World Health Organization, Regional Office for Europe, 1968.

PRIMARY READINGS

Agarwala, Ramgopal, *Planning in Developing Countries: Lessons of Experience*, Washington: World Bank, 1983. Provides an in-depth review of developing-country experience in planning, noting that most plans have failed to live up to expectations. Steps to remedy this situation are outlined. Prepared as a background paper for *World Development Report 1983*.

Cook, W. D., and T. E. Kuhn (eds.), *Planning Processes in Developing Countries: Techniques and Achievements*, New York: North-Holland, 1982. Part of the series Studies in Management Sciences, offering a number of perspectives and insights derived from planning experience.

Djuikanovic, V., and E. P. Mach, *Alternative Approaches to Meeting Basic Health Needs in Developing Countries*, Geneva: World Health Organization, 1975. Report from a major WHO/UNICEF study that paved the way for primary health care.

International Health Perspectives: An Introduction in Five Volumes, Association of American Medical Colleges, New York: Springer Publishing Co., 1977. A self-instructional course in five volumes for students interested in pursuing a career in international health or involved in the health care system of a developing country.

Primary Health Care, Geneva: World Health Organization, 1979. Report of the landmark International Conference in Primary Health Care held in Alma-Ata, USSR, in 1978. First volume in the Health for All series.

Primary Health Care Bibliography and Resource Directory, Washington: American Public Health Association, 1982. Comprehensive annotated bibliography and directory of resources. Headings include planning and management, manpower training and utilization, community participation and health education.

Roemer, Milton I., *Health Care Systems in World Perspective*, Ann Arbor, MI: Health Administration Press, 1976. The author has carried out comparative analyses of diverse health systems worldwide.

SECONDARY READINGS

Blum, Henrik, L., *Planning for Health: Development and Application of Social Change Theory*, Berkeley: University of California Press, 1974.

Gish, O., *Guidelines for Health Planners: The Planning and Management of Health Services in Developing Countries*, London: Tri-Med Books, 1977.

Golladay, F., and B. Liese, *Health Issues and Policies in the Developing Countries*, Staff Working Paper No. 412, Washington: World Bank, 1980.

National Health Planning in Developing Countries, WHO Technical Report Series No. 350, Geneva: World Health Organization, 1967.

Reinke, William A. (ed.), *Health Planning: Qualitative Aspects and Quantitative Techniques*, Baltimore: The Johns Hopkins University, 1972.

Schofield, Frank, "Health Planning in Developing Countries," *Impact of Science on Society*, 25,3:181-257, 1975.

Spiegel, Allen D., and Herbert H. Hyman, *Basic Health Planning Methods*, Germantown, MD: Aspen Systems Corp., 1978.

Training in National Health Planning, WHO Technical Report Series No. 456, Geneva: World Health Organization, 1970.

2

Management Analysis

WILLIAM A. REINKE

Objective appraisal of many health plans quickly reveals the unlikelihood of success-ful implementation. It is both easy and satisfying to propose improved service cover-age through an expanded network of well-equipped and well-staffed health facilities directed by highly motivated primary care physicians. Without realistic consideration of costs of construction and operation, time required for implementation, augmented supervisory and support services needed, and indeed feasibility of attracting compe-tent staff to underserved areas, these proposals are not likely to move beyond the stage of paper exercises.[1]

Granted the essential need for planning to be conducted so as to facilitate imple-mentation, the present chapter is intended to provide a checklist of major manage-ment issues requiring attention if planning is to be meaningful.[2] Consideration of specific methods and techniques of management within each of the areas discussed is a large undertaking beyond the present scope of concern in spite of its obvious importance. For example, we emphasize that a well-functioning basic health services system requires a simplified, well-controlled drug list.[3] We do not, however, elabo-rate upon specific stock control schemes. Selected techniques for implementation are described in greater detail in Part III of this volume.

In order for the list of management issues to be most useful, it should be developed within the context of current thinking about the organization and delivery of essential health services.[4] The attention given in recent years to expansion of services through primary health care has important management implications, as we have already suggested. To illustrate further, if the notion of community participation is to be taken seriously, traditional practices in top-down hierarchical management must be carefully reconsidered. Accordingly, the next section outlines certain features of health systems that are increasingly emphasized and giving direction to health planning and management. These basic features form the backdrop for the discussion of specific management issues that follows thereafter.

RECENT DIRECTIONS IN HEALTH PLANNING

Health planners are intent upon devising means to improve service coverage in more efficient and effective ways. In recent years the notion of coverage has taken on added significance as issues of equity have been highlighted through such slogans as "health for all."[5] Concern for efficiency has directed attention to competency-based training of peripheral workers, including community members, employing appropriate technology. Finally, considerations of effectiveness have led to the search for improved measures of program impact that encompass community desires and satisfaction.

These considerations have been embodied in three important developments: (1) specification and provision of basic health services to currently underserved populations, (2) decentralization of decision making in accordance with varied local needs and desires, and (3) increased community participation in the planning, management, delivery, and evaluation of services. The broadening of both the delivery system and the decision bases places a premium on the development of an expanded system of competent and coordinated management.[6] Moreover, the increased need for qualified managers arises after a long period of relative inattention to training needs in health services administration, apart from hospital management. In spite of their scarcity, doctors have been assigned major administrative responsibilities with little or no prior management training.

Balance of Essential Services

Apart from traditional organizational and management considerations the key to effective provision of primary health care is balance. Services must be selectively provided in response to community need with balanced attention to curative and preventive care. Facility-based care must be balanced against the need for outreach services. Finally service and educational efforts must be balanced with the aim of promoting community self-reliance. There is a natural tendency for health professionals, from their perspective as the sole providers of health care, to remain in their clinics to respond to whatever curative needs may present themselves. An industrial management with this concept of "marketing" is doomed to failure. Such imbalance in the public service field is even more unconscionable.

Decentralization

Actual cases are all too common in which vehicles at remote outposts remain in inoperative disrepair awaiting approval for spare parts from a high official at the provincial or national capital. Many top administrators jealously guard this course of power. Other public servants may be more enlightened but are forced to act similarly because of the absence of trained managers to whom responsibility can be safely delegated, coupled with the lack of a viable system of accountability. While decentralization of decision making has many obvious advantages in principle, it is unworkable in practice in the absence of a broadly based cadre of competent managers working within a well-organized framework that promotes coordination, communication, and control based upon adequate flow of selectively useful information. Just as peripheral service providers require competency-based training in line with clearly specified standing orders and referral procedures if they are to provide safe and effective care, local managers must receive practical instruction and operate under well-established management systems and supervisory procedures, combined with provision for passing on exceptional cases to superiors for resolution.

Community Participation

Although concern is often expressed over the total lack of health services coverage for large segments of the population, the fact of the matter is that most communities have access to some kind of care, often in the form of traditional midwives and untrained indigenous healers. The issue, then, is the more effective utilization and supplementation of existing resources. The community can do much for itself if its resources are appropriately mobilized and organized. The private sector cannot be ignored, especially in regard to provision of curative services. There is a role for the public sector. These three elements must be integrated into an overall system that functions better as a whole than its separate parts have in the past.

This is a significant management challenge. The supervision of health workers who are employed by and responsible to the ministry of health is difficult enough. But how does one motivate and supervise volunteers who are responsible to the community and are not a part of the classic system? In the ultimate case where the community itself is the "boss," management becomes even more complex.[7]

SPECIFIC MANAGEMENT ISSUES

We have stressed the need for plans that facilitate implementation. We have further observed that recent directions in planning have, if anything, heightened the importance of carefully designed strategies for program implementation and management.[8,9] We now outline a number of specific management issues that result. As already noted, space does not permit a full elaboration of management techniques required. Indeed, these must be adapted to local circumstances. The following commentary should, however, provide a convenient checklist of management issues to keep in mind in the process of planning and subsequent implementation, monitoring, and evaluation.

Synchrony of Resources Development

Experience suggests that facilities are the easiest element to plan. Thus examples of empty hospitals and unused health centers are numerous. Training seems to be the next easiest task, especially in the case of minimally trained workers or volunteers. There is a satisfaction gained in being able to cite the quantities of personnel who have been trained and are currently in place. Seldom is there evidence, however, that the personnel are doing what they were trained to do, that they are adequately supervised or able to make appropriate referrals (such capacity may not yet exist), or that the personnel are adequately supported by a functioning supply and transportation system.

The lesson learned from these experiences is that synchronization of resources development is critical. Management of the resources allocation function is essential to efficient operation. The more complex and time-consuming tasks must be initiated first, rather than postponed simply because they are difficult. Only under such conditions will the personnel and other resources be available at a time when the overall infrastructure is in place to utilize the resources efficiently.

A corollary to this principle is that it is often necessary to begin with a relatively narrow scope of services selectively based upon community priorities and system capabilities. Planned, phased expansion can take place thereafter. Regardless of the initial scope of services, their ultimate expansion and integration must be anticipated to ensure flexibility. For example, it is difficult to reorient malaria workers to broader responsibilities if they have been too narrowly trained initially.

Direct and Indirect Control

The control function is central to management. As the roles of the community and the private sector are expanded and explicitly recognized in planning, control by health professionals becomes a potentially ambiguous blend of direct and indirect responsibility. Moreover, authority and responsibility must be in balance for effective action to take place. It is essential, therefore, that responsibility for and authority to control be clearly and harmoniously incorporated into program planning. Planners themselves must clearly distinguish between their roles in planning for public sector direct interventions and in regulating private sector initiatives.

To the extent that services are community-directed, as well as community-based, health professionals take on more of a technical supportive role than one of direct leadership. Distinctions among line, staff, and functional management have always complicated organizational relationships. The importance of these distinctions, and of the difficulties associated with them, is increasingly manifested in community relationships as well.[10]

Services Organization

Integration of basic health services is widely accepted, but integration means different things to different people. From the client's perspective the ideal is contact with a single provider who has a wide range of services to offer according to individual needs at the time. Operationally, however, there are economies associated with specialization. Furthermore, there is a limit to the range of capabilities for which a minimally trained health worker can be prepared.

These varied and sometimes conflicting considerations lead to the notion of technical and administrative integration. Multipurpose workers combine several skills, in contrast to the system in which malaria workers perform functions which are distinct from those of sanitarians and vaccinators. Even where workers are specialized, they may function within an administratively integrated multifaceted program in contrast to organizations with separate categorical programs for malaria control, tuberculosis control, family planning, and so forth. The resulting combinations, each vaguely labeled "integrated," are numerous. Frequently one finds that most services are administratively integrated, while a few major programs remain organized categorically. At the community level, where services are ultimately delivered, several supervisory links are in effect. Multipurpose workers may receive direction and technical supervision from several sources. At the other extreme one supervisor may direct the efforts of several differentially specialized workers. Other intermediate combinations could be cited.

In planning it is obviously necessary to provide for the form of organization that makes most sense in the local context. In doing so, planners must bear the following in mind: consequent criteria for personnel recruitment, worker training needs and potential, administrative leadership requirements and training implications, and organization relationships and management structure once the workers and supervisors are trained and functioning.

A significant management challenge arises from the fact that remote, sparsely populated areas are least able to take advantage of the benefits of specialization and are the most difficult to supervise. As a result, workers in these areas are called upon to function quite independently as generalists; yet personnel in these areas are likely to be the least skilled. Utmost selectivity in task assignment becomes crucial, along with exceptional stress on competency training in carrying out the limited tasks.

Even in less remote areas there is much to be said for teamwork and the generalist approach.[11] If flexibility is not provided in carrying out the functions of workers on leave or otherwise not available, those tasks will be unattended. Uncertainties of services availability, in turn, discourage the community from seeking them. Furthermore, the logistical problems in field supervision through a number of functional specialists make such arrangements ineffectual in most cases. In short, the generalist approach to management and dedication to team effort do not receive the endorsement they deserve.

Human Resources Development

The preceding sections have related to overall concepts of organization and management. Management issues arise as well within specific segments of the health care system. Perhaps the most important of these issues relate to personnel development.[12]

First, it is necessary to specify clearly the *tasks* and *skills* appropriate to individual workers and to define working relationships among personnel. What kinds of auxiliaries would be best in the particular context? What objections can be expected from professional associations? How can the ratio of preventive to curative services be optimized and maintained? To what extent should outreach and educational activities be fostered? What contact should frontline workers have with householders and how often? What collaboration should auxiliaries have with other workers?

A corollary consideration is career mobility. Worker categories should be sufficiently unique to avoid overlap and damaging connotations such as "near doctor." On the other hand, there are definite advantages in placing the rungs of the career ladder sufficiently close together so that more competent workers have continuing opportunity for advancement.

Once worker categories and numbers needed are defined, criteria for selection must be established. What are the prospects for retraining in contrast to fresh recruitment? Should recruits be selected from and returned to the same community? How important are community status and acceptance in contrast to more objective criteria such as educational qualifications and aptitude?

Next come training considerations. What should be the length, content, and form of training? Where should it take place? Who are the best trainers? What is the appropriate balance between didactic and practical components? What mix of initial and in-service training should be provided?

A much-neglected follow-up to training is the assessment of job performance.[13]

Are workers doing what they were trained to do? Are they doing it well? Are skills not utilized really needed? Should these subjects be dropped from the curriculum? Are workers called upon to perform tasks for which they were not trained? Should these subjects be added to the curriculum? Are workers aware of their limitations and properly referring cases they are not prepared to handle? In short, establishment of congruence among community needs, worker performance, and their training is a continuing aim of any health care system.

It follows that continuing education should be an integral part of any personnel development program. Supportive supervision, an essential element of effective management, is perhaps the best form of continuing education. While the policing, controlling, warning, and disciplining actions of supervisors unfortunately tend to dominate, the supervisor role in supporting, counseling, teaching, and motivating workers can contribute much to better job performance. When auxiliary workers face a problem in patient management, the temptation is great for the supervisor to take over, thereby undermining the status and confidence of the auxiliary. The supportive supervisor, on the other hand, serves as consultant and teacher in such a situation. Training for supportive supervision is therefore an important element of planning to facilitate implementation.

Regardless of how well trained a worker may be, performance may be impaired by low morale. Monetary compensation is important in this regard, but it is not sufficient in itself, notably in the case of volunteer workers. Other incentives must be devised. We have already mentioned the quality of supervision and collegial relationships, as well as opportunities for advancement. The challenge to devise other means of promoting morale is as important as it is difficult.

Physical Environment

Large facilities concentrate higher-level technical personnel, ancillary services, and resources, thereby pleasing and facilitating the work of doctors and inspiring the confidence of nearby communities. Such facilities likewise stand as visible monuments of support from ministries of health and international donors. On the other hand larger facilities quickly absorb the limited curative budget so that far fewer small facilities can be built close enough to communities to be available for primary care. Hence, building one larger unit instead of several smaller units raises the clinical standard of care for a privileged minority by depriving the less-well-off majority of minimal care. Furthermore, sophisticated facilities anywhere tend to emphasize clinically based curative services while discouraging preventive and promotive outreach services.

Determination of the number, distribution, and capabilities of facilities is a major planning task with significant management overtones. Rational planning tends to favor a multifacility system in the interests of improved access and coverage, but it also mandates careful attention to the hierarchy of services to be offered, requires a well-functioning referral system for successful implementation, and significantly broadens and complicates the base of supervision.

Provision of adequate supporting services is an important management problem in any case and becomes a more complex issue in a multifacility system. Simple standardized drug lists must be prepared at each level of the system, along with provision for control over drug dispensing which balances safety and flexibility. The need for a supply system free of bottlenecks calls attention to restrictions on importation, licensing, and foreign exchange; prospects for local compounding of imported raw materials; and provision of warehousing and inventory control mechanisms. While, ideally, decision making in drug control should be widely dispersed, this is such a profitable enterprise that control in practice typically is jealously maintained centrally.

Laboratory services present a somewhat different management problem. Since they require special equipment and skills, the question arises as to where specimens will be taken and where they will be analyzed. When service points are widely dispersed, the resulting logistical problems are horrendous. Inadequate management of laboratory services can jeopardize the effectiveness of workers throughout the system and result in underutilization of expensive personnel and equipment.[14]

Transport support is another element of the health care system that can either facilitate or impair its functioning as intended. Transport is needed for supervision, outreach, and referral. Optimal forms of transport differ according to local conditions and according to its varied purposes. Determination of appropriate transport requirements and methods for ensuring that they are met and maintained are important management issues.

Referral systems are chronically ineffective, and the fault goes beyond lack of transport and communication. The "bypass" phenomenon, in which patients pass a nearby facility enroute to a crowded hospital or health center in town, is common. For the referral system to be truly effective, confidence in the local facility must somehow be attained and meaningful flow of patient information to the referral point and back must be established.

Finally, maintenance of both vehicles and equipment is a frequently unresolved management problem. Foreign equipment is often supplied without provision for maintenance services. Where local maintenance is possible, bottlenecks still occur because of the lack of skilled mechanics or because of a rigid, centralized decision making structure which precludes prompt, timely action.

Financial Management

The creation of physical resources and skilled personnel requires budget allocations in the first place, of course, and productive use of these resources depends upon well-oiled fiscal machinery for recurrent expenditure and control.

Too often planning and budgeting are carried out as essentially independent functions as if the former were merely an idle paper exercise. Even when funds have been authorized, their actual disbursement is frequently delayed by a cumbersome bureaucratic process requiring multiple layers of approval. As a minimum, these delays damage service morale. More than this, they can bring program operations to a virtual standstill.

Success in decentralization is based, in large measure, on a meaningful system of accountability. Financial accountability is a major component of this system. Frequently the associated administrative capability simply does not exist, or, if it does, it is so cumbersome and rigid that it is of little value. Attaining appropriate control while maintaining adequate flexibility is an important management task.

Information Systems

Communication and coordination are central to effective management. These in turn require efficient information flow. As in the case of fiscal management, information management is often excessively cumbersome, devoid of useful data meaningfully analyzed and interpreted, or a little of both. In fact, information systems are typically characterized by a superabundance of data and a dearth of useful information. As a result, much time and effort are devoted to report preparation, but the reports are seldom used for decision making.

Information is needed for client management, program monitoring and management, and evaluation. Ultimately the information should contribute to program improvement or redesign. Thus, information systems must be detailed and highly specific to current conditions and actions while providing cumulative summarization for purposes of management decision making and evaluation.

The principles of "management by objectives" and "management by exception" must be borne in mind. Program objectives and progress toward those objectives need to be understood, along with the associated decision points. One must determine who needs what information when in order to take what kind of action.

While concern for timely and rational decisions is at the heart of information system design, personnel other than decision makers must be considered as well. It is necessary to establish who should gather information, who should receive it for decision purposes, and who needs to know the decisions made. Although these roles may be filled at different organizational levels, it is important to keep in mind that data gatherers are not likely to perform their job very well if they fail to see the value of the information provided and receive no feedback on decisions made as a consequence.

The "management by exception" principle suggests that routine information systems should provide a comprehensive survey of all potential problem areas, that is, "exceptions" that could arise, but realistically they cannot be complex enough to supply solutions to all contingencies. Problems (exceptions) identified by the routine information system can be investigated selectively by more intensive data gathering and analysis at a second stage. Thus, management information systems and operations research go hand in hand.

REFERENCES

1. *Primary Health Care: Progress and Problems*, Washington: American Public Health Association, 1982.

2. *Managerial Process for National Health Development: Guiding Principles*, Geneva: World Health Organization, 1981.

3. *The Selection of Essential Drugs*, WHO Technical Report Series No. 641, Geneva: World Health Organization, 1979.

4. Kleczkowski, B., R. H. Elling and D. L. Smith, *Health System Support for Primary Health Care*, Public Health Papers No. 80, Geneva: World Health Organization, 1984.

5. *Primary Health Care*, Geneva: World Health Organization, 1979.

6. Coombs, Philip H. (ed.), *Meeting the Needs of the Rural Poor: The Integrated Community-Based Approach*, New York: Pergamon Press, 1980.

7. Korten, David C., "Community Organization and Rural Development: A Learning Process Approach," *Public Administration Review*, September 1980, pp. 480–511.

8. *Strengthening Ministries of Health for Primary Health Care*, WHO Offset Publication No. 82, Geneva: World Health Organization, 1984.

9. *Managerial Analysis of Health Systems: Technical Discussions of the XXI Pan American Sanitary Conference*, Washington: Pan American Health Organization, 1983.

10. Korten, David C. (ed.), *Population and Social Development Management: A Challenge for Management Schools*, Caracas: Population and Social Development Management Center, 1979.

11. Korten, Frances, and David C. Korten, *Casebook for Family Planning Management: Motivating Effective Clinic Performance*, Chestnut Hill, MA: The Pathfinder Fund, 1977.

12. Bechtell, Rosanna M. (ed.), *Low-Cost Rural Health Care and Health Manpower Training: An Annotated Bibliography with Special Emphasis on Developing Countries*, Ottawa: International Development Research Centre, 1980.

13. Katz, F. M., and R. Snow, *Assessing Health Workers' Performance: A Manual for Training and Supervision*, Public Health Papers No. 72, Geneva: World Health Organization, 1980.

14. Cheesbrough, M., and J. McArthur, *A Laboratory Manual for Rural Tropical Hospitals*, Edinburgh: Churchill Livingstone, Robert Stevenson House, 1976.

PRIMARY READINGS

Bainbridge, J., and S. Sapire, *Health Project Management: A Manual of Procedures for Formulating and Implementing Health Projects*, WHO Offset Publication No. 12, Geneva: World Health Organization, 1974. A basic work on health programming for developing country managers.

Kleczkowski, B., R. H. Elling and D. L. Smith, *Health System Support for Primary Health Care*, Public Health Papers No. 80, Geneva: World Health Organization, 1984. A wide-ranging discussion of issues that includes personnel planning; cost and financial options; health care facilities, equipment, supplies; management systems; community participation; and intersectoral linkages.

Korten, David C., and Felipe B. Alfonso (eds.), *Bureaucracy and the Poor: Closing the Gap*, Singapore: McGraw-Hill International Book Co., 1981. Must reading for those interested in new, more workable approaches to management of social development. Also discusses trends in management training in response to changing perceptions regarding development.

Managerial Process for National Health Development: Guiding Principles, Geneva: World Health Organization, 1981. No. 5 in the Health for All series, this is a seminal work on formulation of national health policies, broad programming, program budgeting, master plan of action, detailed programming, implementation, evaluation, reprogramming, and information support.

McMahon, Rosemary, Elizabeth Barton and Maurice Piot, *On Being in Charge: A Guide for Middle-Level Management in Primary Health Care*, Geneva: World Health Organization, 1980. Practical, down-to-earth guide on how to manage a health care program.

SECONDARY READINGS

Baumslag, Naomi, et al., *AID Integrated Low Cost Health Projects*, Washington: U.S. Agency for International Development, 1978.

Bechtell, Rosanna M. (ed.), *Low-Cost Rural Health Care and Health Manpower Training: An Annotated Bibliography with Special Emphasis on Developing Countries*, Ottawa: International Development Research Centre, 1980.

Coombs, Philip H. (ed.), *Meeting the Needs of the Rural Poor: The Integrated Community-Based Approach*, New York: Pergamon Press, 1980.

Katz, F. M., and R. Snow, *Assessing Health Workers' Performance: A Manual for Training and Supervision*, Public Health Papers No. 72, Geneva: World Health Organization, 1980.

Korten, David C. (ed.), *Population and Social Development Management: A Challenge for Management Schools*, Caracas: Population and Social Development Management Center, 1979.

Korten, Frances, and David C. Korten, *Casebook for Family Planning Management: Motivating Effective Clinic Performance*, Chestnut Hill, MA: The Pathfinder Fund, 1977.

Morley, David, Jon E. Rohde and Glen Williams (eds.), *Practicing Health for All*, New York: Oxford University Press, 1983.

O'Connor, Ronald W. (ed.), *Managing Health Systems in Developing Areas: Experiences from Afghanistan*, Lexington, MA: Lexington Books, 1980.

Peters, Thomas J., and Robert H. Waterman, Jr., *In Search of Excellence: Lessons from America's Best Run Companies*, New York: Warner Books, 1982.

Primary Health Care: Progress and Problems, Washington: American Public Health Association, 1982.

Strengthening Ministries of Health for Primary Health Care, WHO Offset Publication No. 82, Geneva: World Health Organization, 1984.

3

Health Systems Research in Relation to Planning

WILLIAM A. REINKE

Planning connotes change, and change often produces unpredictable or unanticipated results. It would seem natural, therefore, to require that the expected effects of new health programs be confirmed through systematic research prior to wide endorsement and implementation. Certainly it would be considered poor business practice if a private manufacturer introduced a new product that had not been adequately re-searched, developed, and test-marketed in advance. Similarly, in public health matters the planning, research, demonstration, and routine implementation phases must be consciously and closely linked.

The fact that these links are frequently not forged stems in large part from the attitude that the problems to be tackled are obvious and the solutions are simple. The bulk of controllable morbidity and mortality occurs in infancy and early childhood. Much of the ill health at these ages is due to diarrhea, respiratory illnesses, and immunizable diseases that make such an exceptional impact because of underlying conditions of malnutrition. Vaccines, antibiotics, and oral rehydration therapy of proven cost-effectiveness are available to deal with these problems. Thus, the attitude is, Give us the needed money, materials and personnel so that we can get on with the job. To be effective, however, resources must be properly organized and managed. This raises a number of perplexing dilemmas along even the most well-defined paths to action. Consider the following:

- How can knowledge of appropriate health practices be most effectively imparted to parents?
- Given the knowledge, to what extent can the family engage in proper self-treatment, for example, in preparing oral rehydration solutions?
- How many of the individually simple tasks can be reasonably assigned to village-level workers without overburdening them?
- In view of transport and other constraints, how can supportive supervision and continuing education for these workers be ensured?
- How can availability of vaccines and drugs be ensured; for example, is kerosene for refrigerators readily available or must other mechanisms be used to prevent spoilage?

In short, research has provided the technology that permits us to plan affordable solutions to many of our most pressing health problems. To achieve the possible, however, often requires systematic problem solving through field-based investigations in the form of health systems research.

SCOPE AND FEATURES OF RESEARCH

We need to examine more closely the range of circumstances in which research questions arise, so that we may discern the underlying features of health systems research. We will then have the necessary framework for categorizing the content of investigations and describing the relevant approaches and methods of study.

Research questions can arise at the planning stage when the choice among alternative interventions remains unclear. For example, what is the most appropriate balance between outreach and clinic-based services? Demonstration questions form a second category. To illustrate, although the effectiveness of village health workers in home visiting may have been established in one district, feasible means of providing ongoing supervision, training, and resupply throughout the entire province or nation may have to be investigated and demonstrated. Finally, specific questions worthy of special study may arise in the course of routine implementation and monitoring. It may be noted, for example, that the monthly schedule of field supervisory visits is inadequate for some personnel and excessive for others. What objective performance criteria might be employed to determine the need among certain workers for more intensive supportive supervision?

Although research issues can arise at any stage of program planning or implementation, they have certain common characteristics. First, aims should be clearly defined, even if the means of achieving the intended outcomes are uncertain. The research can be evaluated only in the presence of measurable objectives. Second, the investigation is inevitably designed to test alternatives and leads to comparative analysis. The effects of two or more interventions may be compared, or a trial intervention may be compared with a designated standard, with "present practice" elsewhere, or with prior achievements in the area in which change has been introduced. Thus, research involves more than casual observation of experience; it requires rigorous, objective, comparative appraisal. Nevertheless it is pragmatic in addressing daily problems in the operational setting in which they occur. This leads to another characteristic that distinguishes health systems research from classical research. Whereas classic research designs tend to focus only on effects or outcomes, the problem-solving research that interests us here must consider the use of resources (i.e., inputs) as well. As a minimum we must ask whether the contemplated intervention is affordable in practice; frequently we go so far as to ask whether it is cost-effective, that is, whether it is able to achieve the most that can be gained with limited resources.

The comparative measurement of inputs, as well as results, is especially important in connection with replication. A service program is sometimes introduced on a small scale with the intention of eventual wider replication. This aim displays naïveté in that it is unlikely that a program should be exactly duplicated everywhere. Programs are seldom good or bad; rather, some components work in some settings better than others. The nutrition education component may not be very effective, whereas the immunization component is; the feeding centers may produce some nutritional improvements but only at excessive cost; the mobile teams may be useful in some sections of the country but not in others. Only through careful measurement of individual program effects and inputs can the comparative analysis succeed in carrying out the fine-tuning that is necessary to achieve increasing efficiency and effectiveness over time and over wider geographical areas.

Health systems research is complicated in another way. Because it is carried out in the community, it includes multiple variables not easily controlled. This means for one thing that the research is multidisciplinary. To illustrate, causal factors in the behavior of clients must be considered, along with the basic efficacy of treatment. A second ramification of the multivariate nature of the investigation is the consequent importance attached to statistical analysis. Where variables can be controlled in advance, study design for exerting that control becomes crucial and subsequent analysis of findings is relatively straightforward. To the extent that the sorting out of variables can only take place in analysis, however, the choice of analytical method becomes paramount. It follows that there is no fixed methodology associated with health systems research. A wide range of techniques from varied disciplines is employed as circumstances dictate.

Matched against the seeming complexity of field research is the need to provide program managers with timely information for decision making. Researchers generally value quality of findings and search for optimum conditions. Administrators, on the other hand, seek prompt solutions that are "good enough," even if not fully optimal. Health systems researchers must therefore take seriously the need for timeliness, even at the sacrifice of some sophistication. There are times when comprehensive new programs need to be tested, and in these cases adequate time must be allowed for the full effects and interactions to emerge. More often, however, research should be limited to sharply focused questions that can be answered satisfactorily in a matter of weeks or months, not years. Even then, the number of variables to be considered is likely to make the analysis quite formidable.

We have referred to *health systems research*. We prefer that to the term *health services research* to emphasize concern for the entire system, not only the delivery of services. Others have spoken of action research, operations research, or operations analysis.[1] While the terms have caused some confusion, together they convey the notion that research as a necessary adjunct to health planning is accomplished successfully only if it is practical, action-oriented, and based upon real operational issues. It will be endorsed by planners and administrators only if designed to produce prompt solutions to recognized problems.

ILLUSTRATIVE RESEARCH ISSUES

In order to emphasize the practical nature of health systems research, we highlight in this section a number of specific topics currently receiving investigative consideration. While the list is not intended to be exhaustive, it is organized by themes that generally cover the range of system concerns.[2]

Associations of Causality and Consequent Interventions to Be Considered. Research is primarily necessary to identify priority problems and to create a better understanding of the forces impinging upon them.[3] The problems may be disease problems, or they may relate to health behaviors. Why, for example, are certain providers utilized or not utilized for certain conditions? The research may also test the efficacy of interventions intended to alleviate the problems identified. Again, the interventions may relate to specific health conditions, as in the case of nutrition surveillance, or they may address behavioral concerns, as when village health workers are introduced in the hope that their physical and social proximity to the client population will enhance service utilization.

Personnel Development and Deployment. Because personnel is the most costly and important resource in the labor-intensive health sector, it presents numerous needs and opportunities for research.[4] Intensive efforts in recent years to extend services further into the periphery have led to studies of worker role reallocations. The realignments, along with increased use of minimally skilled personnel, have called attention to the need for innovative methods of training. The broadened base of care has likewise focused attention on inadequacies in supervision and the need to examine alternative supervisory schemes.

Community Participation. Community resources must be considered in parallel with providers formally associated with the health care system. The role of village health committees, the selection and training of community workers, and cost recovery through various community financing schemes are all subjects that have been studied widely.[5]

Physical Resources. Essential as human resources are, they can be only as effective as the physical environment allows.[6] Criteria for the siting of health facilities to promote access deserve study, along with schemes for providing outreach from the fixed facilities. Chronic shortages of drugs and supplies prompt systematic review of replenishment cycles and procedures. Similarly frequent cases of vehicle breakdowns and misuse cause investigation of maintenance policies and schedules.

Financing. Reference has already been made to community financing schemes.[7] More generally, improved service coverage leads to increased cost and consequent demand for cost recovery. How can services be paid for without inhibiting utilization by the needy? This is a critical research question that has led to consideration of a variety of payment schemes, including forms of prepayment and insurance.

Organization and Management. Apart from concern for the resources themselves, problems with their organization and management are legendary.[8] The concept of decentralization is endorsed, but the search for effective ways to achieve it continues. Integration of services is likewise supported in principle, while operational meanings remain ambiguous and deserving of systematic investigation. Management information systems are widely discussed, but decisions continue to be made on the basis of limited or faulty data. What does it take to get minimal information in the right form to the right place at the right time? The question has received some attention from statisticians. Like so many other questions, it needs more research attention from the clients themselves, the managers who need the information for better decisions.

APPROACHES AND METHODOLOGY

We have already observed that the methodologic approach to health systems research is eclectic. A system of classification is possible, however, and offers further insights into the nature of research. As the various categories are outlined, bear in mind the one constant in all of them. It is necessary to establish measurable objectives and then to evaluate associated outcomes in comparison with one another, with other empirical findings, or with hypothesized results.

Natural Experiments

Frequently alternative interventions are already employed in different places, so that comparative analysis of existing data is possible. For example, there may be some health centers with two nurse-midwives, some with only one, and a few with none at all. Thus it is possible to compare work patterns and utilization levels under these naturally varying circumstances. The advantage of natural experiments is that the duration of the study is short; in effect it has already taken place. Moreover analysis can be relatively inexpensive inasmuch as some or all of the data may already have been collected. The danger, of course, is that the underlying reasons for the observed variation may not be fully understood and incorporated into the analysis. The need to identify and account for the effect of uncontrolled factors is especially critical here if misleading or erroneous conclusions are to be avoided.

Synthetic Analyses and Simulations

Synthetic analyses are one level of sophistication above natural experiments. Comparison is made among a range of existing conditions in order to predict outcomes under related, perhaps more favorable, circumstances. To illustrate, village health committees may vary in the amount of money collected from local families to support village workers either through fixed salary or fee for services. Analysis of the varied experience may suggest optimal arrangements somewhat different from any tried thus far. The projected ideal should then be tested and confirmed in practice, of course.

Beginning with a sample of real data, computers can simulate in seconds several years of additional "experience" to establish patterns and to draw inferences about optimal conditions.

Systematic Program Monitoring

The longitudinal monitoring and analysis of events is not very different qualitatively from the assessment of past experience. The longitudinal aspect, however, permits more careful observation of the host of factors and changes that may affect results in addition to variables of direct experimental interest. To illustrate this approach, consider the question of the effect of age and marital status on acceptability and performance among providers of maternity care and family planning. If both young, single girls and older, married women are employed, they can be followed systematically over time in order to detect outcome differences of interest. The systematic appraisal would also include measurement of community and other differences that could confound the findings if their presence were ignored.

Focused Testing of Interventions

The prospective testing of a specific intervention comes closest to the classical research design. Consider the matter of selective supervision. Workers in one group of villages receive supervisory visits on a fixed, bimonthly cycle. Workers in an experimental group of villages are visited selectively according to recent performance. In particular, suppose that those who have had fewer than eighty antenatal contacts or fifty well-child visits per month are visited monthly, whereas other workers are visited quarterly.

The study design is simple and straightforward but requires that the intervention be unambiguously defined and uniformly applied, that the intended outcome be specified (improved average performance, reduced variance in performance, or reduced cost of supervision), and that possible effects of nonexperimental factors be accounted for.

Testing of Comprehensive Programs

We have emphasized the importance of sharply focused research questions that give program managers quick answers to current problems. There are times, though, when incremental change and piecemeal solutions are inadequate; more fundamental change is called for. Primary health care is a case in point. While the principle of "health for all" represented a fundamental change in commitment to health care, questions of feasibility in practice have been raised. It has been argued that attempts to provide all components of primary health care to entire populations will fail to mobilize the needed critical mass of resources in priority areas such as malaria control, immunization, or family planning. These concerns have led to calls for selectivity of services and designation of high-risk groups for focused attention.[9]

Others have pointed out possible administrative efficiencies in providing several services together, as well as possible synergisms in effectiveness, for example, in connection with interactions between infection and malnutrition. Such considerations have led to calls for more effective integration of services.[10]

The need clearly exists for more fundamental research that investigates alternative service mixes. Such research is complex and does not produce objective conclusions easily or quickly. The effort would certainly be more productive, however, than current rhetoric and undocumented opinion.

Mathematic Models: Operations Research Techniques

The term *operations research* has been used rather loosely in reference to studies of operational problems. More technically, the field has come to be associated with certain techniques of mathematical modeling.[11] As already noted, health status is difficult to quantify and even more difficult to relate precisely to specified levels of service inputs. Thus mathematical techniques of operations research have limited applicability in health matters. Nevertheless a brief discussion of them is useful in offering insight into the value of careful structuring of problems, even when precise definitive solutions are not possible. Linear programming, one of the best known of the techniques, is illustrated first in some detail to provide better understanding of the mathematical modeling approach. Briefer reference is then made to other major classes of analysis through operations research.

The *linear programming model* has three distinct features. First, there is an objective function to be optimized. For example, an organization providing a variety of services seeks to establish the service mix that is most beneficial in a defined sense. Second, there are constraints on the resources (inputs) available to produce the desired results (outputs). To illustrate, some of the services in the contemplated mix may require specific skills that are in short supply. Finally, it is assumed that all relationships are linear and additive. In particular, if five units of input are required to produce twelve units of output, then ten units of input will yield twenty-four units of output. Moreover, the increase from twelve to twenty-four units of output of type A is assumed to produce the same benefit regardless of the amount of output B also provided.

Suppose that a nutrition education program is to be undertaken with the aid of government health educators, community health workers, or a combination of the two. Each government health worker (G) can make 1,000 service contacts (S) annually, whereas each part-time community worker (C) can be expected to make only 300 contacts per year. The annual cost of maintaining a government worker is $2,000, compared to $400 per community worker. The personnel budget for the program totals $72,000 per year. On the face of it, therefore, community workers would seem to be preferred. Each would provide 300 services for $400, or $1.33 per unit of service, compared to $2.00 per unit of service with government health workers.

Before launching the program one year hence, however, it is necessary to train the workers to provide the new service, and in this regard government workers have an advantage because of their previous experience with health matters. In particular, the capacity exists to train 120 government workers, whereas only half as many community workers could be trained with currently constrained resources.

How many of each category of worker should be trained, and what service level should be achieved as a result? The situation described satisfies conditions of linearity. An objective function,

$$S = 1,000G + 300C,$$

is embedded in the scenario. The service level (S) is to be maximized, subject to the constraints:

$$2,000G + 400C \leq \$72,000 \text{ and } G + 2C \leq 120.$$

The conditions are depicted graphically in Figure 3.1. Limitations on budget are shown by line DC; those on training are shown by line CB. The budget, for example, will accommodate as many as 36 government workers, 180 community workers, or

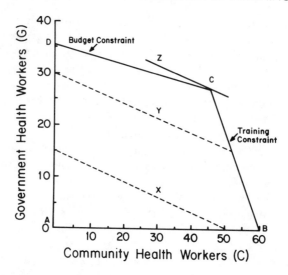

Figure 3.1   Graphic portrayal of linear programming

any combination of the two falling on or below line *DC*. Thus, any feasible solution to the optimization problem must lie within the boundaries of *ABCD*.

Lines *X*, *Y*, and *Z* depict combinations of workers that would yield selected service levels. Any combination on line *X*, for example, would result in 15,000 service contacts, whereas all combinations along line *Y* are associated with 30,000 contacts. Other lines parallel to *X* and *Y* could be drawn for different service levels. Higher service levels are associated with lines above and to the right of *Y*. The highest feasible service level is that which is barely within the constrained boundary *ABCD* at point *C*. This point relates to 26 government workers and 47 community workers. Such a combination would provide 40,100 service contacts at a cost of $1.77 each. This, then, is the optimal solution.

A major advantage of the linear programming approach is that it permits evaluation of existing constraints. In the preceding illustration it was determined that the potential benefits from reliance upon community workers was partially thwarted by constraints in training capacity. What if $2,000 from the personnel budget could be reallocated to increase training capacity by 25 percent?

Application of linear programming techniques to the revised model reveals that it would be optimal to train and employ 22 government workers and 64 community workers. This combination would provide 41,200 service contacts at an average cost of $1.69 each. The expected benefits to be gained from relaxation of the training constraint would be clearly worth the cost.

Conditions encountered in practice typically contain many more variables and constraints than we have illustrated. In such cases graphic techniques are no longer feasible. Computerized algorithms have been devised, however, to accomplish the more complex purposes through application of the principles illustrated.

A more serious problem in practice lies in the formulation of an objective function. The relative value of various services cannot be readily quantified in most cases.

Moreover, client acceptance of available services cannot always be taken for granted, as was done in the illustrative case. Valuation of benefits is necessarily made implicitly, if not explicitly, however, and the implications of value judgments and constraints must be assessed in a manner similar in principle to the linear programming approach, even if mathematical elegance is not possible.

In addition to linear programming, distribution and queuing models have been widely applied and deserve brief mention in relation to health systems. *Distribution models* were originally formulated to determine the least costly means of supplying several distributors from existing supply depots or production facilities. They answer the question, Which depot or manufacturing plant should supply which distributor? The possible application to drug supply systems should be apparent. Likewise these models could serve to determine which clinics should use which referral points. The question is a significant one when referral points have insufficient capacity to accept all patients from the nearest referring centers.

Queuing models are employed in the analysis of waiting lines, whether they be people waiting for service or hospital beds available for use. An obvious application in the health field is an analysis of the flow of patients through a health center or through various hospital services. In particular, a clinic accepting walk-in patients must allow for the random nature of arrivals. Paradoxically, random arrivals tend to occur unevenly in clusters. If long patient waits for service are to be avoided, extra service capacity must be maintained in readiness for the chance occasion when patients arrive in rapid succession. Queuing methods can be employed to establish the appropriate balance between patient waiting time and personnel idle time. The methods can be used as well to ascertain the potential benefits of an appointment system. Similarly, in the case of hospital admissions, queuing methods have been applied to the scheduling of elective procedures.

INSTITUTIONALIZATION OF RESEARCH

By now the value of research in relation to planning should be clear. Moreover, a number of specific problems worth investigating should have become apparent. What remains is the need to provide an environment conducive to productive research. Meaningful investigation is not likely to proceed on an institutional scale until operating agencies exhibit genuine commitment to research by rewarding research productivity and offering career advancement opportunities for competent researchers.

The way in which research is institutionalized varies. Some ministries of health establish working relationships with universities and research institutes for carrying out individual studies under contract. In other cases separate research divisions are set up within the ministry of health itself. Some ministries combine planning, research, and evaluation in a single unit. The important point is that the problem-solving capability be as close to the source of the problems and decision-making responsibility as possible. Where the problems are in the field and the research competence is in the university, a dilemma exists. Effective linkages must be forged, and those in the academic setting must be made to appreciate the importance of practical, timely solutions to real-world problems. Especially in health systems research, the motto "learning by doing" has meaning, and competence is more readily gained in the field than in the classroom. Operating agencies should therefore make a determined effort to develop in-house research capability as quickly as possible. Because of the multidisciplinary nature of the research, however, associations with disciplinary specialists in the academic world should be maintained, and indeed multidisciplinary networks need to be strengthened.

Ultimately ministries of health must establish and maintain community laboratories in support of public health activities just as medical schools have affiliations with teaching hospitals. The community laboratories should reflect the best that is routinely available in health care delivery, so that they can provide high-quality training for service providers and program managers. They should also offer a pioneering climate for seeking practical routes to further health system improvements.

It is sometimes argued that the community serving as the laboratory soon becomes oversurveyed and takes on an artificial character that limits generalization of findings from any studies carried out. There is some merit to this concern, but it serves only as a challenge to public health comparable to the pressure continually exerted on curative services to ensure that practice in teaching centers is appropriately transmitted to community hospitals and to general practice.

REFERENCES

1. Grundy, F., and William A. Reinke, *Health Practice Research and Formalized Managerial Methods*, Public Health Papers No. 51, Geneva: World Health Organization, 1973.
2. Taylor, Carl E., *The Uses of Health Systems Research*, Public Health Papers No. 78, Geneva: World Health Organization, 1984.
3. Ghana Health Assessment Project Team, "A Quantitative Method of Assessing the Health Impact of Different Diseases in Less Developed Countries," *International Journal of Epidemiology*, 10,1:73–80, 1981.
4. Reinke, William A. (ed.), *Functional Analysis of Health Needs and Services*, New Delhi: Asia Publishing House, 1976.
5. Metsch, Jonathan, and James Veney, "Measuring the Outcome of Consumer Participation," *Journal of Health and Social Behavior*, 14:368–374, 1973.
6. Llewelyn-Davies, Richard, "Planning Health Facilities in Developing Countries: Some Case Studies and Their Lessons," *World Hospitals*, 12,3:159–163, 1976.
7. Stinson, W., *Community Financing of Primary Health Care*, Primary Health Care Issues Paper No. 4, Washington: American Public Health Association, 1982.
8. Were, Miriam K., *Organization and Management of Community-Based Health Care*, New York: UNICEF, 1980.
9. Walsh, J. A., and K. S. Warren, "Selective Primary Health Care: An Interim Strategy for Disease Control in Developing Countries," *Social Science and Medicine*, 14,2:145–163, 1980.
10. Kielmann, Arnfried A., et al., *Child and Maternal Health Services in Rural India, The Narangwal Experiment; Vol. 1: Integrated Nutrition and Health Care*, Baltimore: The Johns Hopkins University Press, 1983.
11. Halpert, Harold P., William J. Horvath and John P. Young, *An Administrator's Handbook on the Application of Operations Research*, Washington: National Institute of Mental Health, 1968.

PRIMARY READINGS

Fisher, Andrew, John Laing and John Stoeckel, *Handbook for Family Planning Operations Research Design*, New York: The Population Council, 1983. A simple, practical handbook that details research steps using concrete examples from family planning, with description of methods that are readily generalizable.

Grundy, F., and William A. Reinke, *Health Practice Research and Formalized Managerial Methods*, Public Health Papers No. 51, Geneva: World Health Organization, 1973. Discussion of basic research concepts and description of principal methods followed by a series of case studies.

Taylor, Carl E., *The Uses of Health Systems Research*, Public Health Papers No. 78, Geneva: World Health Organization, 1984. A comprehensive presentation of the subject that includes several illustrative applications.

SECONDARY READINGS

Brownlee, A., et al., *Health Services Research Course: How to Develop Proposals and Design Research to Solve Priority Health Problems*, Brazzaville: WHO Regional Office for Africa, 1983.

Halpert, Harold P., William J. Horvath and John P. Young, *An Administrator's Handbook on the Application of Operations Research*, Washington: National Institute of Mental Health, 1968.

Reisman, Arnold, *Systems Analysis in Health Care Delivery*, Lexington, MA: Lexington Books, 1979.

Research for the Reorientation of National Health Systems, WHO Technical Report Series No. 694, Geneva: World Health Organization, 1983.

4

Health Services Program Evaluation

WILLIAM A. REINKE

Evaluation is more often discussed, less understood, and less practiced than virtually any other concept associated with planning and providing health services. The need to evaluate program performance is readily accepted in principle. On the face of it, then, one might be surprised that so little conscientious, systematic evaluation is observed in practice. Too often what takes place is little more than a superficial *ex post facto* justification of whatever actions have been taken.

On closer examination, the gingery approach to evaluation is not so surprising. Sensitivity arises from the focus on retribution for *past* failures or reward for accomplishments; in either case, these are events over which the program manager no longer has control. Since programs usually produce mixed results, the inevitability of some failure seems to weigh more heavily on management than the elements of success. To be genuinely useful, evaluation must be viewed as a means to improved decision making for *future* action.[1]

SCOPE AND PURPOSE OF EVALUATION

What, precisely, does this imply? Evaluation is not simply a before-and-after comparison of program impact. It begins at the planning stage with appraisal of alternative courses of action; it extends through the process of implementation as progress is monitored through *formative evaluation* and remedial actions are taken as indicated; and it includes end-stage *summative evaluation* of overall program impact. Even the latter should be forward-looking; successful features of the program are highlighted for continuation and replication elsewhere, and failures are identified in an effort to avoid their repetition.[2]

The movement of a ship between ports presents an apt analogy. Before departure a travel plan is carefully prepared after evaluation of alternative routes. The ship's captain and navigator do not then retreat to their quarters, only to emerge several days later to determine whether they have reached their destination as scheduled. (Absurd as this sounds, it is not uncommon for evaluators to collect baseline data and then wait for project completion to undertake their evaluation.) In actual practice, the ship's officers realize that unanticipated weather conditions, traffic, or other factors are likely to require modification of the original navigation plan, or occasionally even the intended destination. Constant monitoring of progress is necessary if prompt action is to be taken to keep the ship as nearly on course as possible. Assured that this is the case, the officers need not be unduly apprehensive about judgments of performance that might be made after the voyage is completed.

MAIN FEATURES OF MANAGEMENT DECISION MAKING

Considering the direct link between evaluation and decision making, we should pause to elucidate the essential features of the decision process before proceeding with a more detailed discussion of evaluation.[3] Since we all engage in decision making daily, the need for elaboration might be questioned. In recent years, however, a formal body of methodology known as *decision analysis* has evolved in an effort to make decisions more rational and less intuitive. Decision analysis is now a fundamental part of formal management training, and it is this formalized process that deserves to be outlined.[4] A more detailed description is given with the aid of a concrete example in Chapter 14.

Essentials of Decision Analysis

Since decisions are designed to produce one or more desired results, the process begins with specification of clearly defined objectives. Typically, a number of different paths exist to the possible achievement of the objectives; that is, there are many means to a given end. Hence the need exists to spell out various courses of action, or strategies, in a way that permits rational evaluation of alternatives leading to selection of the one that is best according to designated criteria.

Although several alternatives may be available, the outcome actually attained through any one cannot be assured because of the element of uncertainty. A vaccination team can decide to visit a particular village on a given day, and indeed the team may choose a market day as the most favorable alternative, but it cannot determine in advance precisely how many children of what ages will be brought for immunization, much less how many measles deaths will be averted as a result. Thus, the existence of several alternatives, each coupled with multiple possible outcomes, complicates the decision process considerably.

In particular, comparative value judgments must be made regarding each of the possible outcomes. These judgments may include intangibles. Suppose, for example, that one method of screening a specified population for hypertension will cost one thousand dollars and yield between twenty and forty false-positives, whereas a second method will produce from fifteen to twenty-five false-positives at a cost of two thousand dollars. The value judgments to be made must include not only direct costs of screening and treatment, but psychologic costs and degree of uncertainty as well.

Even after the value judgments have been made, criteria for their appraisal must be defined. What if the recovery rate associated with Treatment A for a specified condition is 60 percent, whereas Treatment B produces recovery in ninety-nine cases out of one hundred but leads to permanent disability in the other case? Is the decision regarding treatment to be based upon the probability of success or the possibility of failure?

To summarize, the decision process has five key elements:

1. specification of objectives,
2. elaboration of alternative strategies for possible achievement of the objectives,
3. measurement of uncertainty associated with the strategies,
4. valuation of all possible outcomes, and
5. designation of explicit criteria whereby the differentially valued outcomes and degrees of uncertainty will be combined in selecting a preferred strategy for implementation.

From this process clearly emerges the notion of evaluation as comparative analysis of measured achievements in relation to intentions. We also recognize that in spite of the importance of quantification, important intangibles cannot be ignored but rather must be given explicit consideration.

The way in which uncertainty enters into evaluation merits further emphasis. First, it colors both the setting of objectives and the gathering of data concerning their achievement. To illustrate, important as maternal mortality may be in an area, success in reducing the rate may be virtually impossible to evaluate in a population as small as a half million. If at most twenty maternal deaths can be expected and the actual number could range from ten to twenty by chance, a reduction in deaths from seventeen in the year before program initiation to fourteen a year later could hardly be considered definitive.

A second consideration involving uncertainty is the distinction between actions under the control of the decision maker and what must be left to chance. Given the knowledge of hindsight we can readily identify a strategy that might have been more successful. The critical question, however, is whether that strategy was similarly attractive in the face of uncertainty and will be inevitably as successful in the future.

Management by Objectives and by Exception

Integral to the concepts of decision analysis are the central principles of management by objectives and management by exception. Their roles underlying evaluation must also be borne in mind. The stated objectives should indicate what effects are to be achieved in what target population by what time. For example, two years hence 80 percent of all children one year old in a specified district are to be immunized against measles, and that level of coverage is to be sustained thereafter. Intermediate objectives regarding, for example, the availability of vaccines, refrigerators, and trained personnel are also specified. Then procedures for tracking progress are instituted such that scarce management resources are focused only on exceptional conditions that arise, that is, those areas in which progress is lagging.

It follows that the evaluation system must be designed first to identify which among the many potential problems that might arise do, in fact, emerge in practice. The decision maker must then determine whether the necessary corrective action is immediately evident in these exceptional cases or whether further investigation (perhaps through health systems research) is required to establish causal relationships and effective solutions. Routine evaluative information need not provide immediate answers to all questions, but it should be sufficiently comprehensive to ensure that all emerging problems are flagged.

This raises the corollary issues of when and how often information should be gathered and analyzed.[5] Clearly, the timing of reporting should be consonant with the time at which decisions need to be made. This is likely to vary with the course of program implementation. Initial efforts will probably center on the training of personnel, establishment of adequate logistical support, and in general on decisions regarding the capacity to provide services. After problems in this respect are worked out so that unanticipated exceptional circumstances are less likely, attention will undoubtedly shift to the utilization of available services. Finally, questions of service impact will become paramount with a consequent shift in emphasis on information requirements and timing. It should not be concluded, of course, that concerns about capacity, utilization, and impact are transient and strictly sequential. All are of continuing interest, but the intensity and frequency of data collection and reporting vary.

Whereas timing depends upon the locus of decision making, frequency depends primarily upon rates of change. Levels of family planning acceptance (services utilization) can change quite rapidly, for example, whereas birth rates (impact) change slowly. Thus, in a family planning program, reports on contraceptive utilization must be initiated early and updated frequently, whereas the importance of birth rates increases only as the program matures, and even then analyses need not be as frequent.

CAPTURING THE DYNAMICS OF EVALUATION

Distinguishing Input, Process, Output, and Outcome

Underlying the preceding background discussion has been the characterization of evaluation as an ongoing process. In turning to a consideration of specific features of evaluation, we first reflect its dynamic nature by distinguishing program inputs from process, output, and outcome indicators.[6] The distinctions are illustrated in Figure 4.1 in relation to a hypothetical program for improving the effectiveness of basic health services coverage to a defined population.

First, it is necessary to develop personnel with requisite skills and to provide for

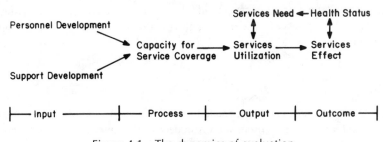

Figure 4.1   The dynamics of evaluation

their support. This involves recruitment and/or training, development of supportive supervision, and organization of logistical and other support mechanisms.

Development of individual system components does not ensure their functional coordination in practice. The process whereby resources are mobilized to produce the intended services capacity must also be evaluated. In the illustrative case, process accomplishments might be measured according to the extent to which the target population has been identified, contacted, and registered and has access to services. The *process* aspect of evaluation might be included under resources input, or it might be thought of as output potential. Its separate identification is advisable, however, to distinguish capacity for action from actual utilization of that capacity.

Output is to be distinguished from outcome in that the product (output) of a health care system is services, which may have differential impact on health status (outcome), the ultimate concern of the system. Outputs are generally easier to measure than outcomes and frequently must serve as proxies for the latter. If a high rate of immunization against measles (output) is achieved, for example, it can be assumed that morbidity and mortality from the disease will be reduced. The simplifying assumption can be unsatisfactory, however, in noting that certain disadvantaged malnourished groups have a higher case-fatality rate than others. This becomes important in considerations of equity discussed later.

Logical Framework

Slightly modified, the format of Figure 4.1 has been embodied in the *logical framework* used by the United States Agency for International Development in project formulation.[7] It is outlined in Figure 4.2 and described more fully in Chapter 15 as a tool for planning.

What we have labeled *outcome* is referred to as *project purpose* in the logical framework and the project, in turn, is related to a broader program. Process indicators are omitted, but each phase of the project is linked by a set of specified assumptions. Likewise, inputs, outputs, project purposes, and program goals must be made explicit through objectively verifiable indicators. Means of verification in each case, for example, service statistics or special surveys, are to be documented.

To illustrate use of the framework, suppose that an intended project output is provision of a designated level of antenatal care to pregnant women in the target area. The indicator might be the proportion of such women seen by a trained midwife during the second trimester of pregnancy. Clinic records, perhaps supplemented by a spot-check of a sample of patients, provide the means of verification. An assumption is that antenatal care serves to identify high-risk pregnancies and thereby improves the likelihood of favorable outcome at delivery.

Pinpointing Difficulties

These evaluative formats reveal the inadequacy of simplistic classifications of success or failure. End results are a composite of predecessor events, any of which could be a source of difficulty. A hierarchy of possibilities for failure accordingly exists:[8]

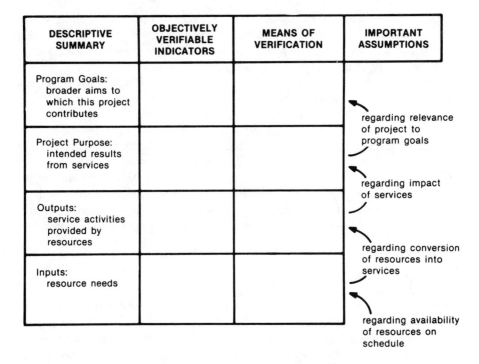

DESCRIPTIVE SUMMARY	OBJECTIVELY VERIFIABLE INDICATORS	MEANS OF VERIFICATION	IMPORTANT ASSUMPTIONS
Program Goals: broader aims to which this project contributes			
Project Purpose: intended results from services			regarding relevance of project to program goals
Outputs: service activities provided by resources			regarding impact of services
Inputs: resource needs			regarding conversion of resources into services
			regarding availability of resources on schedule

Figure 4.2   Logical framework format

1. inadequate resources were planned;
2. planned resources were not actually provided;
3. resources provided were not properly organized into meaningful service activities;
4. activities undertaken did not have the intended effects.

Apart from the vertical hierarchy of possibilities, there is usually a horizontal linkage among various subobjectives, project objectives, and ultimate program objectives. A successful diarrhea control program, for example, requires knowledge of dehydration and how it can be avoided, availability of certain materials and utensils for mixing, ability to prepare the necessary salt solution, proper utilization of the solution, and simultaneous application of appropriate feeding practices. Since ultimate success is jeopardized by failure at any point in the vertical hierarchy, or among the horizontal linkages of objectives, the sooner these problems are identified and remedied, the more complete ultimate success is likely to be.

EVALUATION MEASURES

Potential Appropriateness and Adequacy

In coming to grips with practical measurement issues, we must consider a number of dimensions in potential and actual performance.[9] We must first question whether the actions to be taken are appropriate to the problem at hand. Is malnutrition, for example, most appropriately combated through health interventions? To the extent that health sector involvement is relevant, should efforts be directed toward village feeding centers or home gardens?

Assuming appropriateness, the question arises whether the contemplated program is adequate in size and scope to make a meaningful difference. Is a day-care center designed to attract high-risk children from ten scattered villages likely to draw enough clients to be worthwhile? It is frequently true that unless a certain critical mass of resources is effectively and visibly mobilized, those resources that are allocated will be essentially squandered. Rural health centers in many countries are so inadequately staffed and supported that utilization is minimal, with the result that the time of the limited staff actually provided is largely wasted. This leads to the critical issue of whether under particular conditions it is more advantageous to concentrate severely limited resources on a few major problems rather than to spread resources thinly over all fronts.

Effectiveness and Efficiency

Measures of effectiveness and efficiency are so commonplace that they are some-times considered the sole basis for evaluation of program performance. Even so, their meaning is not always clearly understood. Program *effect* is generally stated as absolute level of accomplishment, whereas *effectiveness* is accomplishment in rela-tion to need or to intentions. In either case, it is important to distinguish program accomplishments from what would have been achieved in the absence of a program. Consider, for example, two communities with 1,000 infants and toddlers each. In the first community 100 children are brought for immunization in the normal course of providing health services. In the second community a campaign is launched with the objective of immunizing 800 children but succeeds in reaching only 600. Assuming that without the campaign in the second community 100 children would have been immunized, as in the first, the campaign effect was to reach 500 additional children. Effectiveness might be measured in one of three ways. It might be simply the dif-ference between the 60 percent rate of achieved immunization and the 10 percent "control" level. A second possibility would be to compare the 500 additional children reached with the 900 target children not covered by regular services. Finally, the comparison could be made between the 500 additional children reached and the 700 (800 − 100) additional children that were intended to be covered. Obviously it is important to define clearly the measure used in a particular case and to be sure that comparisons between programs use the same measures.

In the engineering world efficiency is generally viewed as the ratio of *output* to input. With regard to social services, measures of efficiency, or cost-effectiveness, frequently relate *outcome* to input, for example, in considering program cost per death averted. Thus, ambiguities exist in defining even the most basic terms of evalua-tion.

The issue is more than a semantic one, for population groups that are most difficult to serve, because of physical, social, or economic barriers, are frequently those which stand to gain most from use of the services. For example, it may be costly to motivate rural couples of low socioeconomic status to accept contraception, yet because of their high fertility, the impact of contraceptive use on the birth rate may be large. Specifically the relation between output and input for this group, for example, cost per acceptor, may be unfavorable in comparison with others, whereas the relation of outcome and input, for instance, cost per birth averted, may show a much different picture.

We are led to suggest that the outcome-input relationship of ultimate interest be clearly separated into its two components. The ratio of output (OP) to input (IP) is a measure of efficiency. The ratio of outcome (OC) to output, that is, effect per unit of service, might be designated *impact*. Then the overall OC/IP ratio, *cost-effectiveness*, is the product of these two components:

$$\frac{OC}{IP} = \frac{OP}{IP} \times \frac{OC}{OP},$$

or

$$\text{Cost-effectiveness} = \text{Efficiency} \times \text{Impact}.$$

The choice of terms might be questioned inasmuch as others will continue to define them in different ways and ambiguities will persist. Nevertheless, bearing in mind the two separate components of cost-effectiveness, however they may be labeled, should contribute to clarity in program evaluation. The measures take on additional importance when we introduce notions of equity.

Equity

Primary health care and associated concerns for distributive justice have brought considerations of equity to a level where they parallel notions of efficiency and effectiveness. We are now advised that services are to be provided both cost-effectively and equitably. For the most part, however, the principle of equity has not been translated into concrete measurement terms. As a result, possible incompatibility between cost-effectiveness and equity has not been faced realistically.

To underscore the dilemma, consider a population of 100,000 preschool children, 30 percent of whom are socioeconomically disadvantaged. As indicated in Table 4.1, 60 percent of the latter can be expected to suffer from severe diarrhea during a specified time period, whereas a 40 percent incidence rate is anticipated among the more advantaged children. Because of differences in nutritional status, 2 percent of the disadvantaged cases result in death, compared with a case-fatality rate of 1 percent in the rest of the population. Among the advantaged, five cases can be brought to treatment for $1, whereas only two disadvantaged cases can be reached for this amount.

From these circumstances we derive the measures of efficiency, impact, and cost-effectiveness shown in Table 4.1. The advantaged can be served more efficiently, but impact among those served is greater for the disadvantaged. Combining the two factors, we find that the advantaged can be served more cost-effectively than the

Table 4.1

ILLUSTRATIVE DATA FOR DETERMINATION OF COST-EFFECTIVENESS AND EQUITY

Population Group	No. Children	No. Diarrhea Cases	Deaths if Cases Untreated	Cost per Treated Case	Efficiency OP/IP	Impact OC/OP	Cost-Effectiveness OC/IP
Advantaged	70,000	28,000	280	$.20	5	.01	.05
Disadvantaged	30,000	18,000	360	$.50	2	.02	.04

disadvantaged. In particular, one death can be averted for $20 among the advantaged compared to $25 for the disadvantaged.

What is the most equitable approach? Equal input per capita would seem to be less equitable than equal input per case. Even the latter approach could be considered inequitable because fewer deaths would be averted as a result among disadvantaged because of considerations of cost-effectiveness. Perhaps the most equitable approach would be to equalize the death rates in the two groups. This would require allocation of considerably more resources per capita to the disadvantaged than to the advantaged because of both the higher incidence and severity of disease among the disadvantaged and the relatively unfavorable cost-effectiveness ratio in dealing with the problem in that group.

We see the importance of assigning operational meaning to the concept of equity and clearly establishing trade-offs between cost-effectiveness and equity. In the illustrative case (and others in practice) the two aims cannot be fully satisfied. Whereas all program managers are likely to argue in favor of equity in principle, they may or may not be prepared to argue that some lives are worth more ($25 versus $20) than others, even though that is what is implied by equity in the present case.

EVALUATION PRINCIPLES AND PRACTICE

The subject of evaluation is wide-ranging, and we have viewed it from many perspectives. This concluding section is designed first to summarize, crystallize, and reinforce major principles of evaluation that have emerged from the discussion. We then comment on organizational arrangements best suited to apply these principles in relation to planning, management, and research issues considered in previous chapters.

Principles

1. As a key to improved decision making, evaluation is forward-looking and action-oriented.
2. Evaluation is comprehensive and dynamic, concerned with the examination of policy and plan alternatives, monitoring of progress in the process of implementation, and summative appraisal of final outcomes.

3. Evaluation is founded upon the principle of management by objectives and begins with clear, definitive enunciation of what effects are to be achieved in what population in what time period.
4. Strategies for meeting the stated objectives should be examined for appropriateness and adequacy.
5. Conforming to the principle of management by exception, evaluation plans should provide a broad range of information designed to signal promptly any emerging problems.
   a. Whereas the routine information system identifies problems, it cannot be expected to provide immediate solutions; evaluation must be coupled with special analyses and health systems research.
   b. In the interests of timeliness and parsimony in data collection, the evaluation focus will shift from inputs to process to outputs and outcomes in the course of program implementation.
6. The timing and locus of evaluative reports should conform to the need for timely decisions.
7. The frequency of reporting depends largely upon the pace of change in conditions requiring action.
8. Since evaluation is comparative, it relies on indicators expressing appropriate rates and ratios, rather than absolute levels of accomplishment.
9. Appraisals should distinguish between outcomes subject to decision control and those that occurred as a result of uncertainty and chance.
10. Efficiency, effectiveness, and equity should be clearly defined and trade-offs made explicit.

Practice: Organization of the Evaluation Function

By its very nature evaluation connotes detached objectivity. Yet we have seen how directly it relates to planning and implementation. To be meaningful it must be integrally related to both.

In one respect evaluation is an internal accounting of program operations. In another respect it is an external, post facto audit of program performance. As in financial accounting, the first aspect of evaluation is designed to provide management with a dynamic view of operational progress, serving as an early warning system for detecting impending problems. It must be based upon a sound management information system. On the other hand, the performance audit requires independent, outside appraisal. Analogously to the way in which the accounting function is carried out, it is advisable to unite evaluation and research in a unit that directly serves management and is either within or closely related to the planning unit. In addition, as in the auditing function, periodic provision must be made for independent, external review. The bulk of attention and effort, however, should go into the former function.

REFERENCES

1. *Health Programme Evaluation: Guiding Principles for Its Application in the Managerial Process for National Health Development*, Geneva: World Health Organization, 1981.

2. Anderson, S. B., *The Profession and Practice of Program Evaluation*, San Francisco: Jossey-Bass, 1978.

3. Veney, James E., *Evaluation and Decision Making for Health Services Programs*, Englewood Cliffs, NJ: Prentice-Hall, 1984.

4. Raiffa, Howard, *Decision Analysis: Introductory Lectures on Choices Under Uncertainty*, Reading, MA: Addison-Wesley, 1968.

5. Hageboeck, Molly, *Manager's Guide to Data Collection*, Washington: Agency for International Development, 1979.

6. Donabedian, Avedis, *Medical Care Appraisal*, Vol. 2 of *A Guide to Medical Care Administration*, New York: American Public Health Association, 1969.

7. Office of Program Evaluation, *Evaluation Handbook*, 2nd ed., Washington: Agency for International Development, 1974.

8. Deniston, O. L., I. M. Rosenstock and V. A. Getting, "Evaluation of Program Effectiveness," *Public Health Reports*, 83:323–335, 1968.

9. *Statistical Indicators for the Planning and Evaluation of Public Health Programmes*, WHO Technical Report Series No. 472, Geneva: World Health Organization, 1971.

PRIMARY READINGS

Attkisson, C. Clifford, William A. Hargreaves, Mardi J. Horowitz and James E. Sorensen (eds.), *Evaluation of Human Services Programs*, New York: Academic Press, 1978. A comprehensive treatment of evaluation for a variety of social service programs in which objectives and results are not readily measured.

Clark, Noreen and James McCaffery, *Demystifying Evaluation*, New York: World Education, 1979. Initially prepared for a workshop conducted in Kenya, this simply written manual offers guidelines for training seminars on evaluation for staff members of community development programs.

Health Programme Evaluation: Guiding Principles for Its Application in the Managerial Process for National Health Development, Geneva: World Health Organization, 1981. As Publication No. 6 in the Health for All series, this volume offers the basic perspectives of the World Health Organization on evaluation of primary health care.

Schulberg, H. C. and F. Baker (eds.), *Program Evaluation in the Health Fields*, Vol. 2, New York: Human Sciences Press, 1978. Drawing from many contributors, this publication provides both methodological insights and several case studies.

Suchman, E. A., *Evaluative Research*, New York: Russell Sage Foundation, 1967. One of the early publications in the field, this concisely written treatise on evaluation is a classic and continues to be a useful reference.

SECONDARY READINGS

Anderson, S. B., *The Profession and Practice of Program Evaluation*, San Francisco: Jossey-Bass, 1978.

Application of Epidemiology to the Planning and Evaluation of Health Services, Copenhagen: WHO Regional Office for Europe, 1974.

Hageboeck, Molly, *Manager's Guide to Data Collection*, Washington: Agency for International Development, 1979.

Litsios, Socrates, "Developing a Cost and Outcome Evaluation System," *International Journal of Health Services*, 6,2:345–360, 1976.

Mushkin, Selma J., "Evaluations: Use with Caution," *Evaluation*, 1,2:30–35, 1973.

National Assessments of Health Care Coverage and of Its Effectiveness and Efficiency, Geneva: World Health Organization, 1983.

Shortell, S. M., and W. C. Richardson, *Health Program Evaluation*, St. Louis: C. V. Mosby, 1978.

Statistical Indicators for the Planning and Evaluation of Public Health Programmes, WHO Technical Report Series No. 472, Geneva: World Health Organization, 1971.

Veney, James E., *Evaluation and Decision Making for Health Services Programs*, Englewood Cliffs, NJ: Prentice-Hall, 1984.

II

The Planning Process: Concepts, Methods, and Strategies

The breadth of the issues that planners and administrators face requires understanding of principles and methods from a number of disciplines. If a changing population is to be served appropriately, its demographic characteristics have to be assessed. Knowledge of the nature and distribution of health problems in the client population is based upon principles of epidemiology and biostatistics. Assessment of resource needs and availability requires expertise in economics. How the resources are directed is in part, at least, a political consideration. How the available services are actually utilized by the public is a matter of concern to behavioral scientists. Even this partial list of examples should make clear the multidisciplinary nature of planning.

In addition, of course, there are certain methods of planning per se. Planners, for example, must be able to translate service requirements into specific facilities configurations, staffing needs and training programs.

Part II begins with an overview that elaborates more fully and systematically these and other interrelated components of the planning process. Each element is then covered in detail in a separate series of chapters. The intent is to distill from the various disciplines those principles and methods that are directly useful in health planning and programming. The presentations in digest form are essentially conceptual; specific techniques of analysis are described in Part III.

5

An Overview of the Planning Process

WILLIAM A. REINKE

At the heart of all health planning methodology is the desire to improve health system performance. To begin with, then, we need a clear perception of that system and its component parts. Second, in line with concern for improvement, we examine the hierarchy of goals and objectives that drives the process of planned change. In addition to a conceptual understanding of the system and its purposes, planning in practice requires an analytical framework for concrete appraisal of the various functions of the system; a third section of this chapter is therefore devoted to the development of the essential features of functional analysis. Finally, considering that information is needed to carry out the process of planning, we outline the principal types and sources of data to be drawn upon.

CONCEPTUALIZATION OF THE HEALTH SERVICES SYSTEM

Conceptually, we take the approach portrayed in Figure 5.1, where we note that health services draw upon resources in response to certain health problems for the purpose of producing an outcome in the form of improved health status.[1] Such a broad conceptualization is, of course, of little practical value in coming to grips with real conditions. We must look more carefully, therefore, at each system component in turn.

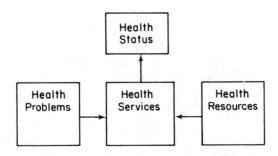

Figure 5.1   Health care system overview

People and Their Health Problems

Health problems (see Figure 5.2) are identified in relation to the population at risk in the planning area. Effectively, then, they have epidemiologic numerators, demographic denominators, and geographic bounds. The last item depends upon the mandate of the planning body, the location of health resources, political jurisdictions, transportation and communication patterns, and population concentrations.

Demographic considerations are based upon the fact that different segments of the population vary in the type and magnitude of their health needs, as well as in their utilization of health services. A planner is especially interested in identifying important population characteristics that are likely to change in relative importance. As a minimum, the population breakdown should include age, sex, and place of residence. Frequently it is advisable to add social class and/or educational attainment, race, and participation in health insurance programs. Precautions must be taken, however, to avoid classifying the population into so many small subgroups that reliable enumeration becomes too costly.

Within each relevant population group the planner must identify the nature and importance of individual health needs, as well as the extent to which these needs are currently translated into demands for health services. Assessment of problems

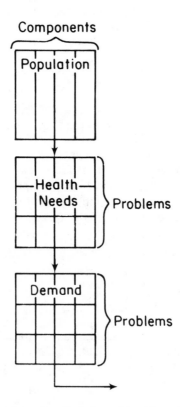

Figure 5.2   Detailed view of health problems

should allow for both cause and effect. It is important, for example, to separate infant deaths during the neonatal period, which can be traced to care of the mother, from post-neonatal mortality that relates to circumstances in the child's care and environment. In general, of course, gross mortality rates provide too crude a measure of health problems. Instead, identification of problems according to the *International Classification of Diseases* may be useful. Furthermore, within this classification system a planner will probably be concerned with morbidity and disability or loss in productive capacity as well as mortality.

Classification of health problems by disease not only provides information on effects in terms of mortality and morbidity but also suggests specific disease agents as causal factors. In addition, more general hazards to health should be identified through reference to water supply sources, sewerage and waste collection systems, feeding practices, food protection mechanisms, housing conditions, and vector control. Table 5.1 summarizes the essential items of information needed under this and the other headings to be considered.

Health Resources

In considering health resources (see Figure 5.3), planners must separate human, physical, and financial components. They must determine the available quantities and locations of different kinds of health workers, inventory existing facilities of various

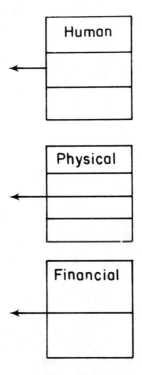

Figure 5.3   Detailed view of health resources

Table 5.1

MINIMAL ELEMENTS OF INFORMATION FOR PLANNING

1. Population Size and Characteristics

    Age-sex distribution
    Geographical distribution
    Transportation and communications patterns
    Educational attainment
    Socioeconomic status
    Health insurance coverage

2. Health Status and Problems

    Disease-specific and age-specific mortality, disability, morbidity rates
    Water supply sources
    Sewerage and waste collection practices
    Child feeding practices
    Food protection mechanisms
    Housing conditions
    Vector control practices
    Fertility rates

3. Human Resources

    Mix of active personnel among major categories
    Attrition rates
    Age-sex distribution
    Type of practice
    Affiliation
    Location of practice
    Training limitations
        Training capacity by location and type of institution
        Enrollment by location and type of institution
        Available teachers
        Available funds for training
        Size of pool of potential applicants

4. Physical Resources and Organization

    Geographical distribution
    Diagnostic and treatment services provided
    Sponsorship
    Organizational relationships and referral patterns
    Political factors influencing organizational authority and responsibility

5. Financial Resources

    Geographical variations in income
    Sectoral distribution of GNP
    Investment patterns contributing to development
    Availability of foreign exchange
    Health expenditures relative to GNP
    Health budget relative to total public expenditures
    Private vs. public expenditures in health
    Current budget vs. development budget

6.   Service Statistics

     Utilization rates
          Annual physician visits per person
          Annual dentist visits per person
          Hospital discharges
          Hospital bed days
          Pre-natal visits per live birth
          Well-child visits per live birth
          Attended deliveries by category of attention
     Coverage
     Demographic and epidemiologic characteristics of population served
     Costs and charges for services
     Sources of payment
     Productivity standards

kinds (public and private), and identify various revenue sources (including insurance schemes, government support of health programs, and private contributions of various kinds).

In some respects an inventory of health resources lacks meaning apart from the services developed from those resources. Knowledge of the number of physicians in a country is of limited value without corresponding information about the number and types of patients seen by these doctors. Still, the fact that a country averages one physician per three thousand population does convey some information about the health potential of that country. Detailed information about the maldistribution of practitioners between the urban and rural areas is likely to be even more relevant for planning purposes.

Human resources must first be viewed with respect to existing supplies and then in terms of the training infrastructure as it could affect future levels. Enumeration of current providers should include community volunteers and indigenous practitioners of local importance, as well as the main categories of professional, paraprofessional, and auxiliary workers employed in the formal health care system. In addition to numbers, the planner is interested in the age and sex distribution, affiliation, and type and location of practice.

In assessing the training base for developing future labor markets, the planner must consider the financial, physical, and teaching constraints of institutions for health training. In some areas it may also prove necessary to survey the potential of general educational institutions, for the health field may be hard pressed in the competition with other professions for scarce secondary school graduates.

As labor data are assembled, the planner has to make some judgment concerning the effect of geographical maldistribution, differences between the distribution of physical and human resources, and relationships among categories of health workers. Suppose, for example, that three regions of equal population have one hundred, fifty, and twenty-five doctors, respectively. Is the effective gap between the second and third region more or less than that between the first two? How much would the judgment be altered if it were learned that the third region has more nurses? How would one look upon the fact that the third region has no hospital to serve additional physicians who might be attracted to the area?

Like human resources, physical facilities fit into a number of categories which must be separately identified and inventoried. These include hospitals, dispensaries, clinics, and private sources of personal care, as well as water, sewerage, and other environmental systems.

The degree of detail embodied in the information depends upon the availability of data and the uniqueness of given resources. Apart from the detail with which records are maintained, the essential criterion of interest to planners is the degree to which facilities can be substituted for one another. Thus, they require a geographical breakdown in order to recognize differences in population groups served. Distinctions are also made on the basis of differences in diagnostic and treatment facilities; consequently information is assembled with respect to short-term general, long-term rehabilitation, and mental institutions, along with the availability of various clinical and laboratory services within the institutions. Frequently distinctions must be made on the basis of the goals of individual health agencies which arise from different sources of sponsorship, and these distinctions may be reflected in the financial structure and organization of the agency; hence health planners are likely to distinguish among government, proprietary, religious, and other types of institutions.

Once the planners have appropriately classified a facility, they must place a value on it, usually in both physical and monetary terms. For example, a hospital might be identified as a two-hundred-bed institution with a certain replacement cost. In looking to the future, the age of existing installations is an important factor, just as the age distribution of physicians is an important personnel consideration.

Although categorization is necessary to the inventorying of resources, attention must also be given to coordination and interactions among categories. Existing referral patterns must be recognized, along with the impact that such factors as increased dependence upon extended care facilities would have upon the need for beds in short-term general hospitals.

Health Services

Figure 5.4 depicts schematically the structure of health services that develops from the organization of resources to satisfy health demands. It also shows the impact of these services upon health status. Health services include diagnostic, treatment, and rehabilitative components. From the standpoint of planning and evaluation, these services should be viewed in functional rather than organizational terms. Thus, these three boxes are each subdivided vertically into the various categories of activity which the services comprise. These activities are directed in varying degrees toward particular health needs which are separated schematically by the horizontal lines. In other words, the planner must understand the present health services structure in terms of the performance of certain functions, each of which is a specific combination of human, physical, and financial resources organized to satisfy to some extent one or more existing health demands.

In viewing the health services structure, explicit recognition should be given to the preventive aspects. Primary disease prevention, such as immunization, has an impact extending beyond the health services box to the basic needs box of Figure 5.2. Secondary prevention as a category of service, such as early detection of cervical cancer, has its major effect at the diagnostic stage, whereas tertiary prevention occurs largely at the treatment stage, as in the case where stroke patients are treated

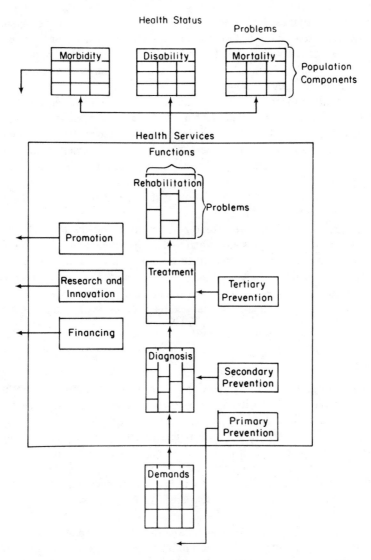

Figure 5.4   Detailed view of health services and health status

in a manner that minimizes muscular deformities and subsequent problems of rehabilitation.

The health field is unique in the extent to which supply and demand interact.
This is exemplified by contentions that physicians largely create a demand for their
own services and that utilization of hospital beds is in large measure determined by
their availability. A complete and realistic appraisal of the health services structure,
therefore, must include factors that influence demand for services. Three such factors
are shown in Figure 5.4. First, we include the various forms of health education and
professional influence that come under the general heading of promotion. Second,
since demand for health services depends in large part upon the extent to which
health problems are vulnerable to attack, we must include medical research and

other innovative activities that affect the state of the art of medicine. Finally, we must recognize the role of the health services structure in extending effective demand beyond what it would be with private financing alone. For example, the health planner must know about training institutions that, in the interests of medical education, offer free services to the medically indigent.

Actual measurement of services rendered should include, to begin with, a compilation of resource utilization data such as the annual number of physician visits and hospital discharges and durations of hospital stay. Recognition of the key role of financial mechanisms in determining the nature and volume of services actually provided is important, and planners must know a good deal about the costs and sources of funding such services. In a broader sense they should be cognizant of the current magnitude of health expenditures in relation to the size of the total economy, along with future trends in both.

Besides recording the mere utilization of services, indices that relate services rendered both to the available resources and to the client population should be created. Examples of the former include hospital bed occupancy rates, average outpatient visits per health center per day, number of deliveries per midwife, and average cost per immunization. Indices related to the client population are illustrated by the proportion of deliveries attended by trained personnel and the proportion of underweight children served by feeding centers.

Health Status

For schematic purposes, health status can be considerd in terms of mortality, disability, and morbidity. Morbidity is linked to population, indicating that the entire health system is dynamic. That is, we are interested in the ability of the health services to modify and improve health status and to return healthy individuals to the population. This suggests, furthermore, that each health status component (mortality, disability, and morbidity) should have the same subdivisions by population groups and health problems (see Figure 5.2). As a result, a planner must identify not only the major causes of health needs but also areas in which these needs are not being met satisfactorily.

Important as health services indicators are, they are not substitutes for measures of health status. This point is highlighted in analyses that show that health status is correlated rather weakly with health expenditures and use of health services.[2] The United States easily leads the world in health expenditures per capita but is surpassed by several countries in life expectancy.[3] Near the other end of the spectrum, Sri Lanka has a notably low infant mortality rate that belies the nation's relatively poor economic status.[4]

Impact of Planning

The health system components and linkages exist regardless of the role that health planning may play. Planning does, however, carry with it the potential for improving the performance of the system (see Figure 5.5). Inherent in the notion of improvement is the specification of goals, or norms, toward which conscious effort is to be directed.

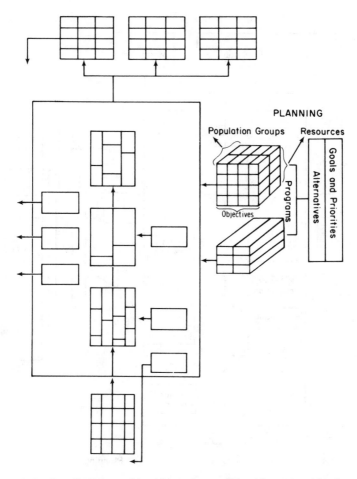

Figure 5.5 Detailed view of health services and health status with planning

The core of planning, then, is the analysis of alternative means of moving toward identified health goals in the light of specified priorities and existing constraints. The selection process results in a variety of program packages. Each program, which is directed at one or more health problems, is designed to achieve specific measurable objectives through a certain combination of resources oriented toward particular population groups. These program packages vary, depending upon whether objectives are limited or more comprehensive, whether the programs are simple or require complex organizations, and whether they are general in scope or directed toward a small population segment, such as mentally retarded children.

The Total Picture

Finally, all the health system components are brought together in Figure 5.6. This figure is a restatement of Figure 5.1, but it is considerably more detailed and expressly incorporates the role of planning into the schematic representation.

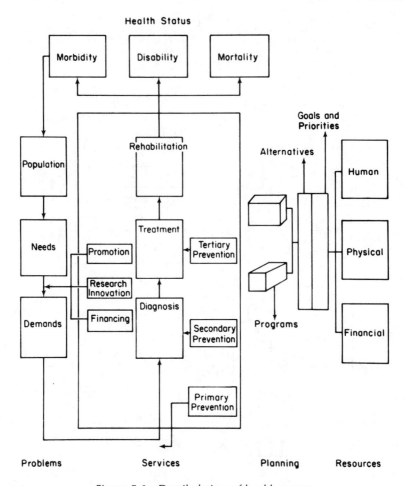

Figure 5.6   Detailed view of health system

THE ESSENCE OF PLANNING

As we focus upon the planning process itself, we reiterate that the core of planning is analysis (in the face of constraints) of alternative means of achieving established goals ranked in some order of priority.[5] The two factors—goals and analysis—form the core of the practical process of planning.

Goals and Priorities

We must first define and distinguish among the terms *mission, goal, objective, target,* and *standard.*[6] Although other terms might be employed, the notions inherent in these five must be a part of rational planning and decision making.

   Mission describes an organization's reason for existence, the general functions of services it performs, and the limits of its jurisdiction and authority. The mission of a state or local health department might be the protection and advancement of the public health of the population of that state or community within certain legally specified limitations.

A *goal* is a long-range specified state of accomplishment toward which programs are directed. It is not cast in terms of current availability of resources or a fixed time for achievement, but it must be consistent with the mission. In the health field, the goal is usually stated in terms of completely overcoming a health problem or reducing it to the extent the state of the art permits.

An *objective* is stated in terms of achieving a measured amount of progress toward a goal.[7] It must include a specification of:

1. *what*: the nature of the situation or condition to be attained,
2. *how much*: the quantity or amount of the situation or condition to be attained,
3. *when*: the time at or by which the desired situation or condition is intended to exist,
4. *who*: the particular group of people or portion of the environment in which attainment is desired, and
5. *where*: the geographic area to be included in the program.

A *target* establishes a measured amount of output to be achieved in relation to a health objective through a specific program activity. Whereas objectives are set with respect to needs in the client population, targets are set with respect to service providers. The targets should be based upon realistic performance standards.

Consider a concrete example to distinguish among objectives, targets, and standards. A population of 1 million with a crude birth rate of 40 per 1,000 population is served by 100 maternity centers, each staffed by a trained midwife who can handle 240 maternity cases per year. Currently only one-third that number are actually seen on average. Because of unsatisfactory delivery practice in the other cases, 640 deaths per year are experienced from neonatal tetanus. The aim is to reduce this number by half through provision of antenatal care, including administration of tetanus toxoid to 60 percent of pregnant women.

The population of one million generates 40,000 births per year. The objective is to reduce the tetanus mortality rate to 320 per 40,000, or 8 per 1,000 births. (In this illustration, pregnancy wastage is ignored.) The target is for the 100 midwives to reach 24,000 women in all with proper antenatal care. As a result, 60 percent of pregnancies will be covered, an accomplishment compatible with a realistic productivity standard of 240 cases per worker. The principle that emerges is that expected outcomes, service targets, and productive capacity must be linked through mutually compatible measures, regardless of what terms are used to describe the measures.

Alternatives and Constraints: A Functional Framework

Targets can be established only after particular programs have been selected from a set of alternatives. Moreover, reasonable objectives can only arise from a consideration of the costs and resources required to achieve the benefits that underlie contemplated objectives. For example, one could not automatically argue that an infant mortality rate of 60 represents a better objective than one of 80. It might be that the reduction from 80 to 60 would require additional nonexistent resources. Specification of aims, then, is intimately bound up with the analysis of alternatives, even though we discuss the two aspects separately.

To be most effective, consideration of program alternatives should proceed within the framework of the health functions of particular concern.[8] To illustrate, one agency has established the following nine study areas: reproduction, nutrition, dental and oral health, infectious and communicable diseases, trauma and safety, chronic diseases, handicapping conditions, mobility, and mental disorders.[9] Other planners might prefer a breakdown in terms of personal preventive, curative, and rehabilitative activities; environmental sanitation; mass campaigns against communicable diseases; and so forth. These functions could be analyzed further with respect to such important dimensions as age or urgency of need (emergency, acute, and chronic conditions).

The framework for functional analysis in relation to goals, objectives, and targets is shown schematically in Figure 5.7. To begin with, broad goals consistent with the overall mission of the enterprise are established. Then, specific quantified objectives are developed with the aim of effective functioning of the health services system. Progress toward the achievement of these objectives is made by means of health programs. These programs, which organize activities for the efficient utilization of combinations of resources, have certain targets. Although a given program may affect more than one health function, individual targets most probably will not. A maternal and child health program, for example, may have both a family planning and a well-child care function, but the program target to immunize 80 percent of the preschool population against measles would apply only to the latter function. Planning takes place, then, in the belief that a measurable correspondence exists between resources expended and activities performed. It further assumes that a meaningful comparison

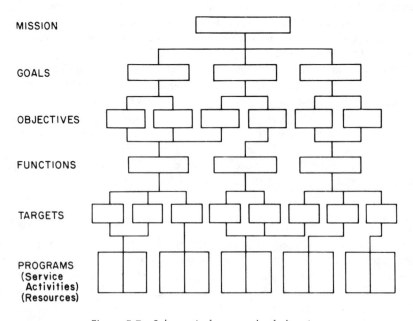

Figure 5.7   Schematic framework of planning

can be made between the activities performed and the degree of attainment of targets and objectives.

The scheme of Figure 5.7 leads at the bottom of the diagram to the appraisal of service activities and resources utilization along the lines indicated in Table 5.2. The intent is to measure levels of effort and resources expended among the designated functions by various functionaries or service points. The total of resources allocated by function (row) is to be compared with the magnitude of existing need. The distribution of functional effort by service entity (column) is to be related to service capacity. Within the body of the table, consideration should be given to the possibility of moving effort toward the left, that is, toward less sophisticated and costly services, without jeopardizing quality of care. To summarize, the functional analysis seeks to establish (1) the level of activities and resources currently devoted to each of the functions, (2) the extent to which community needs remain unsatisfied in various areas, and (3) the potential for modifying or expanding services to meet these needs.

The key to meaningful analysis is to employ measures of need and resource availability that are mutually compatible. To measure need in strictly epidemiologic terms of disease prevalence and mortality rates, while resources are described in economic and financial terms of budgets and staffing patterns, is not very helpful analytically. Rather, needs and resources must both be translated into service terms for the sake of comparability to enable judgments about reallocation of resources to be made rationally. Productivity standards are needed to translate the availability of human resources into services potential. Among the various means of assessing provider effort, work sampling techniques adapted from industry have proved to be especially useful. On the needs side, streamlined community sample surveys have been designed to transcend mere services utilization to measures of fundamental need. For evaluating provider-client interactions, patient flow studies have been developed. These determine the content, quality, and appropriateness of services rendered, as well as the time required, including patient waiting time. Finally, special techniques of cost analysis have been devised to transform cost information into meaningful functional terms.

The functional approach to needs assessment is described in greater detail in Chapter 18, and assessment of personnel effort and costs is covered more fully in Chapter 19. Short of providing the technical detail, brief reference to one or two studies will serve to illustrate the practical application of functional analysis. It has been applied by Yankauer to maternal and child health activities in Latin America.[10] Within the function of well-child care, Yankauer has listed four broad classes of action: (1) screening for early "unrecognized" disease and referral for care, (2) anticipatory guidance for parental education (including nutrition education) designed to prevent future disease, (3) dietary supplementation, and (4) immunization. Each of the four classes of action embodies a series of different tasks; for example, BCG immunization is a specific preventive task of tuberculosis control. Then, "in the context of a health planning framework. . .well child care. . .can be defined as the sum of all specific preventive tasks to be included within a health-care service for mothers and children."[10,p.753]

More generally as increased attention is directed to providing improved coverage with cost-effective services, such analyses make more visible possible impacts upon functional emphasis and demands for scarce resources. For example, one study of

Table 5.2

IDEALIZED MODEL OF THE MEASUREMENT OF EFFORT AND COST BY FUNCTIONS

Functions	Individual Effort and Resources Use					Existing Functional Balance	Functional Balance Based on Need
	Family and Friends	Indigenous Practitioners	Auxiliary Sub-Professionals	Nursing	Physician		
Medical Relief							
Preventive Care							
Family Planning							
Environmental Sanitation							
etc.							
Effort and Cost by Individual Type							
Resources Available							

pediatricians revealed the limited amount of time spent with patients and further showed that one-half of the patient time was spent with well children and another 22 percent treating those with minor respiratory problems.[11] This kind of concrete information gives more solid support to whatever intuitive notions one may have regarding benefits to be derived from the use of pediatric auxiliaries.

THE INFORMATION BASE

Levels of Objectivity

The ability to engage in systematic analysis and to undertake rational planning obviously depends upon the availability of useful information.[12] This is not to say that good planning is based on "hard" data alone. Rather, four levels of meaningful information are to be noted.

The first is in the form of political mandate. If political authorities state that the number of rural health posts must be doubled within five years or that a cardiac care unit is needed in the capital city, planners cannot afford to ignore this information.

The second level of information is expert judgment. While its objectivity may be suspect, we must recognize the fact that the experience of experts generally includes important qualitative aspects of a situation that cannot be captured in quantitative data. Moreover, certain techniques have been developed (notably the nominal group and Delphi approaches described in Chapter 15) which permit group consensus to be established in a reasonably systematic, analytical, and objective manner.

The third level of information is existing records and reports. In principle these should be readily available at little cost and should reflect important trends and emerging problems. In practice, however, they are often incomplete, inaccurate, or out-of-date. They may not be adequately representative, as in the case of hospital statistics that present a biased view of conditions in the community at large. Moreover, the reports are often mere compilations of raw data that have not been subjected to critical analysis. Volumes of services rendered, for example, are seldom related to populations at risk.

The fourth level of information is data collected specifically as a part of the planning process, usually through special surveys. Properly designed surveys can produce relevant and accurate information, but they require skilled professionals and they can be costly and time-consuming.

Thus, each level of information has its values and limitations. In considering the limitations, it is well to recognize that precise data are not as important in planning as in implementation and evaluation. To illustrate, even if the infant mortality rate in a specified area is only known roughly to be in the range of 120 to 180 per 1,000 live births, there can be no doubt that maternal and child health is a major concern. Once a program is mounted to deal with the problem, however, more precise information is needed to determine whether the program is having any measurable effect.

Data Sources

Although the practical importance of qualitative considerations must not be underestimated, sound planning is ultimately dependent upon a solid base of factual data.

Indeed, planning units spend much of their time between planning cycles in maintaining and updating data from various sources. These sources vary according to the particular national or local setting. Likewise, the special features of individual categories of data under economic, epidemiologic, demographic, and other headings need to be understood and are accordingly discussed in later chapters devoted to these specialized topics. In the context of a general overview, however, a review of basic data sources is useful.

Population Censuses

Most countries periodically publish census information which is an invaluable source of data on population size, distribution, and characteristics. The frequency, and therefore currency, of censuses varies, however, along with the degree of detail provided. In particular, needed information about population characteristics may be unavailable for small areas. Even under the most favorable circumstances some underreporting is inevitable, and it is likely to be more severe among certain groups, such as nomads or certain racial minorities.

Vital Registration Systems

Provision for registration of vital events is generally made, but completeness of reporting varies by country and by region within a country. An important consideration is the convenience and motivation for reporting births and deaths in a particular setting. If a birth certificate is required for school enrollment, and primary education is widespread, birth registration is likely to be fairly complete. If the health care system has responsibility for vital registration, motivation for reporting is likely to be low, and convenience likely to be variable. Thus, reporting tends to be more complete in urban areas, where a relatively large proportion of births occur in health facilities and deaths are more likely to occur in association with physician care. A common problem is the failure to report either the birth or death of a child who fails to survive the first week or two of life. This leads to an underestimation of the birth rate and the neonatal mortality rate, both of which are important for planning purposes.

Government Reports

Ministries of health and other public agencies invariably produce voluminous statistical reports. As already indicated, however, quality control over data is generally poor or nonexistent, and the data assembled are often of limited value for planning. Moreover, delays in collecting and processing the data frequently jeopardize the timeliness of the information assembled.

Professional Associations

Medical, nursing, hospital, and other professional associations are a rich source of data with decided limitations. Labor force registration statistics can be useful, but they may not indicate the number of personnel currently active or their location and type of employment. Hospital statistics on numbers of facilities and beds generally do not indicate their quality or service capabilities.

National Surveys

The Health Interview Survey (HIS) conducted continuously by the National Center for Health Statistics in the United States produces a wealth of information on health problems and patterns of health services utilization. The national sample is generally inadequate, however, to provide definitive data for state and regional planning. Such surveys in other countries are even more limited in size or nonexistent. In any event household surveys such as HIS are based upon population perceptions of illness rather than medical diagnoses. This structure has both advantages and disadvantages for planning; the point is that the perspective captured must be recognized. More sophisticated health surveys which include medical diagnoses are occasionally undertaken, but they are extremely costly and cannot be justified on a continuing basis.

REFERENCES

1. Kleczkowski, B. M., et al., *National Health Systems and Their Reorientation Towards Health for All: Guidance for Policy Making*, Public Health Papers No. 77, Geneva: World Health Organization, 1984.

2. Fulop, Tamas, and William A. Reinke, "Health Manpower in Relation to Socioeconomic Development and Health Status," in *Research in Human Capital and Development*, David Salkever, Ismail Sirageldin and Alan Sorkin (eds.), Greenwich, CN: Jai Press, pp. 329–352, 1983.

3. Peterson, O. L., et al., "What Is Value for Money in Medical Care? Experiences in England and Wales, Sweden, and the U.S.A.," *The Lancet*, 1:771–776, 8 April 1967.

4. Gunatilleke, G. (ed.), *Intersectoral Linkages and Health Development: Case Studies in India, Jamaica, Norway, Sri Lanka, and Thailand*, WHO Offset Publication No. 83, Geneva: World Health Organization, 1984.

5. Kleczkowski, B. M., "Matching Goals and Health Care Systems: An International Perspective," *Social Science and Medicine*, 14A:391–395, 1980.

6. Michael, J. M., G. Spatafore and E. R. Williams, "An Approach to Health Planning," *Public Health Reports*, 82:1063–1070, 1967.

7. Deniston, O. L., I. M. Rosenstock and V. A. Getting, "Evaluation of Program Effectiveness," *Public Health Reports*, 83:323–335, 1968.

8. Department of International Health, Johns Hopkins University, *The Functional Analysis of Health Needs and Services*, New Delhi: Asia Publishing House, 1976.

9. *Health Goals for Greater Cleveland: Summary*, Cleveland: Health Goals Committee, 1966.

10. Yankauer, A., "National Planning and the Construction of Maternal and Child Health Norms in Latin America," *American Journal of Public Health*, 57:751–761, 1967.

11. Bergman, A. B., S. W. Dassel and R. J. Wedgwood, "Time-Motion Study of Practicing Pediatricians," *Pediatrics*, 38:254–263, 1966.

12. White, K. L., et al., *Health Services: Concepts and Information for National Planning and Management*, Public Health Papers No. 67, Geneva: World Health Organization, 1977.

PRIMARY READINGS

Development of Indicators for Monitoring Progress Towards Health for All by the Year 2000,
  Geneva: World Health Organization, 1981. No. 4 in the Health for All series, this
  publication proposes four categories of indicators: health policy, social and economic
  factors, health services, and health status.
Elling, R. H., *Cross-national Study of Health Systems, Political Economies and Health Care*,
  New Brunswick, NJ: Transaction Books, 1980. Presents a method, based on contrasting
  case studies, for comparing health systems, using a ten-point scale of regionalization.
*Formulating Strategies for Health for All by the Year 2000: Guiding Principles and Essential
  Issues*, Geneva: World Health Organization, 1979. No. 2 in the Health for All series,
  this document sets forth what countries can do to reorient health systems in line with
  principles of primary health care.
Global Strategy for Health for All by the Year 2000, Geneva: World Health Organization, 1981.
  No. 3 in the Health for All series, this document is the statement on primary health care
  practice adopted at the Thirty-fourth World Health Assembly in 1981.
Kleczkowski, B. M., et al., *National Health Systems and Their Reorientation Towards Health
  for All: Guidance for Policy Making*, Public Health Papers No. 77, Geneva: World
  Health Organization, 1984. Presents a framework for classifying health systems and
  considers reorientation problems in relation to the several kinds of systems.
Roemer, M. I., *Comparative National Policies on Health Care*, New York and Basel: Marcel
  Dekker, 1977. Classifying health care systems as free enterprise, welfare state, underdeveloped, transitional, or socialist, the author examines labor force and health care
  delivery problems in each category.

SECONDARY READINGS

Golladay, F. and B. Liese, *Health Problems and Policies in the Developing Countries*, World
  Bank Staff Working Paper No. 412, Washington: World Bank, 1980.
Gunatilleka, G. (ed.), *Intersectoral Linkages and Health Development: Case Studies in India,
  Jamaica, Norway, Sri Lanka, and Thailand*, WHO Offset Publication No. 83, Geneva:
  World Health Organization, 1984.
Haro, A. Sakari (ed.), *Planning Information Services for Health*, Helsinki: National Board of
  Health, 1981.
McLachlan, G. (ed.), *The Planning of Health Services: Studies in Eight European Countries*,
  Copenhagen: WHO Regional Office for Europe, 1980.
Raffel, Marshall W. (ed.), *Comparative Health Systems: Descriptive Analyses of Fourteen
  National Health Systems*, University Park: Pennsylvania State University Press, 1984.
White, K. L., et al., *Health Services: Concepts and Information for National Planning and
  Management*, Public Health Papers No. 67, Geneva: World Health Organization, 1977.

6

Political Aspects of Planning

WILLIAM A. REINKE AND THOMAS L. HALL

THE POLITICAL PERSPECTIVE

Politics is concerned with relationships of power and influence, generally within the context of government.[1,p.2] At times the association between politics and influence is treated as something that is inherently evil. Political influence, like disease, is an unfortunate fact of life, and in both cases safeguards for prevention of the malady are continually under consideration. Yet those who decry the evils of political influence under certain circumstances can be seen at other times complaining about the inattention to critical needs resulting from a lack of political will.

We would be naive to envision a political process in which political will exists to promote identified legitimate interests, while selfish special interests are thwarted. A clean, healthy environment is obviously in the public interest. The cost of achieving it is equally of general interest. The special interests of groups that contribute to that cost turn out, therefore, not to be so special after all. More accurately, the political process should achieve a reasonable balance in the satisfaction of interests of multiple constituencies with complex value systems. Some planners have tried to remain outside the political process in the interests of objectivity, but such individuals have yet to see their plans carried out. It is the duty of the planner to understand how contemplated actions will affect various health providers, professional associations, clients, public officials, and agency bureaucrats. Such understanding will produce realistic acceptance of certain constraints on action. More importantly, it will enable the planner to utilize the political arena positively in gaining acceptance for a plan framed to balance the needs and concerns of all constituencies involved.

The first level of national political concern is the *will to develop*, that is, the presence of a genuine desire for change. If so, is there a *will to plan*, that is, to bring about the change through systematically considered interventions? Finally, a *will to implement* is required. Political authorities must be willing actually to allocate resources, considering the tax and other sacrificial connotations that carries, and to accept (suffer) the real consequences of change. Countries stand at different points in the sequence of exerting these three wills. The legislature, for example, may have reached the point of authorizing a certain program for the use of nurse practitioners in order to gain the support of program advocates, but funds may have been withheld from the program because of fear of medical association opposition to such appropriations.

In order to assess the state of political will, the planner may examine a number of questions. Is the country's ideological framework congenial to planned change? Which political leaders are committed to change on the basis of what tangible evidence? Do matters of internal politics consume an excessive amount of leadership time? Do graft and corruption siphon off a large proportion of the resources necessary for plan implementation? To what extent have previous plans been oriented primarily toward meeting short-term political objectives or obtaining international assistance rather than toward supporting a continuing developmental effort? What gaps have occurred between the intentions of past plans and subsequent performance? To what extent have the gaps been due to unrealistic goals in contrast to apathy in implementation?

The will to plan is seldom monolithic; wide differences may exist among policy areas concerning the readiness of health and other authorities to consider change. When the overall planning environment is relatively unfavorable, the planner can begin with those policy areas in which the opportunities for improvement are greatest. Conversely, when commitment is generally high, the planner can complement regular activities with efforts directed at concerns not yet widely recognized.

Planners must always be prepared to challenge the status quo. To avoid frustration and failure, however, aims must be realistic, even if this means in an unfavorable environment that objectives can go no further than promotion of the necessary preconditions to successful planning.

If the notion that the health planner is an integral part of the political process, not merely a technician standing above the fray, is accepted, discussion of the political aspects of planning proceeds along two lines. First, we look more closely at ways in which political factors affect the planning process and make it more difficult. Then we develop a series of principles for guidance of the planner in confronting political issues.

CONSEQUENT DIFFICULTIES IN PLANNING

At least five features of the political process are notable as major threats to successful health planning.

1. *Planned change is inherently distasteful to those adversely affected.* Shifting priorities associated with planned change are intended to produce benefits for some segments of the population, but they are likely to be seen as setbacks for other groups. Even potential beneficiaries may be resistant because of the uncertainty of realizing planned effects. Modest benefits widely dispersed may generate limited support, whereas the small group of physicians, nurses, health agencies, or other providers threatened with seemingly adverse changes in their practices can be expected to mount a forceful, focused campaign against the proposed changes. Planners should try to build in compensatory benefits for those adversely affected by the plan, but planners seldom have the ability to offer strong incentives or to impose effective sanctions as means to ensure implementation.[2]

Most people accept the need to plan their own affairs and are reluctant to give up their independence in allowing others to plan for them. As a consequence, planning is unavoidably controversial, and planners tend to underestimate the degree to which the public and politicians oppose planning.[3]

2. *The health perspective of political decision makers tends not to reflect societal priorities.* Attitudes toward health tend to be volatile. As long as they are not personally afflicted with illness, individuals tend to give health matters lower priority than more immediate concerns about food, shelter, employment, and so on. Once illness strikes, however, it surges to the top of the list of priorities for attention. Politicians tend to be relatively healthy, or, if not, they suffer from relatively uncommon diseases that are difficult and costly to treat. It is not unusual for political leaders who have had personal experience with mental illness, heart disease, or polio to give priority to these maladies, even though problems associated with infant and child mortality may be numerically more important in the public at large.

3. *Politicians prefer visible curative endeavors, whereas planners foresee the potential of preventive services.* A hospital dedicated in obvious ways to lifesaving endeavors is a much more attractive monument to political accomplishment than an immunization program that achieves untold benefits for unknown persons at indefinite future times. Even within the curative arena, one costly high-technology organ transplant gains far more media attention than one thousand applications of oral rehydration therapy.[4]

4. *Politicians necessarily face short time horizons, whereas health benefits tend to accrue more slowly.* Because political leaders are continually held accountable by their constituencies, progress must not only be visible but rapid as well. Mortality reduction through treatment of acute episodes of diarrhea is one instance in which political priorities and health concerns are compatible. Over time, however, programs of environmental improvement that bring about drastic reductions in the incidence of diarrhea to be treated may be more cost-effective. The planner must constantly strive to ensure that this and other long-term options involving behavior and life-style changes gain the priority consideration they deserve.

5. *Inherent conflicts among constituencies are ever-present but ever-changing.* In the past, politicians and the public alike have shown considerable deference to the health professions in matters pertaining to health care.[5] Because of the technical nature of medicine, the health administrator has had greater freedom from outside influence to dispose of scarce health resources than has been accorded to other sectors.

Health authorities tended to foster such deference by presenting a public image of dignity and aloofness from controversial issues extending to ethical as well as technical and professional concerns. Their perpetuation of the myth that public health is nonpolitical in character, leading to reluctance to participate in the rough-and-tumble process of interagency politics, meant that opportunities for constructive action were lost and conflicts were needlessly generated through ignorance of the political process.[6]

The situation has changed drastically in recent years.[7] The spontaneous rise in community activism, reinforced in some countries by legislation promoting consumer participation in matters of public policy, has combined with growing awareness of the inability of the health professions to provide comprehensive coverage at reasonable cost to bring the public and politicians into debate on health policies as never before.

IMPLICATIONS OF POLITICAL ISSUES FOR PLANNING

Planning is a mixture of art and science, largely because effective application of the rational techniques of planning depends upon the planner's sensitivity to local political conditions. Despite the individuality of political considerations, however, several general principles are worth noting.

Planning Locus

The health planning unit initially is unlikely to enjoy widespread support or to exercise significant formal authority. It may be both necessary and desirable, therefore, to have a politically prominent and highly placed individual as prime sponsor and promoter of the planning function. While this may ensure short-term survival, it is a tenuous basis for long-term effectiveness.[8] Because political winds change, it is dangerous to have a plan associated with a single political faction. In most organizations, the top jobs are the most vulnerable, so that support limited to this level is especially risky. Perhaps most importantly, because plan implementation requires action throughout an organization, broad participation from the initial stages of plan development is advantageous.

Regardless of how or where the planning function is introduced, the planning unit must constantly seek to broaden its political and organizational base of support. Survival of planning as a viable, ongoing endeavor is more important than gaining acceptance for a specific plan.

Participation by Those Affected

As already suggested, those who are to be affected by planning should be directly involved in the planning process. In this way planners can help ensure that priorities have been properly established, that the plan is feasible, and that the implementation phase will enjoy broad support.

While the principle of involvement is accepted, there is not a clear consensus on means for achieving it. Indeed, in a highly politicized or controversial situation, planners may feel that early involvement of the contending interests would only heighten antagonisms. Although such arguments may be occasionally valid, the planner must realize that controversy is only postponed as a result, not eliminated, and failure to confront the issues early may lead to unrealistic assumptions regarding plan feasibility.

A summary of recent experience in Kuwait is informative in evolving certain guiding principles without pretending to establish a universal formula for action. At the time of the general movement toward primary health care in the late seventies, the Ministry of Health in Kuwait decided to reorganize its health care system along regional lines in ways that would strengthen community primary health care and would also make most effective use of the vastly expanded network of secondary care hospitals then under construction. These policy decisions led to a recognized need for effective planning.

In the absence of a planning unit in the ministry, the obvious suggestion was made to invite an outside consultant group to prepare a single plan of action. More careful reflection, however, led to the realization that a single plan could not begin to address all of the complex dynamics of policy implementation. In the end, therefore, a consultant group from Johns Hopkins University was invited to assist in the development and initiation of a planning process within the Ministry of Health.

Consideration was given first to the establishment of an organizational structure for formulating policy and assessing options for implementation. A policy board was organized directly under the minister, with his active participation. Task forces were formed, in addition, to deal with specific aspects of policy and planning such as epidemiologic assessment, personnel development, and health services research. The task forces were to identify important issues in their respective areas and to process these issues to the point where clear choices and recommendations could be presented to the policy board for action. It was felt that assignment to task force membership would allow key decision makers throughout the ministry to contribute varied expertise and to participate in planning in a more constructive, focused manner than would be possible through one large, unwieldy advisory board. Two-week workshops were conducted for task force members to acquaint them with the philosophy and value of planning as well as specific planning methodology.

Task force members remained full-time managers of various units in the ministry and became part-time planners and policy analysts. The intent was for planning to become integral with management. As part-time planners, however, the task force members found it impossible to develop issues without the aid of a full-time planning unit. A competent secretariat was needed to compile and organize information and to prepare reports for task force response, rather than to expect the task forces to initiate and carry out such activity on their own.

Three features of the Kuwait experience that seemed to be critical to its success can offer guidance elsewhere. First, an influential leader, in this case the minister of health, was the driving force in the development of planning capabilities. Second, an organizational network was set up to facilitate broad participation in the process and provide a mechanism through which the minister's interest and enthusiasm could be conveyed and extended. Finally, a competently staffed planning unit was needed to permit the network of task forces to become more than vehicles for communication and to operate at substantive levels.

Composition of Advisory Bodies

To provide for broad, representative input on planning bodies without inhibiting action excessively is inevitably a difficult task that becomes virtually impossible when consumer representation is considered. Blum contends that U.S. planning councils must include at least thirteen interest categories that cannot be fully accommodated in bodies of fewer than 150 members.[9] Groups of this size must obviously be organized into subgroups, and clear distinctions must be established between advisory roles and decision-making roles.[10] If overall group size is to be limited, it may be necessary to rotate representation from various interest groups in some systematic way. Blum also foresees growing use of polls, surveys, and public hearings as ways to sample the many and changing shades of community opinion on health policy.

Assuming that reasonable balance can be struck in the determination of which interest groups to include on a planning body, the question remains as to how representatives of these groups are to be chosen. Selection of consumer representatives is especially difficult when differences between sociocultural and economic backgrounds of consumers and providers are marked. Unfamiliar with the organization and dynamics of working-class or agricultural communities, the planner tends to assume that persons with leadership roles in schools, religious organizations, businesses, and women's groups are truly representative of both their groups and the greater community of which they are a part. Neither assumption may be entirely correct. Chosen "leaders" are not eager, of course, to challenge the assumptions, but the politics of confrontation in recent years suggests that they are frequently out of touch with the real felt needs of their presumed constituencies and have limited power to affect policy.[11]

It is apparent that meaningful participatory planning requires a balance in membership on advisory councils and policy boards that can only be achieved through intimate knowledge of the interest groups and individual candidates involved. True as it may be that each set of circumstances is unique, this is not very helpful as a generalization. The one principle that emerges is that individuals representing a narrow power base must be included, along with those of modest influence but broader perspective.[12] In the former case, the importance of support from key members of powerful special interest groups is acknowledged. In addition, however, good interpreters of varied group views are needed as valued integrators in the multifaceted planning process.

Staffing the Planning Unit

A priority task for a newly-created planning agency is the recruitment of qualified full-time staff. Competence and integrity must obviously take precedence over other selection criteria, but candidates' political preferences may also have to be considered, particularly in an unstable or highly politicized situation. The top planning job will often be a position of confidence under the chief executive and hence dependent on the party in power. While the political affiliation of staff planners is usually less important, experience suggests that planning effectiveness and continuity will be improved if staff members are drawn from all major political groups.

Politics aside, the main consideration is professional competence in a range of complementary disciplines. Medical knowledge is essential, of course, especially as reflected in the community perspective of epidemiology. Some planning bodies carry this to the extreme in loading the planning unit with physicians. While physician-planners may be at an advantage in gaining the respect of colleagues in the ministry of health, they are at a distinct disadvantage in dealing with economists and statisticians, who usually dominate the planning units in other sectors and in the national planning commission. Consequently, the health sector often suffers in the setting of priorities and the allocation of development funds under national health plans.

Having experienced such setbacks, some health planning units have recruited health economists. Because physicians continue to dominate the entire management structure of the ministry of health, however, the economists find themselves in an obviously subordinate position. Because opportunities for career development are clearly more favorable in other sectors, the ministry of health finds itself able to attract only the less competent nonphysicians. This tendency serves to reinforce their subordinate status. Thus, the planning unit in health is especially challenged to develop a competent multidisciplinary staff of individuals who truly complement one another and can function as a team.

Posture of Studied Objectivity

The planning unit is charged with the responsibility to analyze current and emerging issues, to formulate options for dealing with them, and to present the options clearly, fully, and objectively to decision makers. If this is to be other than an idle, sterile exercise, the planner must be fully cognizant of existing political forces, formal and informal decision processes, and the different value systems that are operative in selecting among alternatives. Yet planners cannot become so immersed in political reality that they are merely the proponents of a narrow partisan viewpoint. They cannot shun the hard choices, but they must maintain reasonable objectivity with regard to them. This is a difficult and narrow path to follow, but the role is essential to a viable planning process.

Planners have experimented extensively with the organization chart in an attempt to find an administrative location with the utopian combination of proximity to the sources of power as well as independence from "politics." Waterston's response to this attempt is that "it is impossible for a planning agency to be both autonomous and effective. . .the very essence to planning, indeed the very decision to begin planning, is political. There is no way of avoiding this, even if it were desirable."[8,p.477]

While remaining fully cognizant of conflicting political values, the planner must accept the impossibility of simultaneously satisfying all values present in any political system. The extreme expression of the planner's ultimate value (that no proposal should be compromised) must inevitably clash with those of radicalism (all proposals should be adopted), conservatism (no proposal should be adopted), checks and balances (the distribution of authority should be wide), and democracy (all participants are autonomous).[2,p.323]

The importance of political factors to the planning process is never so apparent as when a hotly contested election or other governmental change draws near. This was illustrated several years ago in Chile when a three-way presidential race involving candidates of widely differing views coincided with completion of the first phase of a health personnel plan for the country.[13] The planning approach taken stressed the use of flexible models in which several input variables could be modified easily in assessing the implications of alternative actions. The plan outlined the probable course of events—resource requirements and consequent effects of health services on specified problems—under several different sets of hypotheses, only one of these being the continuation of existing policies. Thus the winning party could refer to this useful compilation during its early days in office without the reports being tainted as the prescription for action of the previous administration.

In planning to facilitate implementation, knowledge of decision processes in the health system bureaucracy can be as important as understanding of political influence. Relationships depicted in organization charts provide only a partial introduction to how the system really functions. Numerous persons and interest groups can be cited whose influence is disproportionate to their positions on an organization chart.[14]

Sensitive planning staff will detect many valuable clues as to who counts in the decision process within a given organization. Senior staff of a division or section may have as much of a role as the chief executive in setting agency policy and in ensuring successful implementation. The differential proximity of senior staff to the director's office, particularly in less established bureaucracies, may reflect their current standing in the hierarchy. Those frequently asked to prepare background documents, policy drafts, and speeches, or to accompany key authorities on trips, are in a favored position to influence action. The ease with which different interest groups can gain access to top executives also suggests their relative importance in the system.

The preceding commentary has pictured planners essentially as observers of the decision process. They have a more active role as well in educating decision makers. This role is strengthened as consumer participation is highlighted. According to Lewis, the first step in developing a functional advisory council is to convert all consumers into semiprofessionals, so that all sides are equipped with equal weaponry in the debate over health policies.[15]

In summary, planners cannot be separated from the political process and the health system bureaucracy. Indeed, to be effective, in contributing to conflict resolution and informed decision making they must be closely attuned to differing political values and decision processes. Their role, however, should always be that of facilitator and mediator, never that of partisan participant.

Planning Rationality

Have we not presented an impossible dilemma? The planner is to add light to the heat of controversy, present rational choices, and generally lend an air of objectivity to the political decision process; yet diverse subjective value systems and responsibilities for decision making are to be respected. Can credibility and rationality come to the planning process under such circumstances?

In his classic work *Political Influence*, Banfield postulates five distinct bases for exercising influence, only one of which is "rational persuasion."[2] The other four are friendship, obligation, selling (other than that based on rational persuasion), and coercion, or inducement. Mott distinguishes between two principal models of community health planning in the United States.[16] The *rational decision model* follows the "textbook" sequence of problem solving according to objective and rational procedures. The *community action model* calls for the active participation of all groups affected by the planning process. Because this becomes an essentially nontechnical and subjective endeavor, it is felt to be realistically incompatible with the rational decision approach.

Mott contends that consensus among contending groups is not likely to be achieved spontaneously because contention arises from differing interpretations of health data and consequent divergence in response to potential changes in the health system. On the basis of his detailed study of one of the more influential coordinating councils in the United States, Mott concludes that the only way to induce an organization to accept a decision that runs contrary to its interests is to bring such pressures to bear on it as to make it more costly to the organization to resist than to accept the decision.

Herein lies the key means whereby planning units can serve as effective bridges between the general welfare and special interests. They compile information that permits objective appraisal of existing conditions. They develop rational responses to these conditions. They test the feasibility of these responses in view of their sensitivity to diverse interests and value systems. Finally, they consider how the positions of interested parties might be modified if their perceptions of the conditions changed. Can certain rewards be introduced to offset sacrifices being sought, or are penalties for noncompliance feasible? The aim is to alter the perceived utilities of alternative courses of action in such a way that all, or at least a substantial majority, of the interested parties find it in their own interests to accept the same plan of action.

Information and Communication

Functions of the planning unit already described suggest the importance of its further role as an information clearinghouse. Considerable time and effort must be devoted to the gathering, organizing, processing, and disseminating of data and written documents. Apart from the preparation of routine reports and special studies, planning units have made effective use of periodic bulletins and newsletters, conferences, workshops, presentations, and hearings.

The more important a planning unit becomes as a source of information, the greater is the danger of misuse, for information is a genuine source of power. Consciously or inadvertently, data can be withheld, distorted, improperly filtered, or distributed to the wrong people at the wrong time. An experience in Chile clearly illustrates the problem.[13] Several months before completing preliminary analyses and projections of health personnel requirements, a planning group was asked to make a presentation before the National Health Advisory Council. In an effort to provide the council with a dramatic example of study findings, the planning group reported an impending surplus of midwives that had already been discerned. Invited leaders of the midwifery profession were shocked at the findings, which seemed to contradict the conclusions of earlier studies. The disbelief led to inaction and antagonism toward the planning group, whereas a more diplomatic, carefully documented presentation could have helped direct energies toward a common understanding between the planners and the profession.

The first principle that emerges from this scenario relates to timing. Premature presentation of a problem before it is fully understood and before decision makers are prepared to accept and act upon it is a waste of time. Equally wasteful is the failure to identify a problem until simple solutions are no longer viable.

A second principle is that presentation of bad news must always be coupled with suggestions for overcoming it. Faced with unwelcome information, that is, evidence of a seemingly insurmountable problem, an individual's natural reaction is to disregard the problem and to discredit the bearer of the tidings.

A final risk to be noted in relation to the planning function is the temptation to use planning information for partisan purposes. No clear lines exist between types of information use that are acceptable and those that are not. Moreover, an agency subject to overall direction from the government (and political party) in power cannot ignore selective requests for special analyses, tabulations, or other presentations of potential political value. Nevertheless requests to construct information in support of predetermined conclusions must be resisted in the interests of the integrity of both the planning unit and the individual planner.

SUMMARY

The central arguments of this chapter have been that the political process is often of decisive importance in determining the outcome of planning, and that there is no effective way of isolating planning from the political process. Good planning is inevitably controversial since it introduces technical analysis into a process which heretofore has relied largely on personal judgments and the politics of power. The challenge is to add rationality while still accommodating the interests of diverse constituencies and value systems.

In order to take root, the planning body may require the initial support of a highly placed political patron. Conscious effort should be made, however, to broaden that base of support. Advisory and decision-making responsibility should be divided among advisory groups, policy boards, and task forces in a way that encourages broad participation in the planning process without blocking action. In the interests of broad representation, including consumer participation, planning bodies can easily become nothing more than debating societies.

Assuming that the organizational potential for effective action exists, that potential can be fully realized only with the support of a competently staffed multidisciplinary planning unit. That unit must maintain an adequate base of information that is used judiciously in portraying health conditions, as well as policy and program options and implications.

REFERENCES

1. Key, V. O., *Politics, Parties and Pressure Groups*, New York: Thomas Y. Crowell, 1942.

2. Banfield, Edward C., *Political Influence*, Glencoe, IL: The Free Press, 1961.

3. Feingold, E., "The Changing Political Character of Health Planning," *American Journal of Public Health*, 59:803–808, 1969.

4. Knowles, John H. (ed.), *Doing Better and Feeling Worse: Health in the United States*, New York: W. W. Norton, 1977.

5. Elling, R. H., "The Shifting Power Structure in Health," *Milbank Memorial Fund Quarterly*, 46:Suppl. Part 2:119–143, 1968.

6. Bernstein, B. J., "Public Health: Inside or Outside the Mainstream of the Political Process?" *American Journal of Public Health*, 60:1690–1700, 1970.

7. Holmes, Chris, "Bioethical Decision Making: An Approach to Improve the Process," *Medical Care*, 17,11:1131–1138, 1979.

8. Waterston, Albert, *Development Planning: Lessons of Experience*, Baltimore: The Johns Hopkins University Press, 1967.

9. Blum, Henrik L., *Planning for Health: Development and Application of Social Change Theory*, Berkeley: University of California Press, 1974.

10. Brieland, D., "Community Action Boards and Maximum Feasible Participation," *American Journal of Public Health*, 61:292–296, 1971.

11. Werner, D., "The Village Health Care Programme: Community Supportive or Community Oppressive?" *Contact*, 57:1, 1980.

12. Williams, Glen, and Satoto, "Sociopolitical Constraints in Primary Health Care: A Case Study from Java," *World Health Forum*, 2,2:202–208, 1981.

13. Ministerio de Salud Publica y Consejo Nacional Consultivo de Salud, Republica de Chile, *Recursos Humanos de Salud en Chile: Un Modelo de Analysis*, Santiago: National Health Service Press, 1970.

14. Parston, G., *Planners, Politics, and Health Services*, London: Croon Helm, 1980.

15. Lewis, C. E., "The Thermodynamics of Regional Planning," *American Journal of Public Health*, 59:773–777, 1969.

16. Mott, B. J. F., "The Myth of Planning Without Politics," *American Journal of Public Health*, 59:797–803, 1969.

PRIMARY READINGS

Conant, Ralph W., *The Politics of Community Health*, Report of the Community Action Studies Project, National Commission on Community Health Services, Washington: Public Affairs Press, 1968. Presentation of five case examples of successful health planning largely attributable to the ability of the planners involved to use the political process to their advantage.

Lindenberg, Marc, and Benjamin Crosby, *Managing Development: The Political Dimension*, West Hartford, CT: Kumarian Press, 1981. Synthesis of a wealth of practical experience in various development sectors.

Litman, Theodor J., and Leonard S. Robins (eds.), *Health Politics, Policy and Public Interest*, New York: John Wiley & Sons, 1984. Recounts experience from a number of countries.

McKinley, John B. (ed.), *Issues in the Political Economy of Health Care*, New York: Tavistock Publications, 1985. The provocative views of several authors are presented.

SECONDARY READINGS

Agu, U. U., and G. M. Walker, "A Proposed Method for the Analysis of Public Health Policy in Less Developed Countries," *Socio-Economic Planning Sciences*, 18,2:97–116, 1984.

Banfield, Edward C., *Political Influence*, Glencoe, IL: The Free Press, 1961.

Hawley, Willis D., and Frederick M. Wirt (eds.), *The Search for Community Power*, Englewood Cliffs, NJ: Prentice-Hall, 1968.

Marmor, T., and D. Thomas, "The Politics of Paying Physicians: The Determinants of Government Payment Methods in England, Sweden, and the United States," *International Journal of Health Services*, 1:71–78, 1971.

Parston, G., *Planners, Politics, and Health Services*, London: Croon Helm, 1980.

Seder, Richard H., "Planning and Politics in the Allocation of Health Resources," *American Journal of Public Health*, 63,9:774–777, 1973.

Turshen, Meredeth, *The Political Ecology of Disease in Tanzania*, New Brunswick, NJ: Rutgers University Press, 1984.

7

Economic Aspects of
Health Planning

ALAN L. SORKIN

The purpose of this chapter is to consider those principles of economic analysis which are most relevant to health planning. After briefly defining the scope and content of economics, the discussion focuses on the basic concepts of microeconomics. *Microeconomics* is concerned with the economics of the firm, household, or industry. Next, the principles of macroeconomics are presented. *Macroeconomics* considers the aggregate economy as a whole. Such topics as inflation, unemployment, and the business cycle are within its scope. The relationship between macroeconomics and the theory of income determination is then presented. The chapter concludes with a discussion of the way in which both microeconomics and macroeconomics can be helpful in understanding various aspects of financing health care.

GENERAL ECONOMIC CONCERNS

Economics is fundamentally concerned with the scarcity of goods and services in relation to human wants. If goods and services were not scarce, there would be no economic problem. Given this relative scarcity, certain choices must be made. Thus, to have more of one product (e.g., missiles), we must give up some of another product (e.g., health facilities). Moreover, choice is important because resources can be employed in various alternatives. The land, labor, and capital necessary to build more health centers could be used alternatively to build housing developments. Physicians may be employed in medical school teaching and research, in providing services in offices, or in reviewing health insurance. [1]

Regardless of the type of economic system a country chooses or has imposed by political leaders, three basic issues must be considered: What goods and services are to be produced? How are these goods and services to be made—that is, what techniques of production are to be employed? How is the output of a society to be distributed among individuals? The ability of the system to produce goods and services is constrained by available resources and by technological limits on our productive capabilities. However, within these constraints, the operation of the system is determined by the behavior of individual economic agents (persons, business firms, organizations), as well as by governmental policy decisions.

The first two questions relate to the relative efficiency of the allocation of resources. The last question is concerned with the equity of the income distribution that is obtained.

MICROECONOMIC CONSIDERATIONS

Demand, Supply, and Market Equilibrium

The most fundamental concepts of microeconomics in a market economy are those of demand and supply. What does the economist mean by the concept of demand? *Demand* for a good is defined as the various quantities of a commodity consumers will purchase at all possible alternative prices, other things being equal. The quantity consumers will buy is affected by a number of factors, including (1) price of the good, (2) consumers' taste and preferences, (3) consumers' incomes, and (4) prices of related goods.[2]

The demand comes from individual consumers or household units that are assumed to be maximizing their utility or satisfaction subject to an income constraint and the prices prevailing in the markets for the goods and services among which they may choose.

A *demand curve* is shown in Figure 7.1. The vertical axis of the graph measures price per unit. The horizontal axis measures quantity of the commodity purchased per unit of time. Note that the inverse relationship between price and quantity sold makes the demand curve slope downward to the right.

A clear distinction must be made between movement along a given demand curve and a shift in the curve itself. The former is termed an increase or decrease in the *quantity demanded*, while the latter is known as a *change in demand*. A change in the quantity demanded results from variations in the price of the good, with all other factors affecting the quantity purchased remaining unchanged. For example, in Figure 7.2, a decrease in price from P to P_1 increases the quantity demanded from X to X_1. When the factors held constant in defining a given state of demand change, the demand curve itself changes. Thus, in Figure 7.2, an increase in consumers'

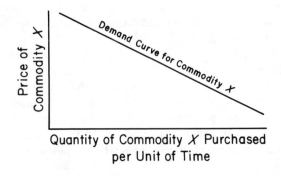

Figure 7.1   Demand curve for commodity X

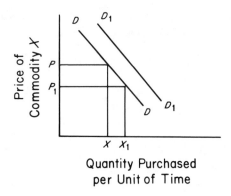

Figure 7.2   Change in demand for commodity X

incomes shifts the demand curve to the right from *DD* to D_1D_1. A shift in consumer preferences to commodity *X* and away from other goods has the same result.

Elasticity

Price elasticity refers to the responsiveness of the quantity demanded to changes in the price of the product, all other factors being held constant. It is defined as the percentage change in quantity demanded divided by the percentage change in price, when the price change is small.[3] In terms of algebra, the elasticity definition appears as:

$$\epsilon = \frac{\Delta X}{X} \bigg/ \frac{-\Delta P}{P}$$

When the elasticity coefficient is less than one, demand is defined to be *inelastic*; when the coefficient is greater than one, demand is *elastic*; and when the coefficient is equal to one, demand is considered to be of *unitary elasticity*.

The Engel Curve

A demand curve indicates the different quantities of one good that the consumer will purchase at various possible *prices*, other things being equal. An *Engel curve* shows the different quantities of one good that the consumer will purchase at various levels of *income*, other things being equal.[4] Engel curves for two different types of commodities are shown in Figure 7.3.

Engel curves provide useful information regarding consumption patterns for various commodities and for different individuals. For basic items such as food, as consumers' income increases from very low levels, their consumption may increase considerably. However, as consumers' income continues to rise, the increases in consumption become less than proportional to the income gains. This is illustrated in Figure 7.3A. For other items such as recreation or luxury goods, expenditures tend to increase in greater proportion than income. The Engel curve presented in Figure 7.3B reflects this situation.

Income elasticity refers to the responsiveness of the quantity purchased to changes

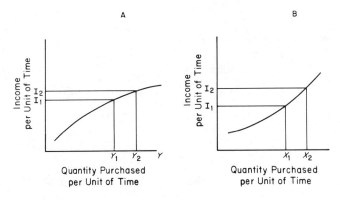

Figure 7.3   Engel curves

in income. When the percentage change in the quantity purchased is smaller than the percentage change in income, the commodity has an income elasticity coefficient that is less than one, an indication of income inelasticity. A percentage change in the quantity purchased that is greater than the percentage change in income produces a coefficient greater than one that is considered evidence of elasticity. If the percentage change in the quantity purchased is equal to the percentage change in income, the income elasticity coefficient is equal to one, a condition of unitary elasticity.

Price and income elasticities are important for health planning. Changes in the price of health services (e.g., due to expanded health insurance or government subsidized care), as well as the growth in consumer incomes, are important in forecasting future utilization of health services. Thus, if planners expect income to grow by 10 percent during the next five years, and the income elasticity of demand is 0.6, then they must be prepared to accommodate an increase of 6 percent in health expenditures apart from attempts to satisfy presently unmet needs. Some estimates of price and income elasticities of demand for health services are presented in Table 7.1. Notice that the bulk of both price and income elasticities are highly inelastic.

Supply and Market Equilibrium

A *supply curve* indicates the relation between market prices and the amounts that producers are willing to supply. Producers are assumed to be maximizing their profits subject to the constraints imposed by the technology available, the market demand, and the prices they face in obtaining resource inputs.

A shift in supply to the right could occur as a result of lower production costs or the discovery of more fertile land. A shift to the left in the supply could occur because of higher production costs or, in the case of agricultural products, natural calamities which reduce the total level of output. A movement along a supply curve is termed a *change in quantity supplied*, while a shift in the curve itself is termed a *change in supply*.

The equilibrium of supply and demand is indicated in Figure 7.4. P_0 represents the equilibrium price and Q_0 represents the equilibrium quantity. In the absence of shifts

Table 7.1

ELASTICITY ESTIMATES, SELECTED STUDIES

Study	Type of Care	Price	Income
Holtmann and Olsen	Dental	-0.127	0.293
	Physician	-0.121	0.057
	Uninsured	-0.164	0.067
	Insured	-0.097	0.056
	Medicare	-0.145	0.133
	Child Physical	0.02	0.048
M. Feldstein	Inpatient Hospital	-1.12	0.54
Davis and Russell	Outpatient Care	-1.03	0.72
	Inpatient Hospital	-0.46*	0.35
		-0.15**	
Phelps and Newhouse	Physician	-0.10	0.08
	Hospital Outpatient	-0.13	0.15
P. Feldstein	Dental	-1.43	1.71
Phelps and Newhouse	Hospital	-0.08	
	Physician	-0.14	
	Dental	-0.16	

* admissions
** length of stay

Source: A.G. Holtmann and E.O. Olsen, Jr., The Economics of the Private
Demand for Outpatient Health Care, John E. Fogarty International
Center for Advanced Studies in the Health Sciences (Washington, D.C.:
U.S. Government Printing Office, 1978), DHEW Publication No. (NIH)78-
1262, pp. 76-77.

in either the demand or supply curves, price would tend toward P_0 in a competitive
market.

Production Theory and Cost Analysis

It has already been noted that the ability of the economic system to transform resources
into goods and services is constrained by technologic limitations on our productive

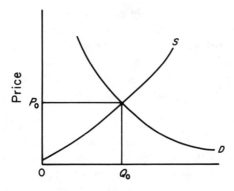

Figure 7.4   Equilibrium of demand and supply

capabilities. Economists use the concept of a production function to describe these limitations. A *production function* is the mathematical relationship between the quantities of various resources used to produce a good and the maximum quantity of that good which they will yield. It is of the form $Q = g(X_1, X_2, ..., X_n)$ where Q is the quantity of output and X_i is the quantity of the ith resource input.[5]

Empirical estimates of production functions provide several types of potentially useful information. First, they can be used to calculate the *marginal products* of specific resource inputs. The *marginal product* of an input is the additional output obtained when the quantity of that input is increased by a small amount while the quantities of other inputs are held constant. Second, production functions indicate the degree to which one input can be *substituted* for another in the production process. For example, for a given decrease in any one input, the function shows the increase in other inputs necessary to maintain the same level of output. Finally, production functions reveal the presence of economies or diseconomies of scale. *Economies (diseconomies) of scale* are said to exist if a K percent increase in all inputs leads to an increase in output of more than (less than) K percent. The absence of both economies and diseconomies of scale (i.e., a K percent increase in all inputs raises output by exactly K percent) is referred to as *constant returns to scale*.

If the unit prices of various inputs are known, one can calculate the total cost of input quantities as $P_1X_1 + P_2X_2 + ... + P_nX_n$ where P_i is the price of the ith input. Furthermore, if one examines all possible combinations of input quantities which according to the production function will yield a given level of output, one can determine that combination of inputs which produces this given output level at the lowest possible cost. Thus, for any level of output we can determine the minimum cost of producing that output. A graph of each output level and the associated minimum cost is called a long-run *total cost curve*. If total cost is divided by quantity we obtain the long-run *average cost curve*. Like the production function, this curve can be used to detect the presence of economies or diseconomies of scale. If it slopes downward (upward) over any given range of output, economies (diseconomies) of scale exist over this range.

One way in which these concepts can be useful for planning purposes is in determining the optimum size (scale) of facilities. Thus, planners would want, for example, to provide for hospitals large enough to take advantage of economies of scale but not so big that diseconomies (increases in long-run average costs) occurred.

Table 7.2 summarizes the results of eight studies of returns to scale in hospitals. While this research does not permit conclusions about the optimal size of a short-term general hospital, it does indicate that economies of scale do exist for a substantial range of output beyond the current average size (135 beds) of nonprofit general hospitals in the United States.[6]

The long-run total cost curve may also be used to derive the long-run *marginal cost curve*, which shows—for every output level—the increase in total cost resulting from a one-unit increment in output. Finally, if we assume that over the time period under consideration some input quantity (or quantities) is fixed while others are variable, one can derive *short-run* total, average, and marginal cost curves analogous to the long-run curves just described. In the short run, total costs may be separated into *fixed costs* (the costs for inputs whose quantities are fixed) and *variable costs* (the cost for inputs whose quantities can be varied).[7]

Table 7.2

FINDINGS OF EMPIRICAL STUDIES ON HOSPITAL COSTS

Investigator	Adjustment for Service Capability	Findings
P. Feldstein	None	Declining average cost
Berry	Analysis of groups offering	Declining average cost
Carr and P. Feldstein	Eight measures of service capability and number of services	U-shaped curve; minimum cost at 190 average daily census
Ingbar and Taylor	Four measures of service activity	Inverted U-curve; maximum cost at 190 beds
M. Feldstein	Nine case-mix proportions	U-shaped curve but coefficients not statistically significant; minimum cost at 300 beds
Francisco	Index of available services and facilities	Declining average cost
Francisco	Analysis of groups offering identical services	Declining costs for small hospitals*
Cohen	Weighted output measure	Constant costs for larger U-shaped curve; minimum cost at 290-95 beds

*Those offering relatively few services and ranging in size up to about 100 beds.

Source: Thomas R. Hefty, "Returns to Scale in Hospitals: A Critical Review of Recent Research," Health Services Research, Vol. 4, No. 4, Winter, 1969, p. 278.

MACROECONOMIC CONSIDERATIONS

As indicated previously, macroeconomics is concerned with those issues and problems relevant to the economy in the aggregate. The most fundamental macroeconomic variable is the *gross national product* (GNP). The GNP comprises the sum of consumption expenditures, gross investment, and government spending. For planning purposes, the allocation of resources to the health sector depends on the total amount of goods and services produced. The relationship between gross national product and the share of public funds devoted to the health sector is presented in Table 7.3 for

Table 7.3

GROSS NATIONAL PRODUCT AND PUBLIC EXPENDITURES ON HEALTH,
SELECTED COUNTRIES, 1978 (millions)

Country	GNP	Public Health Expenditures	Health Expenditures as Percentage of GNP
United States	2,132,900	74,490	3.5
Canada	200,478	11,030	5.5
France	474,503	29,090	6.1
West Germany	642,462	21,466	3.3
Norway	38,675	2,570	6.6
U.S.S.R.	967,820	21,330	2.2
Poland	127,560	3,960	3.1
Brazil	187,260	3,090	1.7
Chile	15,750	367	2.3
Paraguay	2,488	9	0.4
India	117,218	1,360	1.2
Nepal	1,654	11	0.7
Malaysia	15,099	272	1.8
Benin	783	11	1.4
Chad	600	7	1.2
Ethiopia	3,476	43	1.2

Source: Ruth Sivard, World Military and Social Expenditures, 1981 (Leesburg, Virginia: World Priorities, 1981), pp. 25-27.

selected countries. While the developed countries spend a larger fraction of GNP on publicly provided health services, the range, for all countries, is fairly narrow.

The Theory of Income Determination

The core of macroeconomic policy is based on the theory of income determination. The *theory of income determination* in a mixed enterprise or capitalistic economy emphasizes the importance of high levels of savings and investment in order to obtain a rapid and sustainable level of economic growth. Limited savings and investment opportunities result in a low level of economic growth, causing a rise in unemployment. In advanced economies savings are usually undertaken by households, while investment is the result of business decisions.

Developing countries generally lack a sound banking structure which provides a medium for channeling savings into productive investment. For this reason, as well as chronic political instability, many persons hoard gold, silver, and other precious metals. While hoarding may seem rational for the individual, by limiting financial resources for the loanable funds markets, it acts to hinder savings and investment and ultimately development.

One approach which some nations have undertaken in order to supplement limited domestic investment is to encourage the foreign inflow of capital. A high level of foreign investment, under optimal conditions, can lead to an expansion of output and employment at a rate sufficient to lead the country into a more advanced stage of development.

However, foreign investment has a number of potentially negative consequences. First, this activity is often concentrated in a number of extractive industries such as copper or tin mining or petroleum. These industries have limited linkages with other sectors of the economy so that a country with heavy foreign investment in these industries is unlikely to achieve balanced growth. Second, many of these investments are in capital-intensive industries. Thus, the foreign investment enables a few local people to obtain wages above the average, but the *total* employment gain is quite limited. What is really needed in many poor countries is investment in labor-intensive enterprises, but foreign firms are reluctant to engage in this activity because of low expected profits. Third, foreign firms often exhibit a reluctance to hire local personnel for managerial or supervisory positions, reserving these jobs for expatriates.

Given the limited availability of private domestic funds for savings and investment, and the reluctance of many poor countries to suffer the loss of independence that foreign investment (particularly by United States-owned firms) is felt to entail, the primary agent for investment often becomes the central government.

Public Finance

The government obtains funds for investment in health or development projects through taxation. In developed countries the major fraction of government revenues is obtained through an income tax on the earnings of individuals and corporations. However, in developing countries such a tax is often limited to large corporations and their employees as well as the employees of public organizations. This is because of the difficulty of obtaining tax payments from others. Moreover, since developing countries often have a large subsistence sector, many persons are exempt from such a tax.

Because of these constraints, governments often obtain the bulk of their tax revenues from other sources of taxation. One tax frequently used is the sales tax. Such a tax is relatively easy to collect but is generally *regressive*—that is, its incidence falls primarily on the poor. Another source of taxation widely used in developing countries is taxes on imports and exports. Such a tax is fairly easy to collect since it is levied at the time when the commodities enter or leave the country. However, a tax on imports increases the cost of the item to the consumer; and a tax on exports, if passed on to the overseas purchasers, may reduce the overseas quantity demanded. More importantly many developing countries have a foreign trade sector which is quite unstable. Thus, considerable fluctuation in tax revenues frequently occurs, making sound fiscal planning difficult.

Another source of revenue utilized in developing countries and some developed ones is *deficit financing*—that is, a situation in which government expenditures exceed revenues. This frequently results in a phenomenon known as *inflation*, a general rise in consumer prices. When the government operates at a deficit, prices are bid up by the government in order to win resources away from existing users.[8] In effect, inflation is a form of general taxation which no one can entirely avoid. It is perceived by governments, in both developed and developing countries, as being more painless than direct taxation. However, its burden is uneven, falling most heavily on the elderly with fixed incomes and others with inflexible wages.

How does the government finance its deficit? In most cases it simply prints the money. The government exercises its constitutional powers over the currency and thus is able to finance the deficit.

If deficit financing were used with some discretion and the development projects financed in this manner were highly productive, such a policy would be worthy of consideration in countries undertaking considerable public investment. However, countries often lack the administrative discipline necessary to keep the level of inflation under control.

Monetary and Fiscal Policy

One of the implications of the theory of income determination is that particular macroeconomic variables (e.g., savings and investment) can be influenced by governments to achieve particular public policy objectives.

In developed countries the central government uses the tools of both monetary and fiscal policy in order to stimulate economic growth, control inflation, and minimize fluctuations in the level of economic activity. Monetary policy impacts on the growth of the nation's money supply with implications on the ease or tightness of credit and the level of interest rates. If economic activity is declining and unemployment is rising, monetary policy is expansive partly to reduce interest rates and stimulate investment. On the other hand, when inflation is rising and unemployment is low, monetary policy becomes restrictive in order to increase interest rates and discourage investment.

Fiscal policy is the process of using public taxation and public expenditures to help dampen the swings of the business cycle and contribute to the maintenance of a growth economy free from excessive inflation or deflation.[8] Thus, during periods of recession or depression the government level of expenditures exceeds revenues in order to stimulate the economy. In contrast, during times of prosperity the government may operate with a budget surplus in order to exercise a restraining effect on demand.

As indicated previously, the banking system in many developing countries is in an embryonic state. Thus, most developing countries use fiscal policy as the primary agent to control price levels, economic fluctuations, and economic growth. This means that the government budget and the level of revenues play a key role in the process of fiscal planning.

HEALTH CARE FINANCING

Public Financing of Health Care

A number of different methods are available to governments to finance health and social development programs. These include general tax revenues, import and export duties, sales taxes, lotteries, social insurance, and external assistance. Each of these will be discussed in turn, particularly in terms of its distributive effects.

General tax revenues are the single most important source of health care support. The proportion of total national income collected as general tax revenues varies widely among developing countries, however. In a sample of forty-seven such countries, whose tax rates were studied by the International Monetary Fund, this proportion— known as the *tax ratio*—varied from 4 percent to 31 percent. Developed countries in Western Europe and North America have an average tax ratio of 26 percent, excluding social insurance contributions. Developing countries with low tax ratios are completely unable to provide a sufficient level of health care support by relying solely on general tax revenues, even though, as indicated previously, this typically is the largest source of funds.[9]

Although general tax revenues tend to be the single most important source of health care financing in most countries, they may be an unstable source in developing nations because of the fluctuating relationship between budgeted funds and their actual availability and disbursement. Budget projections often include overestimates of tax collections. When funds actually available for disbursement fall short of expectations, changes in priorities may occur. The health sector, often lacking strong political support, may then receive proportionately lower appropriations than had been initially projected. Moreover, the allocation of general tax revenues within the health sector may be affected by political pressures that reduce the efficiency and equity of health care delivery.[10]

Although retail sales taxes are not presently major sources of public revenue in most developing countries, they are frequently used to finance specific programs, such as health care, in which case they may be a significant source of funds for that particular sector. The practice of earmarking sales tax revenues has some advantages. It clearly assigns priority to certain sectors, such as education, health, and other social services, and may thus make the tax politically noncontroversial. Earmarked taxes are often imposed on the sale of beer, liquor, and tobacco products, and on recreational activities, such as sports events and movies.[10] Thus in Colombia, a share of the beer tax is reserved for public hospitals.[11]

Lotteries and other gambling operations frequently serve as sources of earmarked income for health and other social services, particularly in Latin America. However, in few countries is the income from these sources a major component of total health sector financing.

A *social security* or *insurance system* involves the imposition of special taxes on workers and employers exclusively for the benefit of employees and their families. Social security has been instituted, for example, in most Latin American countries, where it usually covers only the 10 to 15 percent of the population who are industrial workers.[12] For the social security recipients, there is usually a separate and well-developed medical service which operates through a special network of hospitals and health centers.

Similar organized facilities under social insurance have been developed in Iran and Turkey. A different pattern exists in Tunisia, where the social insurance system finances medical care for some workers, but the services are obtained from health centers and hospitals that serve the general public and are provided by the Ministry of Health.

Since these contributions are in a special fund, separate from the national treasury, a high degree of financial stability is achieved. In most countries the social insurance fund cannot be used by other government ministries; it is reserved for benefits to the insured. The inflow does vary to some extent with the level of economic activity, but annual appropriations are not required in competition with other public needs, thus limiting political influence. Moreover the general administrative structure of social security programs gives the workers some influence in the management of funds.

The major difficulty with the use of the social insurance mechanism to finance health services in developing countries is that it results in inequities regarding the quality of health services. In Latin America, for example, it was found that expenditures in social security hospitals were two to three times higher per patient day than in hospitals operated by the ministries of health.[13] This has also been found to be the case in Iran and Turkey. In these countries insured persons receive services from more highly qualified professional staff with better resources than those available to the general population. In other developing countries, such as Tunisia, India, and Kenya, differential expenditures exist even though the social security organizations have not constructed separate hospitals for their beneficiaries (except for some recently in India).[14]

These differences in funding levels can be readily explained. The insured workers and their dependents obtain larger per capita expenditures for care than other persons because the funds are raised through special taxes on the most productive sectors of the economy—industry, commerce, or mining—as distinguished from the least productive sector, agriculture, in which the bulk of the population is employed.

In many poor countries the principal alternative to government financing has been development assistance from bilateral and multilateral agencies and extensive funding by foreign nongovernmental organizations. According to Howard, assistance for health from all external sources totaled $3 billion in 1978—less than one-quarter of the total estimated public and private expenditures on health in the sixty-seven poorest developing countries (excluding China).[15] In view of the economic difficulties facing industrialized countries, it seems unrealistic for developing countries to rely on any appreciable increase in external assistance for health in real terms to compensate for an existing shortage in public expenditures.

The tendency of governments to discriminate in budget allocations against programs with high operating costs in favor of capital-intensive projects is aggravated by the reluctance of many external donors to support operating costs. In general, recurrent costs generated per dollar of capital investment are substantially higher for health than for other major public sectors, such as agriculture or transportation. Moreover, the ratios are particularly high for primary health care programs and rural health centers, in which expenditures are mainly for staff and drugs.[16] This makes these programs very vulnerable to budget cutbacks by government.[17]

In nations where the percentage of general tax revenues allocated to health care has increased in recent years, this has often been the result of counterpart funding requirements associated with the acceptance of foreign aid loans. However, for many countries it is unlikely that governments will be able or willing to continue the proportionately higher levels of funding once the aid loans have been disbursed.

Private Financing of Health Care

Even in countries in which general revenues support health service for the majority of the population—as in Asia and Africa—persons in the higher income levels still finance much of their health care through out-of-pocket payments. As a result, a small proportion of the population who can afford relatively high-priced general practitioners and specialists (who are compensated on a fee-for-service basis) has succeeded in diverting a large proportion of the available physician supply to care for their needs.

Moreover, personal payment provides the income for the majority of the indigenous practitioners throughout the world. The fees of village healers vary greatly, and often they receive payment in kind, but their total earnings are considerable.

Moreover, in all nations self-prescribed drugs are paid for by the user. In Latin America, field surveys have shown such expenditures to be extremely high. For example, in Chile almost one-third of all health-related expenditures were for drugs purchased in the private sector.[18] Obviously self-prescribed drugs constitute in large measure the poor family's medical care.

A major source of nongovernmental funding for health care in the United States is health insurance. About four-fifths of the population under age sixty-five had some form of private health insurance in 1980, and about 40 percent of private expenditures on health care were made by insurance companies on behalf of their enrollees.[19]

Insurance reduces the net price paid for health care by the individual (in some cases to zero) and thus increases the quantity demanded for health and medical care services. Moreover, the aggregate effect of an increase in insurance coverage is to cause an upward shift in the total demand for health and medical care. Thus, when the U.S. Medicare program (health insurance for the aged) went into effect in 1966, there was a sharp increase in utilization and concomitantly a rapid increase in medical care prices.

SOME CONCLUDING OBSERVATIONS

The economist's consideration of choice—which emphasizes the scarcity of resources and the weighing of benefits and costs—offers a coherent perspective on resource allocation. Although this approach may seem intuitively obvious, it is not, in fact, wholly consistent with some descriptions of the decision-making process found in the planning literature. One major difference is that according to the economist's methodology, objectives presented in the first stage of a planning process may have to be modified or even abandoned because the cost of achieving them outweighs the benefits. In short, objectives are viewed as tentative rather than accepted as imperatives. Thus, while planners may emphasize the need to offer a full range of services, or the necessity to give every patient the most sophisticated treatment available, these objectives are costly to achieve, and therefore it seems appropriate to ask what is gained by fulfilling them and what is lost when they are only partially fulfilled.[20]

Because administrators and planners in the health sector must rely heavily on medical and scientific experts for technical advice, there is some concern that the former will also defer to the judgment of these experts on matters of value or preference. A common example is the application of health planning "standards" concerning the minimum population required to support various secondary or tertiary hospital services.[21] Strict adherence to these standards obviously precludes consideration of consumer desires as to the volume and types of facilities and services which they would be willing to support.[22] Another situation where this occurs is in determining acceptable levels of safety or risk for new drugs. While this process usually entails very detailed technical studies of the nature and probability of hazards, little attention is paid to the consuming public's view of an acceptable level of risk.

REFERENCES

1. Fuchs, Victor, *Who Shall Live?* New York: Basic Books, 1975, p. 4.

2. Leftwich, Richard, *The Price System and Resource Allocation*, New York: Holt, Rinehart, and Winston, 1960, p. 27.

3. Marshall, Alfred, *Principles of Economics*, 8th ed., London: Macmillan, 1920, Book 3, Chapter 10.

4. Engel curves are named after Ernst Engel, a German pioneer of the last half of the nineteenth century in the field of budget studies. See Stigler, George J., "The Early History of Empirical Studies of Consumer Behavior," *The Journal of Political Economy*, 62:98–100, 1954.

5. Mansfield, Edwin, *Economics*, New York: W. W. Norton, 1974, pp. 122–123.

6. Hefty, Thomas R., "Returns to Scale in Hospitals: A Critical Review of Recent Research," *Health Services Research*, 4,4:275, Winter 1969.

7. Mansfield, *Economics*, pp. 425–451.

8. Samuelson, Paul, *Economics*, 12th ed., New York: McGraw-Hill, 1982.

9. Chelliah, Raja, Hessel Baas and Margaret Kelly, *Tax Ratios and Tax Efforts in Developing Countries*, Staff Papers Vol. 22, Washington: International Monetary Fund, 1975.

10. Zschock, Dieter, *Health Care Financing in Developing Countries*, American Public Health Association, International Health Programs, Monograph No. 1, Washington: American Public Health Association, 1979, p. 24.

11. *World Development Report, 1980*, Washington: World Bank, 1980, p. 4.

12. Roemer, Milton, "Health Care Financing and Delivery Around the World," *American Journal of Nursing*, 71,6:1159, 1971.

13. Bravo, A. L., and A. P. Ruderman, *Cost and Utilization of Ministry and Social Security Medical Care Facilities in Latin America*, Washington: Pan American Health Association, 1966.

14. Roemer, Milton, "Social Security for Medical Care: Is It Justified in Developing Countries?" *International Journal of Health Services*, 1,4,:355, 1971.

15. Howard, Lee, "What are the Financial Resources for 'Health 2000'?" *World Health Forum*, 2,1:23–29, 1981.

16. Heller, Peter, "The Underfinancing of Recurrent Development Costs," *Finance and Development*, pp. 38–41, March 1979.

17. Evans, John, Karen Hall and Jeremy Warford, "Health Care in the Developing World: Problems of Scarcity and Choice," *The New England Journal of Medicine*, 305,19:1124, 1981.

18. Hall, T. L., and A. P. Diaz, "Social Security and Health Care Patterns in Chile," *International Journal of Health Services*, 1,4:374, 1971.

19. U.S. Department of Health and Human Services, *Health: United States, 1981*, DHHS Publication No. (PHS)82-1232, Washington: U.S. Public Health Service, 1982, pp. 263–264 and 268.

20. Salkever, David, and Alan Sorkin, "Economics, Health Economics, and Health Administration," Washington: Association of University Programs in Health Administration, August 1976, p. 53.

21. Navarro, Vicente, *National and Regional Health Planning in Sweden*, DHEW Publication No. (NIH)74–240, Fogarty International Center for Advanced Study in the Health Sciences, Washington: U.S. Department of Health, Education, and Welfare, 1974.

22. Klarman, H. E., "National Policy and Local Planning for Health Services," *Milbank Memorial Fund Quarterly*, 54,1:11, Winter, 1976.

PRIMARY READINGS

Lee, Kenneth, and Anne Mills (eds.), *The Economics of Health in Developing Countries*, New York: Oxford University Press, 1983. Very comprehensive coverage of virtually every facet of economics as it relates to development planning for health.

Samuelson, Paul, *Economics*, 12th ed., New York: McGraw-Hill, 1982 . The classic in the general field of economics.

Sorkin, Alan L., *Health Economics in Developing Countries*, Lexington, MA: Lexington Books, 1976. An extremely readable volume on the subject.

SECONDARY READINGS

Abel-Smith, B., "Health Priorities in Developing Countries: The Economist's Contribution," *International Journal of Health Services*, 2,1:5–12, 1972.

Heller, Peter, "The Underfinancing of Recurrent Development Costs," *Finance and Development*, pp. 38–41, March 1979.

Lee, Kenneth, *Economics and Health Planning*, London: Croon Helm, 1979.

Newhouse, Joseph P., *The Economics of Medical Care: A Policy Perspective*, Reading, MA: Addison-Wesley, 1978.

Roemer, M. I., "Social Security for Medical Care: Is It Justified in Developing Countries?" *International Journal of Health Services*, 1,4:354–361, 1971.

Sorkin, Alan L., *Health Economics: An Introduction*, 2nd ed., Lexington, MA: Lexington Books, 1984.

Weisbrod, Burton A., *Economics of Public Health*, Philadelphia: University of Pennsylvania Press, 1961.

8

The Demographic Base for
Health Planning

MARGARET BRIGHT

Demography is the study of the size, territorial distribution, and composition of population. It is also concerned with the components of population change—fertility, mortality, and migration—and with the changing characteristics of the population.

This chapter first describes certain features of population change that provide the demographic context within which planning takes place. Second, in the hope that health planners will become more frequent and knowledgeable users of demographic data, attention is given to common sources of these data and to some of their limitations and inaccuracies. Finally, mention is made of some specific uses which can be made of demographic data in health planning.

GENERAL DEMOGRAPHIC CONSIDERATIONS

Patterns of Population Growth

In developing countries the present rate of population growth is without historical precedent. Annual growth rates of 2 to 3 percent are not uncommon, and in a few cases rates approach 4 percent. These rates, if continued, would result in a doubling of present population within a generation. Large declines in mortality have caused the acceleration of population growth in the developing countries, and in many countries it will continue to be a factor in increasing growth rates. Growth rates will continue to be high even when death rates have leveled off, because birth rates remain high and in many developing countries have been resistant to change.[1]

Even in developing countries where birth rates have declined, they so far exceed the death rates that large population increases continue. A case in point is Taiwan. In this country a decline in the death rate has been under way for some time, and the expectation of life at birth now exceeds seventy years, a level approximating that of the developed countries. On the other hand, the birth rate, although declining from 41 to 21 per 1,000 since 1959, is still sufficiently above the death rate to add over 300,000 annually to the current population base of 19 million.

In the already developed countries the present potential of population increase is much less than in the developing countries, although there is considerable variation among developed countries. In most European countries, the annual rate of growth in recent years has been below 1 percent and in some countries below 0.5 percent. Rates for the USSR and for developed countries outside Europe are higher.

All developed countries have low death rates, which may continue to decline slowly but not in sufficient magnitude to affect population growth appreciably in the near future. Fertility levels will thus be the main determinant of population growth, and since childbearing is to an increasing extent subject to control in these countries, population growth may be expected to fluctuate from time to time in response to changing conditions.

It is necessary to recognize, then, that the ability to make accurate projections of the future population in any instance depends on the capacity to assess correctly what the future fertility behavior of the population in question will be. This is difficult at best. Short-term projections are likely to be better predictors than long-term projections. Indeed, there is no past performance to demonstrate accuracy of population projections over a long-term period. The present conventional practice in population projection is to prepare different population projections, based on different assumptions about future fertility levels, and to revise the projections at regular intervals. In the United States in 1970, for example, projections for 1980 ranged from 222 million to 238 million, depending upon assumptions about future fertility.[2] The 1980 census revealed that the population had, in fact, reached the lower end of this range.

The effects of net immigration or net emigration on national growth have not been emphasized here, since in recent years neither has much affected the rate of population growth in either developed or developing countries. If immigration is permitted, however, its importance in national growth will be in inverse relationship to natural increase; that is, the same volume of immigration will contribute more to population growth when birth rates are lower than when they are higher. With birth rates low in recent years in the United States, at least one-fifth of the annual population growth has been attributable to net immigration.

Age Structure

Since health needs are to a large extent age-connected, the age structure of a population is one of the more important features of its population composition to be considered in health planning. In general, the age structures of developing and developed countries are distinctly different. Developing countries characteristically have greater proportions of young and smaller proportions of old than do developed countries. They also have higher dependency burdens, that is, higher ratios of persons in dependent ages to those in the productive ages.

How do countries come to have the kind of age structures they have? A fact not generally known is that the age structure of a population—the proportion of old or young—depends mainly on the birth rate and not on the death rate.[3,47-58] Developed countries have a higher proportion of their population in the older ages because their birth rates have declined from higher levels and not primarily because death rates have declined in the older ages. Persons in older age groups are survivors of the birth cohorts produced when birth rates were higher, and populations become older as members of earlier and larger birth cohorts advance in age. On the other hand, developing countries have higher proportions in the younger ages because their birth rates have remained high. Also, contrary to commonsense notions, mortality declines may even contribute to making a population younger. This is the case where reductions in infant and childhood mortality have occurred and have increased the ranks of the young. Thus, countries which have maintained high birth rates and have at the same time had large reductions in mortality at the beginning of life have the youngest populations of all.

Birth rates and the age structure of a population are therefore related. Where birth rates are high, the young tend to constitute a larger share of the population. In turn, a young population produces more births, for more young women will enter and survive the childbearing period. A young population is, therefore, one with great potential for population increase.

Implications of Population Growth and Age Structure for Health Planning

Typically, the developing countries have demographic characteristics which, in addition to social and economic conditions, reduce their options in health planning.[4] With present rates of population growth, most such countries are faced with the problem of providing services to populations which will be doubling within a period of twenty to thirty-five years. Will they find it possible to provide the same type and volume of health services to such extended numbers? Is it possible to expand present services under the pressure of increased numbers? Will it be necessary to institute further priorities in health planning with the result that some services will be emphasized and others not, some segments of the population provided for and others not? Children predominate in these countries; should health services for children predominate at the expense of services aimed at improving the health status of those in the economically productive age groups? Are increases in mortality, rather than decreases in mortality, a distinct possibility in some countries?[5] Given the rate of population growth and the unfavorable structure (i.e., high dependency ratio), what priority should be given to health as opposed to other needs such as education, welfare, economic development programs, and other public functions?

Recently many developing countries have established national family planning programs, usually in conjunction with health programs, in the hope of slowing birth rates and their population growth. Health planners in these countries should not, however, be overly optimistic about the consequences of these programs in easing the constraints on planning for health services in the several years ahead. With possibly a few exceptions, these programs have not yet had any effect on the birth rates and population growth. Even in Taiwan, which has had one of the earliest successful family planning programs, the potential for population increase has been shown to be very great. It has been calculated, for example, that even under drastic reductions in fertility—that is, if fertility declined so that the two-child family (half its present size) became the average at once for all new families in the future—Taiwan's population would still continue to grow for another sixty years, at which time it would level off at about 60 percent above its present population level.[6] Of course, no evidence indicates that any such substantial decline in fertility is in sight.

The case of India is a dramatic one, since present fertility levels are much higher than in Taiwan, and the national family planning program to date has been less successful. In 1985, India's crude birth rate of 34 was producing an annual population growth of 2 percent, so that the population of 760 million was expected to pass the billion mark near the turn of the century. Even if the two-child family became the average at once, the population would reach one billion before the second decade of the twenty-first century.[5] Such an assumption for India is, of course, ridiculous for prediction purposes, but the figures do illustrate that even under the most successful reduction in fertility, India's population growth in the future would still be enormous. Because of its age structure, India's potential for population growth is still great, no matter what reduction in fertility is achieved.

Thus, while health planners in countries with high fertility levels and age structures conducive to rapid population growth should be aware that family planning programs will not ease the burdens in health planning for many years into the future, they will be ill-advised to ignore the importance of attempting to reduce fertility. The longer the interval before the reduction in fertility begins, the more distant the time when the rate of population growth begins to level off. Farsighted health planning will call for reasonable allocation of resources between the prevention of births and the nurturing and saving of lives.[7]

Developed countries, on the other hand, have social and economic as well as demographic characteristics which provide far greater options in health planning than exist in developing countries. Their greater resources, theoretically at least, may be allocated to providing a wider range of health services to all segments of the population. Thus, as the proportion of older persons has increased, more resources have gone to providing health services for those with chronic diseases, a luxury which few of the developing countries have yet been able to afford. Services for the chronically ill are enormously costly, however, and medical advances and institutional innovations for sustaining the well-being and life of the chronically ill are only in process of development and less often yield the dramatic results which similar resources applied to the health needs of younger populations do. Thus, partly at least as a consequence of the age structure of their population and the generally larger proportions of old people, developed countries face the problem of determining how resources for health shall be allocated among different age segments of the population.[8]

A final point is that health planners will have to take into account the consequences of fluctuations in the birth rate in order to plan for the number of people there will be in the future and in particular age groups. Ample evidence from among the developed countries already shows that even where contraceptive practice is widely diffused throughout the population, birth rates on occasion fluctuate upward and downward. Marriage and child-spacing patterns, as well as changes in family size preference, vary in response to a variety of social and economic conditions and may cause birth rates to fluctuate within rather broad limits. Most developed countries experienced "baby booms" after World War II; in some countries, notably the United States, Canada, Australia, and New Zealand, rises in the birth rate were sustained for a long enough time to affect greatly the size of the total population, the age structure, and the potential for future growth.

There is, therefore, no way of knowing what the unborn portion of the population at some future date will be. For the immediate future the number of women in the childbearing ages can be estimated, but the number of children to whom they will give birth cannot. Probably no one anticipated the fluctuation in the number of live births that took place in the United States after World War II. Just prior to the war (1940), the number was 2.3 million. It rose to 3.7 million in 1947, to a maximum of 4.3 million in 1957, declined thereafter to 3.5 million in 1968, and has rebounded somewhat in recent years to its current level of 3.8 million because of large increases in the number of persons now in the childbearing ages who were born in the baby boom years. The future is problematic because of uncertainties about marriage and childbearing trends.

Fluctuations in the size of birth cohorts create problems for planning which are different from those which derive from consistent increases or declines in the number of births. Under consistent declines, demands for particular services are less with each successive cohort; under consistent increases services are in great demand. When, however, the size of birth cohorts fluctuates greatly, resources and personnel needed for services may be alternatively inadequate and overabundant. Rises in the number of births, for example, call for additional maternal and child health services. By the time they have been provided for, and often at considerable investment in buildings, equipment, and training of personnel, the need may have diminished. Meanwhile, services needed for other age segments, such as school health services, may have been curtailed, but are now in short supply as the births of earlier periods swell the ranks of the school-age population.

Theoretically at least, the greatest impact of fluctuations in the size of cohorts may be felt as survivors move into older age groups. Here the prevalence of chronic diseases is high, the cost of providing services great, and the organization of services most complex. Thus, in the United States, consequences of fluctuations in births may be more acute in the next century than in the present one.

Geographic Distribution of the Population

In the developing countries high proportions of the population generally live in rural areas deficient in modern medical and sanitary facilities. The physical remoteness of the rural population poses serious problems for extending even minimum health services and facilities. Many health planners question the efficiency of using scarce personnel and resources for the small achievements which efforts in such cases would bring, yet there are strong pressures to equalize the geographic availability of health services to all segments of the population.

The rapid growth of population in cities of the developing countries undoubtedly contributed to the neglect and delay in providing health services in rural areas. In many of the developing countries, cities are growing at a much more rapid rate than the rural hinterland. In several Latin American nations, for example, recent population growth has been twice as great in cities as in rural areas, and the most rapid growth has been in the largest cities. Latin American countries tend to have larger proportions of their population in cities than do those in Africa and Asia, and the pace at which urbanization has occurred exceeds that of most developed countries when they were urbanizing. The future pace of urbanization most likely will also accelerate considerably in Asia and Africa.

In the past, public health professionals have traditionally limited their purview of demography to changes in mortality. Analysis of mortality changes represented one means of assessing their achievements. Increasingly, however, health planners must take account of other demographic changes as well. They may from time to time benefit by the assistance of demographers. However, the relevance of population changes for health planning will probably be best attended to if health planners themselves make some attempt to understand in a general way how populations change. The foregoing discussion is an attempt to assist in this direction.

SOURCES OF DEMOGRAPHIC DATA

Demographic data derive from several sources. They are collected both by a canvass of the population and from record systems.[9]

The Population Canvass

Two types of population canvass have evolved for obtaining information on the size and characteristics of the population: the population census and the sample survey.

The *population census* is the older method. Although early censuses were taken in China and the Roman Empire, in various European cities and states in the sixteenth and seventeenth centuries, in certain of the French and British colonies in colonial America, and in French Canada, the first continuous series of reliable reports on population was that of Sweden. Here, however, the system of house-to-house enumeration was soon replaced by a continuous accounting system. Periodic censuses began in the United States in 1790 and in England and Wales in 1801. Between 1855 and 1865, complete census enumerations were carried out in twenty-four countries, and the number rose to forty-nine in the years 1925-1934. The increase in the number of sovereign nations in the period following World War II, together with the encouragement and technical assistance provided by the United Nations, has greatly stimulated census taking. By 1964 over two hundred countries, sovereign and nonsovereign, had undertaken population censuses, some for the first or second time only.

The *sample survey* is a more recent innovation, following the development of sampling theory. The sample survey is presently the main source of demographic data in some of the newly formed African nations, where scarcity of resources and personnel and other factors present awesome obstacles to a complete population canvass and where vital registration systems are virtually nonexistent.

Sampling in conjunction with the decennial census was first employed in the United States in 1940 and has since been greatly extended. Since 1960, a total count of the population has been made on only five items (age, sex, race, relationship to head of household, and marital status). The remaining data have been obtained on a sampling basis.

Governments sometimes conduct periodic sample surveys to obtain demographic data in addition to those data obtained from their regular population censuses and registration systems. Cases in point are the National Sample Survey in India and the Current Population Survey in the United States. Special sample surveys restricted to certain population groups are also undertaken by governmental and other agencies. For example, much of what is known about fertility trends and differences among areas has been derived from information obtained in sample surveys. The advantages of the sample survey are timeliness, economy, and quality. It cannot, however, replace the census in supplying demographic data for small areas.

Population censuses in different countries vary in the information collected and the tabulations published, although the United Nations has encouraged the collection of certain types of data and certain basic tabulations. The United Nations itself publishes in the *Demographic Yearbook* the distributions of population by age and sex available from population censuses of various countries. Recently, where sample surveys have been used in lieu of the total population canvass, the United Nations has published the distribution of population by age and sex estimated from these surveys.

The best source of the basic demographic data available from population censuses is the subject-matter index which appears at the end of *Demographic Yearbook*, published annually. Here are given the types of data tabulations published, the year in which the data appeared in the yearbook, and the time coverage on the item or tabulation under consideration.

Also, introductory remarks in each *Demographic Yearbook* are extremely useful in providing an understanding of definitions used in census taking. Each table showing either frequencies or rates has footnotes which describe the departure from usual procedures in the case of particular countries. For these reasons, it is recommended that the yearbook be consulted in advance of the published census reports of individual countries.

Record Systems

Three major types of record systems providing demographic data are the vital registration system, the population register, and administrative records of government agencies.

Vital registration systems have been established in many countries for the purpose of the legal recording of births, deaths, marriages, and divorces. The first such national system was begun in England and Wales in 1837; that of the United States was among the last of the highly developed countries. In the United States, the first mortality statistics from registration data (including only 40 percent of the United States population) were published in 1899, and the first birth statistics (including 90 percent of the population) were published in 1915. Not until 1933 was the last state admitted to the registration system for births and deaths, and several states still are not included in the registration system for marriages and divorces. Evolving a vital registration system has been an enormous task in the United States, not only because of the size of the country, but also because of the federal system.

Probably at least one-half of the world's population still lives in areas where the registration of births and deaths does not occur or is so incomplete that reliable crude birth rates and death rates cannot be calculated. Records of vital events are needed for many purposes, personal and administrative, as well as for demographic analyses. But the establishment of complete registration of vital statistics requires an extensive administrative apparatus and a thorough reeducation of the public.

The United Nations and its specialized agencies as well as the international organizations which preceded them have all devoted much effort to the improvement of vital statistics. They have specified definitions to distinguish all vital events. They have specified types of information which should appear on certificates. They have given technical assistance to the establishment and improvement of registration systems in various countries. Even so, availability of reliable statistics on vital events improves slowly.

In some countries registration is compulsory only for births and deaths, in others for only part of the population (e.g., "European nonindigenous" population). In other countries no national provision exists for compulsory registration, and municipal or state ordinances do not cover all geographic areas. Still other nations have registration areas which comprise only part of the country, the remainder being excluded because of inaccessibility or other conditions. Vital statistics coverage is particularly incomplete for Africa, having been confined largely to European populations and including only partial statistics or estimates for the indigenous segments. Similarly, coverage is uneven and statistics incomplete and unreliable for much of Asia and parts of Latin America.

The best published single source of data on vital statistics for countries as a whole is the *Demographic Yearbook*. On the basis of information obtained from various sources, the United Nations classifies the reliability of vital statistics data from various countries into three categories: (C) those stated to be relatively "complete," that is, representing at least 90 percent coverage of the events occurring each year; (U) those stated to be "unreliable," that is, less than 90 percent coverage; and (. . .) those concerning which no specific information is available.

As with population census data, it is well to consult the tables in the yearbook before referring to the official reports of individual countries to get some notion of the reliability of the data for the nation in question. The tables in the yearbook also provide numerous footnotes which are useful for evaluating definitions used for determining population coverage, and for ascertaining whether tabulation is by date of occurrence or of registration. Such detail may not be provided in official reports of governments, yet it is necessary for evaluating the usefulness of the vital statistics and for determining comparability among countries.

The yearbook has not yet published mortality statistics for subdivisions within countries, but on occasion has provided birth statistics according to whether mothers were residents of urban or rural areas. When vital statistics data for local areas are needed, the yearbook may provide information about coverage and reliability which will determine whether such data exist for different localities and whether they are worth seeking out in other sources.

In Taiwan and a number of European countries, a continuous *population register* is maintained to serve many legal and administrative functions. Such registers are important sources of demographic information, possibly providing data equivalent to those obtained from population censuses and a registration of vital events. One advantage of the population register is that in the calculation of vital rates (e.g., birth and death rates), the data for both the numerator (i.e., births, deaths) and the denominator (population) are from the same source. In most countries the two types of data are compiled under different systems of collection. Another advantage of the registration system is that it may be used as a source of information on internal migration. One problem of population estimation for intercensal years in local areas is that the extent of in-migration and out-migration is unknown and must be estimated with data other than those on migration.

The problem of maintaining population registers is in many respects not unlike that of maintaining vital registration systems. Procedures must be defined and followed on a continuous basis, government functionaries and the public must be educated, and data must be processed at various levels of government. Continuing studies are needed to evaluate the accuracy of the demographic data.

Various *administrative record systems* from both governmental and private agencies also serve as sources of demographic data. In the United States the Bureau of Immigration and Naturalization is the only source of data on the number of immigrants and emigrants. The Department of Defense is the source of data on the number of persons in the armed forces both in the United States and overseas. Both agencies regularly make these data available to the Bureau of the Census for the preparation of population estimates in intercensal years. Data on school enrollment are sometimes used for estimating migration in making intercensal population estimates in local areas.

Another of the more comprehensive governmental record systems is that dealing with individuals covered by various social security programs, of which those under Medicare and Medicaid are relatively recent additions in the United States. Data from such sources are in some instances useful when the interest is in special populations.

ERRORS IN DEMOGRAPHIC DATA

This section is intended to make health planners aware of the more common types of deficiencies and limitations of these data. Here we emphasize the limitations of data found in a wide range of circumstances.

Type of Errors

The simplest and sometimes hardest errors to detect are those of *omission or inflation of numbers*. Omissions (usually more frequent than inflations) are more common in some biologic and social subgroups than in others. Babies and young children are frequently underreported in censuses and surveys and sometimes those of one sex, usually females, more than the other. In the United States nonwhites (especially young adult males) are more frequently underreported than whites; in certain countries the indigenous populations are more often underreported than other sections of the population.

A second type of error is *placing people in the wrong subgroups*. These errors can occur during the collection of data or at a later stage in the data processing. A common type of such error is age inaccuracy. In some cases people simply do not know their age, and no improvement in the system of data collection will yield accurate age information. Often, however, errors of this type are systematic rather than random ones. For example, people tend to show *digit preference* in reporting age, that is, giving ages ending in zero or five.

A third type of error commonly encountered in census enumerations are those which result from *biased measurements of time*. A substantial body of evidence indicates that the longer the interval of time between the event and the time of the census, the more likely the event will be forgotten and not reported. For example, older women are more likely to underreport the number of children they have ever borne, especially if the children died in early childhood. Also, this error is greater among women who have had a large number of children.

The preceding types of errors occur also in the data on vital events obtained from registration systems. As indicated earlier, the registration system may not cover all areas of the country and all segments of the population within it. Omission will probably be less frequent when the birth or death occurs in a hospital than when it does not. Completeness may vary with the event; that is, birth registration may be more accurate than death registration, even when both sets of data are collected under the same system. Any information about personal characteristics which appears on the certificate may be incorrect—age, sex, occupation, marital status, nationality or ethnic background, and so forth.

Vital events, also, seem susceptible to certain types of errors in classification. Live births may be incorrectly registered as fetal deaths, or as infant deaths. Births may be classified incorrectly according to parity. Vital events may also be registered at the wrong place or time. They may be registered at the place of occurrence rather than at the place of residence. Many events are recorded as taking place at the time they are recorded rather than at the time they occurred.

Cause of death statistics, which are of great importance from the public health point of view, are unfortunately among the poorest data supplied by the vital statistics system. The validity of cause of death is dependent upon the quality of medical diagnosis. The percentage of deaths medically certified varies greatly among countries; moreover, even when these deaths are medically certified, the knowledge upon which the medical certification is based varies. Even though medical certification may yield fairly reliable statistics for the major groups of causes of death, improvement is still needed both in specificity and in accuracy.

The *Demographic Yearbook* publishes the number of deaths by cause and cause-specific death rates for countries in each of its issues. It also indicates the percentage of deaths which are medically certified. The cause of death tabulation is according to the "Classification of the Abbreviated List of 50 Causes for Tabulation of Mortality of the International Statistical Classification of Diseases, Injuries, and Causes of Death." Cause-specific rates are not computed when at least 25 percent of the reported deaths are reported as due to senility, ill-defined causes, and unknown causes (B-45). A cursory glance at the size of this group serves as a rule of thumb barometer for a first evaluation of the quality of cause of death statistics.

Assessment of Accuracy in Demographic Data

A number of rule of thumb procedures may be applied initially in making assessments about the accuracy of demographic data. First, a general knowledge of the circumstances of collection and processing is always valuable. All too often consumers of published demographic data do not bother to read the explanations and footnotes which accompany published data. Previously we have referred to the utility of the United Nations *Demographic Yearbook* in supplying definitions of terms, footnotes explaining the data used, and evaluation of the accuracy of the data published. Second, bizarre and unusual findings—data which depart from expectation—should be viewed with skepticism and carefully checked. Third, if more than one source exists for the same or similar data, consistency checks between series of data may be undertaken. Fourth, the source of error is sometimes easier to locate in detailed tabulations. For example, age reporting may be more deficient in some age groups than others.

Comparative checks used in assessing the quality of demographic data may be external or internal checks. *External checks* are those in which records obtained from separate collection systems (or from different operations of the same system) are compared with one another. *Internal checks* refer to the comparison of various data obtained in one collection process.

The simplest type of *external check* is the comparison of data from two different collection systems, for example, data from a census and a registration system. A case in point would be the comparison of the number of children enumerated in a census as zero to nine years, compared with the number of births recorded in the vital statistics in the ten years prior to the census with allowance for attrition by mortality in the interval. Any great discrepancy would indicate further assessment before either set of data was used.

One method now widely used for estimating errors in the enumeration of a population, or segments of it, is the *survival method* or the *reverse survival method*. For example, the size of the same age cohort is compared at two successive census dates (i.e., those five to nine years in 1970 and those fifteen to nineteen in 1980), with account taken of the attrition from mortality which would occur in the interval between censuses. Large discrepancies indicate differences between the two censuses in the accuracy of enumeration of persons in specific age groups.

Record linkage studies provide external checks for assessing the accuracy of certain types of data. Examples include age and diagnoses entered on hospital records compared to those entered on death certificates. These procedures are time-consuming but may in certain instances justify the effort. For example, preference for coding of the cause of death on the death certificate may be allotted to the cause which precipitates the death. Other diseases present in the individual at the time of death may escape tabulation. These, however, may be of special concern to those interested in the prevalence of certain diseases or to those interested in certain health programs.

Internal checks of the data have been used more commonly in evaluating demographic data because the inconsistencies in a set of data often become apparent to the consumer in the course of using it. Such comparisons do not provide clues as to whether a population is undercounted or overcounted. They do, however, allow for more accurate estimation of distributions and rates. For example, one may question why the number of infants under one year is less than the number between one year and two years, if there appears to be no reason to expect that infant mortality has increased or birth rates have declined.

In many cases internal checks are based upon comparisons with the accumulated experience from many populations. For example, we know that the sex ratio (males per one hundred females) at birth varies within a very narrow range in those countries with reliable birth registration data. If in a birth series which we examine the sex ratio is exceptionally high, we might suspect that female births are underreported.

SPECIFIC DEMOGRAPHIC DATA NEEDED FOR HEALTH PLANNING

A serious gap exists between the quantitative information about populations necessary for all kinds of social and economic planning and the amount and quality of data actually available. Several reports have been prepared by the United Nations outlining the types of demographic data needed for different types of planning.[10,11]

Studies of Health Levels

Health planning requires indicators for evaluating health conditions among different segments of the population. Various measures of mortality have commonly been used for this purpose. The demographic data required for the simplest of these measures are as follows:

Measure	*Demographic Data Required*
1. Crude *death* rate	Total deaths in year; total population at midyear
2. Age-specific *death* rate	Deaths tabulated by age; population tabulated by age
3. Age- and sex-specific *death* rate	Deaths tabulated by age and sex; population tabulated by age and sex
4. Age-, sex-, and cause-specific *death* rate	Deaths tabulated by age, sex, cause; population tabulated by age and sex
5. Infant mortality rate	Deaths under one year of age; live births during year

Obviously, reliable data for even these simple measures are not always available for many national populations. They are, of course, even more deficient if the interest is in rates for particular areas of a country or for different subgroups of the population. Where population data are available for denominators, death registration data may be missing or of poor quality for numerators. Or, as in even a country such as the United States, the death data may be available on an annual basis for different jurisdictions (e.g., counties, cities), but during the intercensal years the population data are either unavailable or of doubtful quality because of poor methods of population estimation. The methodology for population estimation for local areas is as yet poorly developed even in the technologically advanced countries.

It would be optimistic to assume that data collected from routine procedures, such as a population census or a vital registration system, will ever exist in the detail needed by health planners. Such data are costly to collect, and innovations in data collection systems tend to be infrequent. Health planners will need to recognize that, even in the most developed countries, either they make use of the limited data available, or they be prepared for costly expenditures for special surveys to obtain the data needed.

Other indicators of the health conditions in the population are morbidity and disability prevalence rates. Data on morbidity and disability obtained by sample survey can be used in conjunction with census data to determine morbidity and disability rates in different segments of the population. Such data are available in the United States National Health Survey and sometimes from studies done in local areas. Wherever possible local area surveys should be taken around the time of the population census, for at that time the population "at risk" is most accurately known.

Studies of the Availability of Health Services

In planning health services, the extent of match between services and population requires information about the geographic distribution of both. Gross measures for national populations, for example, number of hospital beds or number of physicians per thousand population, have limited use, for they conceal differences in distribution of both services and population. Such measures are needed for smaller geographic areas. If information about services (numerator data) can be coded to the same geographic base as population (denominator data), such measures can be obtained for geographic units which make sense for health planning purposes. Such procedures depend heavily upon the employment of modern techniques of data processing. Eventually, when information in one data system (e.g., birth records) is linked to that of another (e.g., infant mortality records) through standardized geographic coding, it will be possible to identify areas where particular types of health programs (e.g., pre- and postnatal clinics) have to be concentrated.

Studies of Projected Needs for Health Services and Facilities

Estimates of the future population are crucial for projecting the need for future services and facilities. Historically demographers have shown little daring with respect to the preparation of population projections for local areas, though in recent years the United States Bureau of the Census has developed a method for making such projections.[12,13] In addition, the need for these projections and certain underlying principles to be considered in undertaking them have been outlined in a report of the United Nations.[11] Several papers prepared for the World Population Conference in Belgrade in 1965 also considered the problem of projections for smaller areas than an entire country.[14, pp. 6–9,61–65,91–96]

The United Nations has recommended separate projections for the urban and rural population sectors, since this distinction is useful in many types of planning. Also, separate projections should be made for the principal cities of a country and for certain administrative or economic regions involved in national development plans. The United Nations has recommended that projections of the population be prepared for not more than twenty to twenty-five years into the future. Alternative sets of projections should be prepared to include not only what appears to be most likely in terms of past experience but also plausible deviations from the past.

The *component method*, or variations of it,[12] is usually suggested as the method most suitable for making local area projections. At the base year, a distribution of the population by sex and by age (single years preferably; quinquennial age groups alternatively) is required. The number of males and females in each age group at the base date is taken as a basis for estimating the number of survivors in successively higher age groups at successive future dates. The size of each future generation of births is estimated by applying projected fertility rates to the number of women in the childbearing age groups. Estimated net additions or subtractions through migration should also be taken into account. Thus the preparation of the projections requires separate projections of mortality, fertility, and net migration.

REFERENCES

1.   Gwatkin, D. R., and S. K. Brandel, "Life Expectancy and Population Growth in the Third World," *Scientific American*, 246,5:57–65, 1982.

2.   Bureau of the Census, "Projections of the Population of the United States, by Age and Sex (Interim Revisions), 1970 to 2020," *Current Population Reports*, Series P-25, No. 448, Washington: Government Printing Office, 1970.

3.   Freedman, R. (ed.), *Population: The Vital Revolution*, Garden City: Doubleday & Co., 1964.

4.   Olurunfemi, J. F., "Population in Health Planning," *Social Science and Medicine*, 17,9:597–600, 1983.

5.   *1985 World Population Data Sheet*, Washington: Population Reference Bureau, 1985.

6.   Avery, R., "Taiwan: Implications of Fertility at Replacement Levels," *Studies in Family Planning*, The Population Council, 59:1–4, November 1970.

7.   *World Population Trends and Policies: 1981 Monitoring Report*, Department of International Economic and Social Affairs, Population Studies No. 79, New York: United Nations, 1982.

8.   Siegel, J. S., "Demographic Background for International Gerontological Studies," *Journal of Gerontology*, 36,1:93–102, 1981.

9.   Hauser, P. M., and O. D. Duncan, *The Study of Population*, Chicago: University of Chicago Press, 1959.

10.   United Nations, *National Programmes of Analysis of Population Census Data as an Aid to Planning and Policy-Making*, ST/SOA/Series A/36, New York: United Nations, 1964.

11.   United Nations, *General Principles for National Programmes of Population Projects as Aids to Development Planning*, ST/SOA/Series A/38, New York: United Nations, 1965.

12.   Bureau of the Census, "Methods of Population Estimation: Part I. Illustrative Procedure of the Census Bureau's Component Method II," *Current Population Reports*, Series P-25, No. 339, Washington: Government Printing Office, 1966.

13.   Bureau of the Census, "Illustrative Projections of the Population of States," *Current Population Reports*, Series P-25, No. 326, Washington: Government Printing Office, 1966.

14.   United Nations, *Proceedings of the World Population Conference, Belgrade, 30 August to 10 September 1965*, Vol. 3, E/CONF, 41:4, New York: United Nations, 1967.

PRIMARY READINGS

Bogue, Donald A., *Principles of Demography*, New York: John Wiley & Sons, 1969. Both a comprehensive text and a reference work, covering the entire field of population study.

Demographic Yearbook, New York: United Nations. A standard reference for data as well as information on methods, reliability, and validity.

Hill, Kenneth, H. Zlotnik and J. Trussell, *Manual X: Indirect Techniques for Demographic Estimation*, Population Studies No. 81, New York: United Nations, 1983. An important guide for making the best possible estimates from incomplete and inaccurate data.

The Population Debate: Dimensions and Perspectives, Papers of the World Population Conference, Bucharest, 1974, New York: United Nations, 1975. Papers from a seminal conference on the population problem.

World Population Trends and Policies: 1981 Monitoring Report, Department of International Economic and Social Affairs, Population Studies No. 79, New York: United Nations, 1982. National, regional, and global review of trends and policies regarding population growth and its component factors.

SECONDARY READINGS

Age and Sex Patterns of Mortality: Model Life Tables for Underdeveloped Countries, Population Branch, Population Studies No. 22, Series A, New York: United Nations, 1955.

The Concept of a Stable Population: Application to the Study of Populations of Countries with Incomplete Demographic Statistics, Department of International Economic and Social Affairs, Population Studies No. 30, Series A, New York: United Nations, 1968.

Gwatkin, D. R., and S. K. Brandel, "Life Expectancy and Population Growth in the Third World," *Scientific American*, 246,5:57–65, 1982.

Oreglia, Anthony, *Uses of Census Data for Health Services Planning and Management*, Health Services Research and Training Program, Lafayette, IN: Purdue University, 1973.

Preston, Samuel H., "Empirical Analysis of the Contribution of Age Composition to Population Growth," *Demography*, 7:417–432, 1970.

Reinke, William A., Carl E. Taylor and George E. Immerwahr, "Nomograms for Simplified Demographic Calculations," *Public Health Reports*, 84:431–444, 1969.

Urbanization: Development Policies and Planning, Department of International Economic and Social Affairs, International Social Development Review No. 1, New York: United Nations, 1968.

9

Epidemiologic Base for Health Planning

TIMOTHY D. BAKER AND WILLIAM A. REINKE

Defined as the study of the *distribution* and *determinants* of disease frequency in humans,[1] *epidemiology* is obviously of central importance in health planning. Study of the distribution of disease is called *descriptive epidemiology* and is of importance in setting priorities and identifying the target population for service intervention. *Analytic epidemiology* concerns disease determinants, a matter of interest in establishing the focal point for intervention.

SCOPE OF CONCERN

Epidemiologic Questions

More specifically, the planner examines health problems with six questions in mind: 1. What is the magnitude of the problem? 2. What trends are evident? (i.e., Is the problem likely to worsen during the plan period?) 3. What patterns of selectivity are exhibited? (i.e., Are individuals of certain age, sex, occupation, or other characteristics more likely to be afflicted?) 4. Is the problem preventable? 5. How treatable is it? 6. What is currently being done by health providers and those in other sectors, as well as individual members of the target population and their families? Thus planners view epidemiologic assessment very broadly. They look at the distribution and determinants aspects of disease in terms of the potential for concrete actions, and in addition assess population behavior with respect to actions currently available. They may conclude, for example, that present service programs are quite appropriate, but they need to be made more accessible and/or acceptable to the public.

Requisite Types of Information

The epidemiologic questions lead to the need for four categories of information. First, the presence of overt illness must be documented. This requires determination of the number of persons affected (disease rates), the extent of the affliction (acute or chronic), and the intensity of the problem (mortality rates and levels of disability).

Second, information is needed on existing hazards to health, or precursors of disease. These may be environmental or personal factors. Environmental concerns include polluted water and air, inadequate waste disposal, unhygienic food distribution practices, and unsafe conditions in the home, in the workplace, or on the highways. These precursors and their effects may be identified in epidemiologic studies looking into the time and place of morbidity and mortality from specific conditions. Personal factors that are hazardous to health include a host of life-style variables such as high rates of smoking and alcohol consumption, improper nutrition and weaning practices, and unhygienic food preparation. These precursors are identified through carefully planned epidemiologic research on specific forms of illness. Health planners should keep informed on such research findings so that they can design programs to help eliminate the hazards or to reduce their effects on disease incidence.

The third type of information needed involves population characteristics related to disease and its precursors. The value of data on age, sex, socioeconomic status, and occupation is apparent, not only in understanding sources of illness but also in identifying certain risk groups as targets for intervention. Educational attainment is another item of useful information relevant to knowledge of disease and behavior in dealing with it. Regional differences in disease prevalence are also important. Epidemiologic studies in developed countries have shown, for example, that male mortality is often higher in regions that are highly urbanized and where mining and heavy industry are concentrated, whereas in less developed countries rural mortality is apparently universally higher than urban mortality.[2]

The fourth category of information concerns client attitudes and behaviors regarding health care. In spite of considerable attention given to so-called underserved areas, the fact remains that indigenous healers are everywhere, and Western medicines, as well as local remedies, are widely available. As a result, some form of action is taken at considerable cost in treating a large proportion of illnesses. Planners need to know how far people are traveling to what practitioners at what cost and to understand better the rationale for the patterns of behavior. In some cases the planner may find private treatment-seeking behavior for curative care to be satisfactory, so that scarce public resources can be focused on preventive and promotive services. In other cases the planner may determine that the substantial community resources being utilized for health care need to be more efficiently or effectively organized through government channels or otherwise.[3]

Information Uses

The scope and content of epidemiologic assessment in planning are summarized by citing the four principal uses that are made of the information analyzed. In the first place, epidemiologic information is essential in setting program priorities. The priorities are derived from assessment of the magnitude of the problems as well as the feasibility and likely impact of intervention. This leads to the second purpose of epidemiologic analysis, which is to determine the size and form of programs to deal with various diseases. At times the program may be single-disease-specific, as in the case of oral rehydration for control of diarrhea. At other times the program will tackle multiple problems, for example, an antenatal program to deal with a number of conditions of pregnancy and early infancy. The third use of information is in identifying the target population for programmatic intervention. Obviously, if an especially vulnerable high-risk group can be isolated, limited program resources can be employed more cost-effectively. Finally, baseline epidemiologic information is essential, along with comparable follow-up data to evaluate the effects of programs.

Having defined the overall role of epidemiology in health planning, we proceed to a consideration of specific measures that are often employed in epidemiologic assessment, along with ways in which the data are organized to form various rates and ratios to facilitate meaningful analysis. The chapter concludes with reference to common data sources and a discussion of the quality of information likely to be available from them.

EPIDEMIOLOGIC MEASURES

The crude death rate, infant mortality rate, and life expectancy are the three most commonly cited indicators of health status. Although relatively easy to obtain, the crude death rate is of limited value since it relates deaths to the total population and therefore ignores age distribution. As a result, a country like the Philippines, with a very young population, has a crude death rate lower than those of European countries, even though the infant mortality rate is five times as high and life expectancy is nearly a decade less. The infant mortality rate is considered to be the best single indicator for developing countries because the risk of death is especially great during the first year (infant deaths often accounting for one-fourth of the total) and because such deaths are largely preventable. Life expectancy is also a useful measure inasmuch as it is effectively a composite of survival rates at all ages and is therefore not affected by the age pyramid of a particular population. Even so, these measures are not adequate in themselves for two reasons. First, they do not give direct evidence of causation and program interventions likely to be effective. Second, diseases that cause discomfort and disability to large numbers can be as important as those that cause the ultimate disability, namely death, less frequently. Moreover interest for planning purposes extends beyond the manifestation of disease to the access and utilization of needed services, as well as the satisfaction derived from them. Our discussion must therefore cover a wide range of desirable measures and must in addition be realistic in citing practical difficulties to be faced in fulfilling these desires.

Desired Measures

Mortality

Their limitations notwithstanding, measures of mortality are essential. The planner requires basic knowledge of major causes of death by age and place of residence or occurrence, and possibly by time of occurrence if seasonality or other time factors are important. Place of residence of the deceased can be useful in relating mortality to the living environment. In cases of accidental death, however, the place of occurrence can be highly informative.

Attempts to establish mortality levels can be traced as far back as the seventeenth century, and about a century ago efforts were initiated to secure uniformity in the recording of causes of death.[4,5] This has resulted in the *International Classification of Diseases* (ICD), now in its ninth revision.[6] The seventeen major categories listed in Table 9.1 are broken down into three-digit codes (about eight hundred diagnoses) and subclassifications of up to four digits that give the specific diagnosis in greater detail. To illustrate, cholera is given the three-digit code 001 and cholera due to *vibero el Tor* is designated 001.1.

Because the system of classification is largely anatomically based, its value to the health planner is limited. For example, "Diseases of the Respiratory System" include maladies that call for widely differing control measures. To cite a few: *pneumococcal pneumonia*—early diagnosis and treatment and occasionally immunization; *emphysema*—smoking cessation programs; *aspiration pneumonia*—alcohol control programs, for the most part.

Table 9.1

MAJOR INTERNATIONAL CLASSIFICATION OF DISEASES (ICD) CATEGORIES

I.	Infectious and Parasitic Diseases
II.	Neoplasms
III.	Endocrine, Nutritional and Metabolic Diseases and Immunity Disorders
IV.	Diseases of the Blood and Blood-forming Organs
V.	Mental Disorders
VI.	Diseases of the Nervous System and Sense Organs
VII.	Diseases of the Circulatory System
VIII.	Diseases of the Respiratory System
IX.	Diseases of the Digestive System
X.	Diseases of the Genito-urinary System
XI.	Complications of Pregnancy, Childbirth and Puerperium
XII.	Diseases of the Skin and Subcutaneous Tissue
XIII.	Diseases of Musculo-skeletal System and Connective Tissue
XIV.	Congenital Anomalies
XV.	Certain Conditions Originating in the Perinatal Period
XVI.	Symptoms, Signs and Ill-defined Conditions
XVII.	Injury and Poisoning

The 800 ICD diagnoses have been reorganized into various abbreviated (aggregated) lists of 50 to 307 diagnoses that, in general, are more useful for planning purposes. Even more appropriately, the planner may wish to establish programmatically oriented disease combinations that depart from the ICD coding scheme altogether. Thus, immunizable diseases might be placed in one group, fecal-oral contamination diseases might form a second group, vector-borne diseases a third, and so on. The regrouping of immunizable diseases might draw influenza from "Diseases of the Respiratory System," roto virus from "Intestinal Infectious Diseases," tetanus from "Other Bacterial Diseases," and yellow fever from "Anthropod-Borne Viral Diseases."

Whatever classification scheme is used, it should not lose sight of the fact that more than one program is needed for some diseases and on the other hand a single program may combat several diseases. In particular, case-finding and treatment services may be required at the same time that preventive measures such as immunization or vector control are carried out. Water and sanitation programs exemplify the multipurpose approach. No degree of sophistication, however, will produce an ideal, all-purpose system of classification. Moreover, even modest sophistication may be unwarranted when the reported diagnoses are of questionable accuracy in the first place.

Morbidity

An accounting of nonfatal illness is obviously necessary, for morbidity contributes substantially to the burden of disease on society. Morbidity is more difficult to measure than mortality, however, as it lacks the definite end point of death. When respondents in household surveys are asked a general question about recent illnesses in the family, they tend to report considerably fewer cases than when they are questioned about the presence of specific conditions such as headache, fever, nausea, or diarrhea.[7] It is sometimes argued, therefore, that probing is necessary to stimulate recall. It could likewise be argued that the minor headache resulted in little impairment and was not considered an illness in need of attention. At the other extreme no amount of probing is likely to elicit information about a serious disease that remains asymptomatic. Only an expensive survey that includes medical examinations will reveal the full picture of biologic need.

It is apparent that the concept of morbidity is inherently fuzzy. Since health planners assess morbidity with a view to possible remedial actions, they must be clear what needs according to whose perceptions are to be acted upon. In this context a balance must be struck between public desires and professional views of the disease process.

A satisfactory compromise might be reached by limiting attention to illness resulting in time lost from normal activity, including employment, school, and household tasks in the case of homemakers. For some purposes an even more stringent limitation to bed-days is used. The advantage in either case is a reasonably reliable measure of conditions that all would agree represent genuine morbidity. The disadvantage, of course, is that important unrecognized health needs may be overlooked. Besides acute morbidity, the presence of chronic disease and disabilities such as blindness need to be measured.

Utilization and Satisfaction

If planners need to know the public's cognizance of disease, they must also understand patterns of action currently employed when illness strikes. Government health service statistics are usually inadequate for this purpose, for they cover only a small portion of the care received. Visits to private practitioners, indigenous healers and pharmacies, as well as use of local herbs and other forms of self-treatment are important aspects of services utilization that should be documented as to volume of care, adequacy, and appropriateness. It is also useful to know reasons for the use of specific providers, including factors of access and acceptability. Community surveys are likely to be needed for these purposes.

Measurement Problems

Reference has been made along the way to a number of difficulties in measurement. We now catalogue and underscore some of the more serious problems and note in addition some difficulties in interpretation of findings.

Need, Want, and Demand

The concepts of need, want, and demand are overlapping but sufficiently different for each to require consideration. The planner must distinguish among these measures and be clear which is being employed in a specific instance. The term *need* is most often used in reference to professionally determined indications of biologic deviation from the normal state of health. Thus, the presence of worms may be considered a "need," even though the individual or family involved may consider this to be a usual condition. The public, on the other hand, may express certain wants that have no recognized medical basis. Some products are sought for their cosmetic value; certain tonics are used for the sense of well-being they create, regardless of whether they produce any discernible physiologic benefit. Demand represents the subset of wants that individuals are willing to act upon. Demand, therefore, requires a willingness to sacrifice time, money, or goods in exchange for the product or service. The planner seeks to promote congruence between needs and wants, and then to ensure that such congruence is converted into effective demand insofar as possible.

Individual or Composite Measures

Attempts have been made to combine several variables into a single measure of health status, socioeconomic status, or other factor of interest in planning. While this approach connotes a simplification that is attractive, it loses sight of various dimensions of an issue that may be individually important.[8] It is probably worth distinguishing between relatively uncommon diseases with high mortality rates and problems that affect large numbers in relatively minor ways. In keeping the mortality, morbidity, and disability aspects separate, however, the need remains somehow to balance these aspects in establishing overall priorities for the allocation of scarce resources. Mathematically derived composites may be considered unacceptably artificial, but any subjective combining of the multiple dimensions of a problem should be appraised critically for its basic rationality.

Disentangling Cause and Effect

To be meaningful, measurement inevitably leads to analysis, interpretation, and value judgments, including determinations of inequities in service delivery.[9] In particular, the data are likely to reveal that more privileged groups in society are in relatively good health and are frequent users of health services. Are these people healthy because of the care received or are both factors merely the product of broader socioeconomic forces? In contrast the true level of need may be underestimated for segments of the population with limited access to services and consequent low rates of utilization and overt indications of need. Finally to what extent do living conditions associated with low socioeconomic status lead to poor health as opposed to the case in which chronic illness reduces opportunities for work and results in deterioration of socioeconomic status?

These questions are difficult to answer but nevertheless of practical interest to the planner in seeking to identify needs and means of alleviating them. Obviously the information system available to the planner should be as informative as possible in distinguishing cause from effect, but associations that are not necessarily causal should not be misinterpreted as such.

Identification of Risk Groups

Closely related to the cause/effect dilemma is the difficulty in isolating high-risk groups as a focus for programmatic attention.[10] The difficulty arises in part because existing data sets seldom provide the detail needed to analyze differences among various subgroups of the population. Too often, however, information about education, occupation, marital status, and a host of other characteristics is laboriously collected in special surveys as a matter of curiosity but never analyzed for programmatic implications.

INDICATORS

Absolute numbers of deaths or episodes of illness are of limited value. Implicit in the notion of epidemiologic assessment is the presumption that these numbers will be related to defined populations or compared with established standards or experience elsewhere.[11] It is important to make these assumptions explicit in emphasizing that essentially all epidemiologic assessment is based upon the creation of indicators in the form of rates and ratios. Rates relate occurrences in a population to the total population exposed to the possibility of occurrence. As an obvious example, the infant mortality rate compares the number of deaths during the first year of life with the source of those deaths, that is, the number born and at risk of being included in the numerator as well as the denominator. Ratios compare two relative frequencies. To illustrate, disease rates in communities with piped water and those without could be compared by forming ratios of the two rates.

Apart from stressing the general importance of indicator rates and ratios in epidemiologic assessment, we single out certain especially important ones for definition and discussion. A more analytical presentation of major epidemiologic concepts and techniques is given in Chapter 18.

Adjusted Rates

Overall rates of interest may be aggregates of experience within various population subgroups. The *crude death rate*, for example, aggregates mortality experience at all ages. The crude rate effectively weights each of the age-specific rates by the relative size of each age group. Two crude rates can differ, therefore, either because the age-specific rates are different or because the weights given to these rates (i.e., composition of the population) differ. Since interest in comparative analysis usually centers on the first consideration, it is necessary to exclude the latter effect. This is done by using a single set of weights for aggregating experience in each of the populations to be compared. Adjustment need not be limited to age, of course. Two populations with different degrees of urbanization, for example, could be compared after adjusting for these differences.

Incidence, Prevalence, and Duration

In dealing with acute conditions, the number of episodes of illness is of principal concern, whereas chronic diseases cause more concern over the total patient load at a given time. The first concern is expressed in *incidence rates*, the number of new cases in a given unit of time in relation to the total population at risk. The second concern relates to *prevalence*, the total number of cases, new and old, existing at one point in time.

The incidence of nonpreventable illnesses may be unaffected by the health system, but care may be effective in reducing the duration of an episode, and therefore the prevalence rate. In particular, prevalence is the product of incidence times average duration.

Relative Risk

In judging the relative importance of specific causal factors, it is informative to compare disease incidence in one group exposed to the risk factor of interest with the corresponding rate in a nonexposed group. The comparative ratio is known as *relative risk*. Suppose, for example, that 15 percent of bottle-fed infants in a community contract diarrhea in a given month whereas the incidence among breast-fed infants is 5 percent. A relative risk of 3 is therefore associated with bottle-feeding.

Sensitivity and Specificity

Detection of disease may be prohibitively costly if carried out through full-blown diagnostic procedures in an entire population. Therefore, less expensive screening procedures have been devised for the population as a whole or for selected risk groups. Screening for tuberculosis has been accomplished, for example, through X-rays and through sputum examinations. In some cases the screening procedures fail to detect disease (false-negative results); on other occasions healthy individuals may be erroneously suspected of having disease (false-positive results). The ramifications are measured in terms of sensitivity and specificity (see Table 9.2). *Sensitivity* is the proportion of true positive cases screened as such, 90/100, or 90 percent in the illustrative case. *Specificity* is the proportion of true negatives screened as such, 95 percent in the example given.

Given the 10 percent prevalence rate indicated in Table 9.2, two-thirds (90/135) of those screened positive would be deservedly followed and treated. If the prevalence rate were 1 percent, only 15 percent of those screened positive would be correctly classified. Thus, the relative importance of sensitivity and specificity depend in part on prevalence rates. In addition, the benefits of early detection must be balanced against the costs (monetary and psychologic) of unnecessary treatment of false-positive cases.

In the early stages of a disease control program specificity tends to be more important than sensitivity for two reasons. First, because of the backlog of accumulated cases, the health care system is unlikely to have the capacity to treat everyone in need. If some cases are missed in screening, therefore, the consequences are not so serious. The second consideration is that in the interests of gaining credibility for the program, most of those screened positive should truly benefit from intervention. This means that false-positive results should be kept to a minimum through high specificity.

OBTAINING THE INFORMATION

The practical matter of data acquisition requires that the planner become acquainted with available sources of various kinds of information and balance quality against cost and timeliness in each case. Most countries can provide numerous records and reports as low-cost sources of vast quantities of unreliable data of little value. Carefully controlled representative surveys typically suffer the disadvantage of being limited in scope regarding both subject matter and geographic area. Large-scale surveys can be excessively costly and so time-consuming that the data are out-of-date before they are processed. *Rapid epidemiologic assessment* (REA) is a relatively new concept that holds promise for the future but is not a well-defined tool at present.[12] Streamlined sample surveys in general represent a grossly underutilized source of planning information that is discussed in greater detail in Chapter 16.

Table 9.2

ILLUSTRATIVE EXAMPLE OF SENSITIVITY AND SPECIFICITY

| Screening | True State | | |
Results	Positive	Negative	Total
Screened Positive	90	45	135
Screened Negative	10	855	865
No. Individuals	100	900	1,000

In addition to the foregoing general observations, several specific data sources are cited and evaluated in the following paragraphs. [13]

Censuses

Periodic population censuses are invaluable sources of data on population size, distribution, and characteristics as has already been established in Chapter 8. The data provide denominators for the calculation of health indicators. In addition they provide indirect indicators of the nature and magnitude of health problems themselves. For instance, age distributions permit estimates of age-specific mortality rates. Information on population density, occupation, sex, and other distributions suggests the likelihood of certain problem concentrations.

The infrequency of censuses, along with the lack of detail provided, are disadvantages, however. Specifically, needed information about population characteristics may be unavailable for small areas.

Vital Registration Systems

Vital events registration offers a continuous means of tracking births and deaths by age and cause. [14] Completeness and reliability of reporting may be uneven, however. Events in certain age or population groups may be consistently underreported, for example births among nomads or perinatal deaths. Moreover, reported causes of death may be skewed, especially for deaths occurring without medical intervention. Where a birth leads to early death, neither the birth nor the death may be reported and both rates become distorted. Even though the case is omitted from both the numerator and denominator of the death rate, the effect on the numerator is much greater.

In most developed countries an accurate vital registration system was started in a few advanced areas where it could be checked for completeness and accuracy before certification. The system then spread, finally covering the whole country. Developing countries might follow a similar development process.

Communicable Disease Reports

Reports of certain communicable diseases are a major part of the published statistics of most health departments. They tend to be selective in disease coverage, however, and those included are either incompletely reported or erroneously labeled. Doctors in the United States, for example, continued to report malaria cases long after the disease had been eradicated in the country.

There are reasonable systems for establishing sentinel reporting areas to determine the extent of communicable disease. For *sentinel reporting*, an interested and conscientious clinic or practitioner agrees to supply complete reports on all designated diseases and thus serves as a "sentinel" for disease outbreaks in the community. In this situation, as in so many others, carefully monitored special surveys can be more informative than routine reporting.

Service Statistics

Voluminous service statistics are compiled by most service agencies. Health planners in some countries use hospital in-patient statistics as the principal basis for estimating the major causes of mortality. These, along with hospital and health center out-patient reports, become the main source of morbidity estimates. While these sources may be the best available, they are usually far from satisfactory. Because vast quantities of data are derived from many sources, quality control is difficult and delays in data processing frequently preclude timely reporting of results. Even under the most favorable circumstances, cases seen by the reporting institutions are unlikely to be representative of conditions in the population at large.

Publications of the World Health Organization, notably the *World Health Statistics Annual*, are the most important sources of comparative international health data. It must be recognized, however, that the statistics originate with the member countries and therefore raise the same doubts about quality as the country reports themselves.

Professional Associations

Medical, nursing, hospital, and other professional associations can be a rich source of data with decided limitations. Personnel licensure statistics can be useful, for example, but often they do not exclude currently inactive individuals; nor do they indicate the present location and type of employment of those who remain active. Hospital statistics on numbers of facilities and beds generally do not indicate their quality or service capabilities. The Professional Activities Survey (PAS) in the United States provides comparisons among hospitals in volume of surgical procedures by type, average length of stay, and other indicators of utilization, but the survey is limited in its coverage of institutions. Similarly, health insurance agencies usually maintain detailed and accurate records, but only on a highly selective group of clients and providers. In most countries accidental deaths are reviewed in some manner by a medicolegal system, which therefore can be a useful basis for determining the extent and nature of injuries as a cause of death.

While each of these and related sources of information is limited in scope, together they can usefully complement more general data sources, as well as providing clues regarding quality of the main bodies of data.

Surveys

The National Center for Health Statistics (NCHS) in the United States carries out a number of ongoing surveys that have rightly attracted attention as models that might be adapted to circumstances in other countries. Three of the series merit specific citation.

- Series 10: *Health Interview Survey (HIS)*. A sample of geographically stratified households provides data representative of regional and urban/rural differences. Questions elicit information about the household's economic, educational, and other characteristics; recent morbidity experience; and utilization of health services. Additional questions are inserted from time to time to collect information for special purposes.
- Series 11: *Health and Nutrition Examination Survey (HANES)*. A smaller subsample of individuals is surveyed more intensively by means of physical examination to ascertain nutritional status and existence of chronic disease conditions such as anemia, hypertension, and visual problems.

• Series 22: *National Natality and Mortality Survey.* Sample surveys stemming
  from vital records acquire additional data on characteristics of births and deaths
  not available from the records themselves. For example, mortality by socioeconomic class is evaluated.

The NCHS also conducts surveys of the institutionalized population, discharges
from short-term acute hospitals, and experience in chronic hospitals, nursing homes,
and long-term care facilities.

   In addition to such ongoing surveys numerous special surveys are always being
carried out by universities, research institutes, and in some cases by ministries of
health themselves. Information from these studies tends to be underutilized by planners, either because they are not acquainted with the surveys or because they are considered "special." Many such studies deserve closer scrutiny for their generalizability.
As a minimum they might produce tentative conclusions of general interest to be
confirmed by a brief follow-up study instead of a costly, large-scale general survey.

   Finally, we should not underestimate the importance of epidemiologic assessment
by field-workers through systematic appraisals of local conditions. Workers can and
should be trained to interpret data as well as record it. The result is likely to be more
accurate information that is actually used.[15]

CONCLUDING OBSERVATIONS

Seldom is there a dearth of epidemiologic data. Frequently, however, the quality,
and therefore the usefulness for planning, is highly suspect. Health planners are
accordingly advised to promote the development of streamlined and closely monitored
surveillance techniques for rapid epidemiologic assessment. This could constitute a
highly significant and lasting contribution to the planning process.

   In the meantime, they need to draw upon available measures selectively and
cautiously. Whatever measures are employed should be related meaningfully to the target population through formation of appropriate indicator rates and ratios. Undoubtedly
a large dose of judgment based upon experience has to be added. While not an ideal
arrangement, this approach is superior to blind acceptance of "hard" data that are
patently faulty.

REFERENCES

   1. MacMahon, B., and T. F. Pugh, *Epidemiology Principles and Methods,* Boston: Little
Brown & Co., 1970.
   2. "The Inequality of Death: Assessing Socioeconomic Influences on Mortality," *WHO
Chronicle,* 34:9–15, 1980.
   3. Levin, L. S., et al., *Self-care: Lay Initiative in Health,* New York: Prodist, 1976.
   4. Graunt, John, *Natural and Political Observations Made upon the Bills of Mortality,*
Baltimore: The Johns Hopkins University Press, 1939.
   5. Humphreys, Noel A. (ed.), *Vital Statistics: A Memorial Volume of Selections from the*

Reports and Writings of William Farr, London: Offices of the Sanitary Institute, 1885.

6. *Manual of the International Statistical Classification of Disease, Injuries and Causes of Death,* 9th rev., Vols. 1 and 2, Geneva: World Health Organization, 1977.

7. Department of International Health, Johns Hopkins University, *Functional Analysis of Health Needs and Services,* New Delhi: Asia Publishing House, 1976.

8. Chen, Martin K., and Bertha E. Bryant, "The Measurement of Health: A Critical and Selective Overview," *International Journal of Epidemiology,* 4,4:257–264, 1975.

9. Chen, Milton M., J. W. Bush and Donald L. Patrick, "Social Indicators for Health Planning and Policy Analysis," *Policy Sciences.* 6:71–89, 1975.

10. *Risk Approach for Maternal and Child Health Care,* WHO Offset Publication No. 39, Geneva: World Health Organization, 1978.

11. Bice, Thomas W., "Comments on Health Indicators: Methodological Perspectives," *International Journal of Health Services,* 6,3:509–520, 1976.

12. Laukaran, V. H., *Review of the Literature Related to Rapid Epidemiological Assessment,* Washington: National Academy of Sciences, 1984.

13. "Recommendations of Working Group on Data Bases for the Measurement of Levels, Trends and Differentials in Mortality," *World Health Statistics Quarterly,* 36,1:72–77, 1983.

14. Ferrara, Conrad P., *Vital and Health Statistics: Techniques of Community Health Analysis,* Atlanta: Center for Disease Control, 1980.

15. "Use of Epidemiology in Primary Health Care," *WHO Chronicle,* 34:16–19, 1980.

PRIMARY READINGS

Beaton, G., and J. Bengoa, *Nutrition in Preventive Medicine,* Monograph Series No. 62, Geneva: World Health Organization, 1976. Discusses the major deficiency syndromes, epidemiology, and approaches to control of malnutrition.

Chin, J., and F. Morrison (eds.), *Communicable Diseases Control Planning,* International Health Planning Methods Series Vol. 1, Washington: U.S. Department of Health and Human Services, 1979. State-of-the-art summary on surveillance and control of specific diseases, including tuberculosis, malaria, onchocerciasis, schistosomiasis, leprosy, filariasis, and enteric diseases.

Hetzel, Basil S. (ed.), *Basic Health Care in Developing Countries: An Epidemiological Perspective,* New York: Oxford University Press, 1978. Epidemiologic perspective on essential features of planning, programming, implementation, and evaluation of health care in rural areas with particular focus on the Western Pacific Region and India.

Lilienfeld, Abraham M., *Foundations of Epidemiology,* New York: Oxford University Press, 1976. A basic reference on the principles and methods of epidemiology.

Morley, D., *Pediatric Priorities in the Developing World,* London: Butterworth, 1973. Stresses social, economic, and cultural factors affecting the interaction of infectious diseases and nutritional status in children.

The Place of Epidemiology in Local Health Work: The Experience of a Group of Developing Countries, Geneva: World Health Organization, 1982. Reviews the types of epidemiologic questions to be raised and tools for acquiring the requisite data at community level.

Risk Approach for Maternal and Child Health Care, WHO Offset Publication No. 39, Geneva: World Health Organization, 1978. Explanation of a specific method to identify priority health problems by determining the risk to mothers and children.

Sabin, E., and W. Stinson, *Immunizations in Primary Health Care,* Primary Health Care Issues Paper No. 2, Washington: American Public Health Association, 1981. State-of-the-art paper on child immunizations with particular reference to the WHO Expanded Program on Immunization.

Toward a Better Future: Maternal and Child Health, Geneva: World Health Organization, 1980. Examines the causes and risks of maternal, infant, and childhood mortality and morbidity and discusses possible interventions.

SECONDARY READINGS

Austin, J., and M. Zeitlin (eds.), *Nutrition Intervention in Developing Countries: An Overview,* Cambridge, MA: Oelgeschlager, Gunn and Hain, 1981.

Benenson, A. (ed.), *Control of Communicable Diseases in Man,* 14th ed., Washington: American Public Health Association, 1985.

Davis, R., and G. Blevins, *Methods of Malaria Vector Control: A State of the Art Literature Review,* Office of International Health, Washington: U.S. Department of Health and Human Services, 1979.

Epidemiology and Control of Schistosomiasis: Report of a WHO Expert Committee, WHO Technical Report Series No. 643, Geneva: World Health Organization, 1980.

Field Manual of the Expanded Program on Immunization, Geneva: World Health Organization, 1977.

Holland, W. T., and L. Karhausen (eds.), *Health Care and Epidemiology,* London: Henry Kimpton Publishers, 1978.

Knox, E. G. (ed.), *Epidemiology in Health Care Planning,* Oxford: Oxford University Press, 1979.

LaForce, F. M., M. S. Lichnevski, J. Keja and R. H. Henderson, "Clinical Survey Techniques to Estimate Prevalence and Annual Incidence of Poliomyelitis in Developing Countries," *WHO Bulletin,* 58,4:609–620, 1980.

McCarthy, M., *Epidemiology and Policies for Health Planning,* Oxford: Oxford University Press, 1983.

Stallones, Reuel A., "Comments on the Assessment of Nutritional Status in Epidemiological Studies and Surveys of Populations," *The American Journal of Clinical Nutrition,* 35:1290–1291, 1982.

Wallace, H. M., and G. J. Ebrahim (eds.), *Maternal and Child Health Around the World,* London: Macmillan Tropical Community Health Services, 1981.

10

Health Personnel Planning

TIMOTHY D. BAKER

Crucial to any planning endeavor is provision of human resources in adequate quantity and with appropriate competence to deliver and support the needed services. In the labor-intensive health sector where two-thirds of costs may be for personnel, the importance of labor force planning is further underscored, and its urgency is highlighted by the long lead times required. Hospitals can be built in months; it takes a decade to train a doctor. It is especially disheartening, therefore, to observe throughout the world decaying water systems, unstaffed health centers, and empty hospitals as monuments to dismally inadequate personnel planning.

The planning takes place at two levels. At the macrolevel there is need to plan for enough workers to meet, but not exceed, future effective demand for their services, that is, to fulfill perceived needs that are backed by willingness and ability to commit the necessary resources. At the microlevel the functions and task assignments of those workers need to be determined. In practice the two aspects are pursued simultaneously; it is difficult to say precisely how many nurses should be trained until their roles and work loads have been clarified and quantified. Following the logic of presentation in this volume, however, we confine our attention in the present chapter to the basic principles and methods of global planning; a description of specific techniques of job analysis will be found in Chapter 19 as part of the broader discussion of analytical techniques guiding plan implementation.

Because of the multifaceted nature of health personnel planning, a framework for analysis is essential.[1] The one presented here has proved useful in practical tests in countries as varied as Taiwan, Turkey, Peru, and Nigeria, where cooperative labor force studies have been conducted under the auspices of the Department of International Health of Johns Hopkins University.[2-5]

The analytic framework has four parts:

1. Supply analysis and projection of supply: measuring the current supply of all types of health workers in some detail and projecting the supply forward to target dates ten to twenty years in the future, with anticipated additions of new graduates and estimated subtractions for death, migration, retirement, and change of profession;

2. Demand analysis and projection of demand: evaluating the effective economic demand for health services from both the private and public sector and

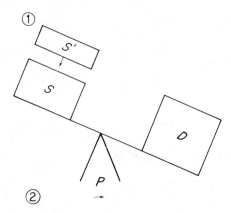

Figure 10.1   Supply-demand balance on the fulcrum of productivity

projecting the effective economic demand forward to the ten- to twenty-year
target dates;
3. Productivity analysis and projection: estimating the average number of services
   per health worker per unit of time and projecting changes;
4. Matching future supply and demand: comparing the projected supply with the
   projected demand and recommending necessary adjustments to effect a balance
   in light of inevitable constraints.

Supply can be brought into balance with demand by either (1) increasing supply
(S') or (2) increasing productivity (see Figure 10.1). Increase in productivity is limited
by standards of acceptable quality. On an economic basis total services may be
increased at the same cost by increasing units of service per health worker, or by
substituting less expensive health workers. This sounds quite simple, and as a concept
it is. Complexities arise in practice, however, as will be discussed later.

SUPPLY ANALYSIS

Current Supply

Categories of Health Workers

The first step in supply analysis is to decide whom to count. The categories which
are costly to society (total numbers x average earnings) should be given the most
attention. Therefore doctors, nurses, dentists, technicians, and pharmacists should be
included. Midwives, herbalists, and similar categories should be counted in countries
where they are numerically important. Other groups may be included for completeness
when planning resources are adequate. It is not generally considered necessary to
count untrained persons who happen to be working for medical institutions. Most
drivers, hospital maids, and hospital clerks should not be studied in detail as they are
part of larger general labor pools.

Definition of categories of health workers is the next step in analysis of supply. Just what will be included under the term *doctor*—should osteopaths, licentiates, grade-B graduates be included? What about chiropractors, herbalists, curanderos? Although definitions vary from country to country, a useful guiding principle is to have one group of doctors comprising all persons licensed to practice modern, scientific medicine. This is not to say that the herbalists and curanderos should not be counted; such groups may be important, but they should be studied separately.

In measuring supply, overclassification of health professions into many subgroups is confusing. For each class of health worker, three groups—professional, assistant, and aide level—should be adequate for most general health personnel planning. Usually a definition based on years of training and income level is most useful in determining these groupings (see Table 10.1).

The importance of measuring the various specialty groups varies from country to country. In any case, information on numbers of teachers in the health professions is important for measuring capacity for expansion of schools.

Counts of Workers

Information on the current supply of health workers varies from country to country and profession to profession as to source and accuracy. For professional health workers who come from the country's training institutions, a count of the past graduates, corrected for migration, deaths, and retirement from the profession, gives the potential number of professionals available. This source is only as reliable as the estimates of deaths, retirements, and migration, however, and obtaining these estimates is difficult.

Health workers in subprofessional categories often have not been formally trained in educational institutions, but have merely taken an examination or, in some cases, simply applied for and received a license. This leads us to the second source of data on current supply, namely the licensing institution. This institution, if its basic registration is complete, can serve as a good source of the maximum numbers of legal practitioners in a given country. This source of data is often out-of-date, however, as most licensing agencies lack adequate methods for removing those who leave the licensing area, die, or stop practicing.

Professional registries, which are maintained in many countries, are a third source of data. Registries maintained by an annual, biennial, or triennial registration system give reasonably current estimates of the total number of active practitioners. In many countries, however, this system misses practitioners who are working in government institutions, for they may not require registration. Combining government payrolls with the registry of private physicians makes estimates of total health personnel possible, but name checks are required to prevent double counting of professionals with more than one job.

In countries lacking a general registration, one often finds a special registration for permission to use narcotics. Since essentially all physicians in private practice require narcotics at one time or another in their practice, this is a reasonably good source of information, if the regulations are enforced. The same problem of enforcement exists with lists of health workers paying professional taxes required in some countries.

Professional societies occasionally have an accurate roster of all members of the

Table 10.1

HEALTH WORKERS BY INCOME AND TYPE OF PRACTICE

Type of Practice	High Income, Long Education (12 Years Basic + 6–13 Years Professional)	Medium Income, Medium Education (10–12 Years Basic + 2–5 Years Professional)	Low Income, Short Education (6–12 Years Basic + 0–2 Years Professional)
Unsupervised independent general clinical practice	Physician (GP)	Assistant medical officer, licentiate, behdar, health officer (Gondar), feldsher, nurse	Dresser
Hospital or group practice	GP and specialist: e.g., surgeon, pathologist, radiologist, physiatrist, orthopedist	Nurses (general duty and specialist), surgical technician, laboratory technician, X-ray technician, physical therapist, etc.	Nurses/aide, practical nurse, dresser, laboratory assistant
Antenatal, delivery, and postnatal care	Physician-obstetrician	Midwife	Auxiliary midwife, dai
Drug compounding and dispensing	Pharmacologist	Pharmacist	Dispenser, compounder
Mental health	Psychiatrist	Psychiatric nurse, psychiatric technician	Psychiatric aide
Dental practice	Dentist	Dental hygienist	Dental aide
Public health	Health officer (M.D.)	Health visitor, public health nurse, health educator	Home health aide, etc.
Environmental sanitation	Sanitary engineer	Sanitarian	Malaria assistant, sanitary inspector, etc.
Average cost of training:	X	1/3 – 1/2 X	1/10 – 1/5 X
Average earnings per year:	Y*	1/5 – 1/2 Y	1/10 – 1/5 Y

*Including consideration of private practice as well as government salary.

SOURCE: Baker, T., "Paramedical Paradoxes—Challenges and Opportunity," in G. Wolstenholme and M. O'Connor (eds.), Teamwork for World Health, CIBA Foundation Symposium, p. 130, London: J. & A. Churchill, 1971.

profession and in some cases even include those who are not members of the society. Complete, accurate, professional society registers are usually found in developed countries.

Census data may prove useful if the general census mechanism is worthy of confidence. The major drawbacks of a general census are that it is usually, on the average, five years out-of-date and that census enumerators accept the statements of informants without verification. Thus, many unqualified practitioners may be listed as qualified professionals.

Pharmaceutical companies occasionally have accurate and up-to-date lists of private practitioners. Our experience, however, has been that these lists are far from complete and that companies are frequently reluctant to release them.

The last and undoubtedly most accurate method of determining the current supply of health workers in the country is to conduct a special survey. Unfortunately, this method is both time-consuming and expensive. If a country has no good source of information on numbers and distribution of professionals, however, a survey could be the starting point for an effective registration system. Such a system is a necessity for rational health planning in any country of the world today.

Characteristics of Health Workers

In addition to the total number in each class of health professional, distributions by age, sex, educational background, income, type of practice, specialization, productivity, and geographic location are important factors.

Knowledge of age composition is essential for making predictions of change in supply. For example, in Taiwan we found almost five times as many doctors aged thirty-five to forty-four as those aged twenty-five to thirty-four.[2] Authorities were unaware of this dangerous gap in physicians, which would not have manifested itself until twenty years after our study, when it would have been too late to institute corrective measures. The sex distribution of health professionals is particularly important in countries where women have a very different working pattern from men. Educational background is especially useful in defining categories of health workers and in comparing contributions of different training institutes to the health sector work force.

Income level is important for all projections, and attempts to change the supply require adequate information on the costs of these changes.[6] Reluctance of professionals, especially in the private sector, to disclose their income hinders the determination of income levels. In many cases disclosure of real income would bring major penalties in the form of increased taxes. In Taiwan we had to approach the problem indirectly.[2] We found the average monthly expenditure for physician services (from sixty-six thousand persons in the random sample), multiplied this average by the total island population, and divided the product by the number of physicians practicing in Taiwan. In this way we derived the average physician income.

Another significant attribute of health workers is their type of practice, that is, the number of hours they work, and those for whom they work (private practice, for the state, for a commercial concern, for a voluntary agency, or for a combination of these). If an adequate method of defining specialists exists, numbers of various types of specialists can be useful.

Some knowledge of productivity—the number of patients seen by the average practitioner per unit of time—is essential.[7] Information on variation in productivity from region to region and among specialties is also useful. Where productivity falls below acceptable norms, supply can be effectively increased without adding a single person merely by increasing productivity.

In order to measure the importance of immigration of health professionals, the number of native-born and native-trained workers is needed. Knowledge of geographic distribution is necessary because a country may have an adequate, overall number of health workers so poorly distributed that corrective action is indicated.[3] Finally, special studies of professional and student attitudes on rural practice, migration, retirement, and so on, can be useful for future planning.

Projections of Supply

Losses

Change of supply may be divided into losses and increases. Losses are primarily by death, retirement, and migration.

Theoretically, the most accurate method of age-specific professional death rate determination is to divide all registered deaths of professionals for each age group by the population of professionals in each age group. If the professional group is small, we must use a period longer than a year. Where professional associations keep accurate records of memberships and deaths and where all professionals are counted in their statistics, these records offer an alternative source of data for direct calculation of professional death rates. Official registration data and professional association data may be combined to secure a more accurate determination of professional deaths. This method has the drawback of being time-consuming if separate classes of health professionals are not distinguished on the death certificates. Where accurate information is not readily available, this direct calculation of professional mortality for personnel studies is not justified.

The second alternative is the use of age-specific death rates for the general population, assuming that the physician death rates equal the general death rates. The assumption is faulty, however, for physician age-specific death rates are uniformly lower than the general population age-specific death rates. The problem can be overcome by applying a correction factor to the general mortality rates. Even if only approximate, the adjustment usually yields satisfactory results, for losses by death are generally small in comparison to losses from retirement and other voluntary withdrawals from employment.

Retirement is usually the greatest source of loss to the profession. Age of retirement from government service can vary from fifty-five to sixty-five, or even seventy in some countries. In private practice, in which usually one does not retire but "fades away," median retirement age is a matter of judgment.

In some countries losses by change of occupation are very significant. In most of Latin America, where the medical degree is as much a mark of an educated person as it is the key to a professional career, many physicians do not practice medicine. Determination of these losses may be made by surveys of one or more cohorts of graduates of professional schools. In some countries many physicians are reported to leave the practice of medicine because they are unable to make a living in medicine.

This is evidence of defective health personnel planning. Special cases of change in profession, such as Taiwanese midwives' going into nursing, also occur. One change of "profession" of particular significance for the female health worker is marriage. One must carefully examine the working pattern of women to determine the extent to which marriage causes an interruption in work, and whether the interruption is temporary or permanent. Studies of this kind can be the basis for planning retraining programs for women or offering flexible work schedules as an inducement to return to work.

The last major source of losses to the profession, migration, differs widely in importance among countries. Migration takes place for both immediate shift in employment and for advanced training. In practice it is very hard to separate the two. If professionals from developing countries undertake a ten-year course in a highly specialized field that has no application to the problems of their own countries, they essentially constitute as much of a loss to their profession as the professionals who migrate directly. Regional or state health personnel planning is difficult in countries with appreciable interstate or interregional migration.

Increases

Increases in supply are primarily from new graduates. Obviously, training schools are a major source of new health professionals, but it is not enough merely to take the number of graduates from each school for the past several years and average them. Evaluation of the plans and proposals of educational authorities in the various health professions gives a better estimate of the increase by new graduates than statistical projection of past performance. Increase of health professionals by immigration is extremely rare in most developing countries (with the exception of most oil-producing countries). The creation of a new group of professionals occasionally occurs when one class of professionals is upgraded in status by governmental decree.

Four basic factors determine a country's potential for increasing its number of trained health professionals. The first is the "raw material," that is, qualified applicants. Training institutions should know the annual number of qualified applicants for admission each year. Correction should be made for multiple applications when multiple training institutions exist. In estimating the number of future applicants, the demands of other sectors of the nation's economy for trained workers must be taken into consideration. Generally, in relation to the number of openings, medical schools have a higher number of qualified applicants per place in class than the other health professional schools.

The second determinant of potential for increased supply is the educational plant capacity, that is, the number of students who can be taught in existing teaching facilities. For clinical fields such as nursing and medicine, this also implies the availability of suitable "teaching" hospital beds, as well as the classroom facilities normally associated with educational institutions. In addition to the study of the existing facilities both the feasibility of new construction and methods of extending the present facilities should be reviewed, so that more students might be handled by using more efficient teaching methods. In particular, removal of factors causing high dropout rates during training can increase output substantially without requiring corresponding increase in input.

The third factor determining potential for increase is capital: the funds available for expanding training facilities and paying for the recurring costs of training and education.

The fourth determinant is the availability of teachers. Because of the long time lag in preparing a teacher, it is also probably the most important. Reviews of existing resources of qualified teachers are needed, as are determinations as to whether salary and prestige are adequate to attract the teachers needed to expand training facilities. As in the problem of limitation of educational plant capacity, existing numbers of teachers could be extended by converting some part-time faculty to full-time. This approach must be planned with care, as exclusively full-time teaching staffs are often divorced from the realities of practice.

DEMAND ANALYSIS

Current Demand

Many different methods exist for determining the demand for health workers. In clinical medicine if one disease has many remedies, one assumes that none of these remedies is really adequate. Such is the case in demand analysis for health workers.

Basic Biologic Need

Determination of the basic biologic need is based on (1) determining the level of mortality and morbidity of a country, (2) estimating the time of health professionals needed to care for each type of case representing the various types of morbidity and mortality, (3) multiplying the time per case by the estimated annual number of cases to get the total professional hours needed, (4) determining the average hours worked per year by the professionals, and (5) dividing total hours needed by hours per professional to determine total required supply of health professionals to meet basic biologic needs. The best known document on this method is the classic report by Lee and Jones.[8]

Although this approach has the seductive appeal of seeming to be the most scientific appraisal, for many reasons it is not practical. First, few developing countries in the world have sufficiently detailed and accurate morbidity and mortality statistics to give the exact figures needed for this type of estimate. Second, no measure of health professional time required by any given level of morbidity or mortality can be accurate when health problems have many alternative solutions that require entirely different types of health personnel. For example, should one equate the morbidity from diarrhea with a sanitary engineer's time to design a water supply system, or with the services of the nurse or community health worker in rehydration? Third, and most important, even if one could calculate the "need," this is not a measure of public "demand" for the services of health professionals. Unused health clinics in areas of continuing health need stand as examples of this, as do physicians unable to earn a living in the larger cities of underdeveloped countries (where there are crying needs for medical attention which the people cannot afford to express in terms of effective economic demand).

The Status Quo

The most common approach to health personnel analysis is the *normative* approach, whereby existing professional-to-population ratios are enshrined as norms.[9,10] The major flaw in this method is that it fails either to determine the suitability of present ratios or to account for changes in demand due to technological innovations or to changed demographic character of the population. Closely akin to the status quo approach is the "Parkinsonian" modification which says in effect, "Our doctors and nurses are busy now; therefore we need more." This was the method used in early efforts to set standards for public health nurse staffing in the United States. Some communities had a ratio of public health nurses to population of 1 to 10,000. In the opinion of authorities, the nurses were overworked, so the ratio was changed to 1 to 5,000.

Comparative Method

The *comparative method* takes the ratios for other countries and reasons that the country under study has effective economic demand for at least as many health workers as the reference country. The flaw in this method lies in the fact that very few countries are truly comparable.

Expert opinion is often used for estimation of demand for health workers. Indeed, in some instances, this is probably the best estimate available, particularly in fields that employ small numbers of health workers for whom there is no real public demand, such as health education, sanitary engineering, and other highly specialized personnel.

Established Standards of Practice

In the Soviet Union, where essentially all medical care is given by government personnel, estimation of demand for doctors has been based on observed norms of practice. On the average, one out-patient doctor sees five patients per hour, works 5.5 hours a day, 240 days a year, and, theoretically, handles about 6,600 visits in a year. Total visits per 1,000 population are observed, and doctors are "allocated" on the basis of total population. Similar methods are used for allocation of medical specialists, nurses, and feldshers. The approach is similar to the basic biologic need approach. The Soviet system is said to work satisfactorily in practice, but it is complex and exacting. Apparently, the full extent of demand has not yet been established, for earlier publications[11] proposed increasing the doctor/population ratio from 1/610 to approximately 1/350, and more recently, targets of 1/280 have been set.

Effective Economic Demand

In countries where the private sector offers an appreciable source of financing for health services, an entirely different approach must be used: measurement of effective economic demand. This is best determined by a random sample survey of patterns of demand for health services throughout the country to be studied. Demand should be quantified by basic demographic and socioeconomic attributes of the population, thus giving a basis for predicting change of demand as the age pattern changes and the population becomes better educated, more urban, and wealthier.

In the public sector, the number of budgeted vacancies may be used as an index of unmet demand.

In countries with both private and public payment for medical care a mixed method of analysis of demand is appropriate. Indeed, since no perfect method for measuring demand exists, one should utilize elements of all relevant methods and arrive at a composite judgment on the current demand for medical services. Where two or more methods are employed, results can be examined for similarity, either to increase confidence in their validity or to establish the need for further appraisal.

Projection of Demand

Changes in Population Size and Composition

The primary factor affecting change of demand in countries with slight to moderate health worker shortages is population increase: the more people, the more services demanded, assuming that economic growth at least keeps pace with population growth. The increase in demand may not be directly proportional to the increase in population, however. If the population gains higher percentages of older people and/or young children, demand for health care increases because these groups universally require more medical attention. The geographic redistribution that often accompanies population increases must also be taken into consideration. Specifically, as the country becomes increasingly urbanized, the demand for health services changes in size and character.

Economic Development

Economic development may also play a major role in increasing demand. Increases in income and in educational attainment lead to raised expectations and greater sophistication in the use of health services. High-income groups demand more medical care at the present time; logically, therefore, as the present low-income groups improve their status, they, too, will be able to afford and demand more medical services. Economic development also increases public sector demand as more tax revenue is available to fund public health programs. Development can further bring about important shifts in the type of demand as well as its magnitude. The use of more highly trained and expensive modern medical practitioners in place of herbalists and indigenous medical practitioners can have important implications for planning.

A related source of change in demand to be considered is alternation of the supply and accessibility of health workers. Effective demand for a physician does not exist in a village where physicians are unknown or unavailable. A new road, however, that fosters village contact with a neighboring town and its medical services is likely to change demand patterns markedly.

Unpredictable Factors

Whereas the previous effects on demand may be predicted with considerable accuracy, the following factors, which can likewise exert significant effects on demand, are virtually unpredictable. These include changes in disease patterns, technologic advances, and organizational change.

Measles has changed markedly in many countries from an extremely severe disease with high morbidity to a far milder condition. Leprosy is thought to have changed considerably during society's experience with it. New diseases, such as acquired immune deficiency syndrome (AIDS), may be introduced where they did not exist previously, distorting the picture of demand for medical care.

With respect to technological change, the demand for radiologists would never have been predicted before the discovery of the X-ray. The discovery of antibiotics has changed the health service demand picture considerably, probably more from the standpoint of shifts within the health professions than from changes in total demand. For example, the discovery of isoniazid and PAS has very definitely reduced the number of chest physicians and tuberculosis hospital nurses required and increased the demand for public health nurses to carry out home care programs.

Modifications in the organization of health services influence both the available supply of health workers and the demand. For example, as health ministries "ruralize" their health services, more demand may develop. Changes in administrative policies now in existence could have marked effects on the demand for medical care. For example, in some clinics only the first twenty patients in line are admitted each day. The people know this and know that they must suppress demands for medical care since it is not available under the present organizational system.

PRODUCTIVITY

Measurement of productivity in the health sector is a special and complex problem. In most instances individuals of different professional background and capability jointly supply widely different services. A simple example is solo practitioner dentists who restrict their practice to filling teeth. In this case, the dentist's productivity would be the number of teeth filled per unit of time, for example, per day. In general, a relatively longer time period is more appropriate, in order to include losses from vacation, time spent in continuing education, administration, and other deviations from normal activities.

The most complex example is a hospital staff offering a range of services from brief out-patient visits to complex surgical procedures and including personnel from janitors to cardiac surgeons. Measuring the productivity of a hospital complex or its individual members calls for modern methods of industrial engineering, systems analysis, and detailed time and motion studies.

After careful measurement of the time actually required for given procedures, and the administrative time which must be allocated to them, equivalency units may be established. For example, one surgical procedure may equal ten out-patient visits, or one medical in-patient day may equal five out-patient visits.

Although not exactly productivity in a strict technical sense, the services produced per monetary unit spent on salaries is an important measure. The problem of measurement of productivity is further complicated by the differing levels of salary of the various members in a complex medical organization. It may well be that a more highly trained, and better paid, technician may be more productive even in terms of cost than a less qualified and less well paid worker. However, major economies usually can be realized as functions are transferred from high-salary to low-salary workers.

Examples from dentistry show the magnitude of increases in productivity that may be expected from use of auxiliaries and aides. An American Dental Association survey showed that each additional full-time auxiliary working with a practicing dentist increased the dentist's productivity by approximately 30 percent.[12,13] A U.S. Navy study showed that each middle-level dental technician, up to three, could boost the productivity of a dentist well over 50 percent.[14]

There are limits to this principle; otherwise, we would have the janitor performing all health sector functions. Downward delegation of functions is limited by (1) quality of care expressed as end results of services, (2) acceptability to consumers, and, perhaps most important, (3) acceptability to the professionals who set standards for care. Physicians in developing countries often state that nothing but physician care is good enough for their people, although, in fact, only a small portion of the people have the benefit of any modern medical services at all.[15]

WILL SUPPLY MATCH DEMAND?
RECOMMENDATIONS TO EFFECT A BALANCE

After one has estimated the future demand and the future supply for periods ten to twenty years in the future, discrepancies between them must be analyzed and resolved. For most professions in most countries this analysis will reveal future potential shortages, more so in some regions of the country than in others. In some cases, however, one might predict surpluses of certain categories of health workers, in respect to the effective economic demand.[16]

Possible Actions

Three types of action are possible to stave off predicted personnel shortages. More workers of a given type might be added through training or other means of recruitment. Role substitution might be contemplated, so that workers who are plentiful are asked to take on functions previously assumed by those in short supply. Finally, shortages might be alleviated through increases in productivity.

Additional Personnel

Increases in numbers of personnel trained can be accomplished either by increasing annual intake per training institution or by increasing the number of institutions. In either case one must determine whether there are adequate numbers of qualified applicants and qualified teachers and sufficient funds to support the increased scale of training. Possibly government subsidies will have to be provided for the students and for the training institutions.

The unique nature of some shortages may require special measures. In particular, difficulties in filling rural posts may call for reserving places in training institutions for candidates from rural areas. In addition, the training itself should be oriented to rural needs, and provision may have to be made for salary supplements and special allowances for rural service.

In the past, the purpose of expanded training efforts has sometimes been defeated because graduates have been lost to migration. Thus, training initiatives may have to be coupled with compulsory service and restrictions on migration for a period of time following graduation. Fortunately, since 1980 the major flow of health professionals from poor to rich nations has markedly decreased.

Substitution

The second general way to avert shortages is to substitute one category (usually less skilled) for another. Such substitutions imply changes in training programs to fit professionals better for their new roles. If, for example, nurses are to act as physicians in rural clinics, they should be trained in elements of diagnosis and treatment rather than only in bedside nursing. Such changes also call for new patterns of supervision and quality control. If the quality of medical care is not to deteriorate markedly when lower-level personnel are substituted for higher-level personnel, good supervision is essential.

Increased Productivity

Increased productivity, the third basis for overcoming shortages, requires creative appraisal of the specific circumstances to identify promising inducements to greater efficiency. Regular sessions of in-service training can enhance morale as well as competence. Group practice or other modified organizational arrangements can be effective in many cases. Of course, good supervision is essential to optimum performance.

Programming the Alternatives in the Face of Constraints

Since all these recommendations have social and economic costs, the ultimate policy decisions will not be in the hands of the health personnel planner, but rather at higher levels of government. These policy decisions will involve such issues as equal distribution of care regardless of ability to pay versus better care for the more "productive" members of society, equal rural-urban distribution of medical personnel versus the efficiencies of group and hospital practice, the pros and cons of governmental support for education, implications of changes in retirement age, the extent of governmental support of medical care, and types of governmental control that may be exercised on the health industry.

While personnel planners cannot make these decisions themselves, they must pose clear and detailed alternatives for implementing programs to alleviate shortages. At the same time they should describe the various constraints in initiating new training programs or new systems to increase productivity. These constraints fall into the categories listed in the following discussion.

Educational concerns. How many applicants with the desired prerequisites would be available? Are the educational prerequisites appropriate for the types of training programs recommended? Are the training programs appropriate for the jobs to be filled?

Social concerns. Would assistant doctors be acceptable in all communities? Are there limitations to the employment of males in certain health professional roles? For females? What limits exist on upward mobility? (e.g., Does the opportunity exist for dressers to become medical assistants, or for medical assistants to become doctors?) Do regional or tribal prejudices block free job mobility of health workers? Does the social level of certain health professions thwart recruitment of qualified applicants?

Economic concerns. What are the total costs of training adequate numbers of a given type of health professional? More important, what are the total earnings in the profession? (For instance, what would be the total annual cost for education and maintenance of replacing all short-trained nurses by university graduates?) Are the short-term education costs and the long-term maintenance costs in keeping with the nation's ability to pay? (Some health professionals are unable to accept the fact that most countries cannot afford to meet all health staff needs.)

Political concerns. Are there imperial decrees that "a medical college shall be established"? What are the political pressures toward centralization or decentralization? Does the existing tax structure favor national, state, or locally financed training institutions? How strongly (in deed, not just word) is the nation committed to equal health care for all?

Professional concerns. Will existing professionals refuse to work with assistants? Are there professional practice laws that bar the use of new types of health workers? Would these laws be difficult to change? How restrictive are present licensing or certification laws? Change can often be instituted more easily through the training of new graduates than through persuasion or reeducation of established practitioners. For example, new dentists can be trained to utilize assistants more successfully than established dentists can be persuaded to change their current habits of practice.

In summary, health personnel planning is a complex analytical process; yet it is not only a mathematical exercise. Important policy decisions must be made, and many obstacles, while seemingly irrational, are nevertheless real and must be faced. The prospect for change always meets with resistance, of course, and is inherent in the planning process. The matter is especially critical in labor force planning, however, for here we are dealing with people's careers and lives.

REFERENCES

1. Hall, T. L., and A. Mejia (eds.), *Health Manpower Planning: Principles, Methods, Issues*, Geneva: World Health Organization, 1978.

2. Baker, T. D., and M. Perlman, *Health Manpower in a Developing Economy*, Baltimore: The Johns Hopkins University Press, 1967.

3. Taylor, Carl, Rahmi Dirican and Kurt Deuschle, *Health Manpower Planning in Turkey*, Baltimore: The Johns Hopkins University Press, 1968.

4. Hall, T. L., *Health Manpower in Peru*, Baltimore: The Johns Hopkins University Press, 1969.

5. National Manpower Board of Nigeria, *Health Manpower Survey 1965*, Lagos: Federal Ministry of Economic Development, 1969.

6. *The Target Income Hypothesis*, Publication No. HRA 80-27, Washington: Bureau of Health Manpower, 1980.

7. *The Current and Future Supply of Physicians and Physician Specialists*, Report No. 79-13, Division of Health Professions Analysis, Washington: Department of Health and Human Services, 1980.

8. Lee, Roger I., and Lewis W. Jones, *The Fundamentals of Good Medical Care*, Chicago: University of Chicago Press, 1933.

9. Bane, G., *Physicians for a Growing America*, Report of the Surgeon General's Consultant Group on Medical Education, U.S.P.H.S. Publication No. 709, Washington: Government Printing Office, 1959.

10. National League for Nursing, *Nurses for a Growing Nation*, New York: National League for Nursing, 1957.

11. Rozenfel'd, I. I., *Planning and Allocation of Medical Personnel in Public Health Services*, Translated from the Russian and published for the National Science Foundation, Washington, Jerusalem: Israel Program for Scientific Translations, 1963.

12. American Dental Association, Bureau of Economic Research and Statistics, "Survey of Dentist Opinion, 1964," *Journal of the American Dental Association*, Nos. 70 and 71, 1965.

13. *Reports of Offices and Councils*, Section on Dental Education, Chicago: American Dental Association, 1965.

14. Cassidy, J. E., *Maryland Dental Manpower Projection*, Doctoral thesis, Johns Hopkins University, Baltimore, Maryland, 1968.

15. Baker, T., "Paramedical Paradoxes—Challenges and Opportunity," In: G. Wolstenholme and M. O'Connor (eds.), *Teamwork for World Health*, CIBA Foundation Symposium, pp. 129–141, London: J. & A. Churchill, 1971.

16. Salmon, M. E., and P. A. Culbertson, "Health Manpower Oversupply: Implications for Nurses, Nurse Practitioners and Physician Assistants," *Hospitals and Health Services Administration*, 30:1, 1985.

PRIMARY READINGS

Baker, T. D., and M. Perlman, *Health Manpower in a Developing Economy*, Baltimore: The Johns Hopkins University Press, 1968. The Taiwan situation analyzed here is notable for the existence of a large private sector.

Fendall, N. R. E., *Auxiliaries in Health Care: Programs in Developing Countries*, Baltimore: The Johns Hopkins University Press, 1972. Providing a thorough discussion of the functions and training of auxiliaries, this is an early classic on the subject.

Hall, T. L., *Health Manpower in Peru*, Baltimore: The Johns Hopkins University Press, 1969. Of obvious relevance to Latin American planners, this study is also of more general interest for its concept of "rationalized demand" and its disaggregated approach to demand analysis.

Hall, T. L., and A. Mejia (eds.), *Health Manpower Planning: Principles, Methods, Issues*, Geneva: World Health Organization, 1978. Principles of health personnel planning are derived from a synthesis of international experience, and key issues on labor force distribution and utilization are raised.

Health Manpower Planning: A Comparative Study in Four Countries, Washington: U.S.

Department of Health, Education and Welfare, 1978. The countries considered are Colombia, Ecuador, Honduras, and the United States.

Hornby, P., D. K. Ray, P. J. Shipp and T. L. Hall, *Guidelines for Health Manpower Planning: A Course Book*, Geneva: World Health Organization, 1980. The Hall and Mejia volume provides an overview; this follow-up self-instruction text is designed for those who are to implement a plan.

Katz, F. M., and T. Fulop (eds.), *Personnel for Health Care: Case Studies of Educational Programs*, Public Health Papers Nos. 70 and 71, Geneva: World Health Organization, 1978, 1980. A two-volume series of case studies of innovative approaches to training many types of health personnel.

Roemer, M. I., and R. J. Roemer, *Health Care Systems and Comparative Manpower Policies*, New York: Marcel Dekker, Inc., 1981. A detailed comparison of Australia, Belgium, Canada, Norway, and Poland.

Storms, Doris M., *Training and Use of Auxiliary Health Workers*, International Health Programs Monograph Series No. 3, Washington: American Public Health Association, 1979. Assembles varied experience in design and management of nonphysician health provider programs in developing countries.

Study on Health Manpower and Medical Education in Colombia, Vols. 1 and 2, Washington: Pan American Health Organization, 1967. A study notable for its extensive appraisal of the incidence of disease and the demand for medical care.

Taylor, Carl, Rahmi Dirican and Kurt Deuschle, *Health Manpower Planning in Turkey*, Baltimore: The Johns Hopkins University Press, 1968. Stresses the distribution of the labor force within the country, a major problem in Turkey.

SECONDARY READINGS

Akhtar, S., et al. (eds.), *Low-Cost Rural Health Care and Health Manpower Training: An Annotated Bibliography with Special Emphasis on Developing Countries*, Ottawa: International Development Research Centre, 1981.

Fendall, N. R. E., "Training and Management for Primary Health Care," *Proceedings of the London Royal Society*, 209,1174:97-109, 1980.

Fulop, Tamas, and Milton I. Roemer, *International Development of Health Manpower Policy*, WHO Offset Publication No. 61, Geneva: World Health Organization, 1982.

Kindig, D. A., and C. M. Taylor, "Growth in International Physician Supply," *Journal of the American Medical Association*, 253,21:3129–3132, 1985.

Lynton, R., and V. Pareek, *Training for Development*, West Hartford, CN: Kumarian Press, 1978.

The Medex Primary Health Care Series, Honolulu: University of Hawaii at Manoa, 1983.

Mejia, A., "World Trends in Health Manpower Development: A Review," *World Health Statistics Quarterly*, 33,2:112–126, 1980.

Sorkin, Alan L., *Health Manpower*, Lexington, MA: Lexington Books, 1977.

Staff, R. J., and D. R. Porter, *Guidelines for Analysis of Health Manpower Planning*, Office of International Health, Rockville, MD: U.S. Public Health Service, 1979.

The Traditional Birth Attendant in Seven Countries: Case Studies in Utilization and Training, Geneva: World Health Organization, 1981.

Training and Utilization of Auxiliary Personnel for Rural Health Teams in Developing Countries, WHO Technical Report Series No. 633, Geneva: World Health Organization, 1979.

11

Planning Health Facilities

TIMOTHY D. BAKER

SCOPE AND IMPORTANCE

Construction of health facilities on the basis of well-conceived plans is important, not only because of the large capital outlays involved but also because of the long-term recurrent cost implications associated with construction decisions. New health facilities in large developed countries can absorb billions of dollars worth of resources each year. Moreover, unneeded facilities can add upward of three hundred dollars per day per patient for costs of unnecessary hospitalizations that occur when the supply of hospital beds is not constrained. Avoidance of these costs can result in savings of as much as 10 percent of the annual health budget.

If savings of this magnitude are important in developed countries, how much more crucial is effective facilities planning in less developed countries with far more critical resource constraints.[1] Hospital operating costs account for the majority of the ministry of health budget in most developing countries. This underscores the need for objective appraisal of the need for additional hospital facilities balanced against the possibility of greater expansion of less sophisticated and expensive forms of care. Whatever the outcome of that appraisal, careful design of the needed facilities to maximize efficiency and productivity can limit operating costs substantially.

This chapter discusses ways of analyzing the need for facilities, establishing the cost of meeting those needs, and preparing for actual construction. Within these three areas our intent is that readers gain competence in dealing with eleven specific questions. They should be able to (1) list types of health facilities, (2) estimate demand for facilities by type and location, (3) plan surveys of existing facilities, (4) estimate the costs of new construction and renovation of old facilities, (5) convert the capital costs for construction and renovation to annual sinking fund or depreciation terms, (6) estimate the costs and benefits of operating new facilities as compared to old, (7) know sources of capital funding, (8) know the importance of operating costs in relation to construction costs, (9) identify the problems and constraints to rational health facilities planning, (10) prepare alternative master plans with cost comparisons for various mixes of health facilities, and (11) identify consultants (project teams) to help plan individual facilities.

NEEDS ASSESSMENT

Types of Facilities

The construction of general hospitals utilizes the bulk of resources for construction of health facilities. The current trend is away from construction of special acute hospitals, such as maternity hospitals and eye hospitals. Special hospitals occupied a vogue in the early part of the twentieth century but have grown increasingly less suitable in view of modern demands for shared services such as X rays, laboratories, and laundry. Also, special-purpose, acute-care hospitals require large populations with easy access for full utilization.

Similarly, special-purpose chronic-disease facilities such as leprosaria and tuberculosis hospitals are declining in importance. The increased use of psychotherapeutic agents has markedly reduced the demand for mental hospitals, which were really more custodial institutions than health facilities anyhow.

As populations age, there has been a marked increase in the demand for construction of another custodial type of institution–the nursing home. With increasing numbers of elderly people who cannot be cared for at home, the construction of new nursing homes, and the conversion of existing buildings into nursing homes have been major thrusts in the health facilities construction industry. In addition rehabilitation hospitals for the chronically disabled have taken an increasing part of the health facilities construction budget. As the population ages in developing countries, and as the trend toward nuclear families increases, they will require more long-term care facilities.

Medical school hospitals are one special example of hospitals requiring special skills in planning to integrate the research and teaching functions of the facilities with the service functions.[2]

In addition to hospitals health facilities include health centers, satellite health posts, group practice buildings, individual patients' and dentists' offices, special free-standing out-patient clinics (such as health department clinics), and free-standing minor surgical, X-ray, diagnostic, and laboratory facilities.[3,4] Planning effective, inexpensive health centers and health posts is a particular challenge for planners in developing countries.[5]

Another way to classify health facilities is by type of ownership. Ownership may be by national, state, or local government; quasi-governmental organizations; nonprofit corporations; profit-making private corporations; religious groups; industrial firms; or individuals.[6]

Demand and Need

Estimation of the demand and need for hospitals rests on several factors. The first and most important is population. However, major differences in hospital beds to population ratios exist. Even within developed countries some are 50 percent higher than others (ranging from roughly four to six short-term beds per thousand population).

The second factor is the economic level of the area planned for. For example, there is a fifteen-fold (1,500 percent) difference in the number of hospital beds per thousand persons in Nigeria and in Canada. Third, the availability of funds for hospitalization modifies the demand on these beds by the population at various economic levels. The general availability of public and private insured hospital care has greatly increased the demand for hospital care in many countries.

Fourth, the accessibility of facilities helps to determine the effective demand. If the facilities are readily available by normal means of transport, they are more heavily utilized. Fifth, the age pattern also affects demand for health care facilities, particularly hospitals. Older populations almost always have a higher use rate. Sixth, past utilization rates and trends are probably the best indicators for short-term changes in demand in the future.

Finally, *Roemer's law*, that there will be a demand for as many hospital beds as are built, applies to a large spectrum of ratios of hospital beds to population. The United States has reached the point of building out of range of Roemer's law, but its continuing applicability in most places cautions facilities planners in developing countries to be wary of overbuilding.

Facilities Surveys

The need for facilities must be judged against current availability. The most easily available sources of information on existing facilities are government records and those of licensing and accrediting agencies. In virtually all of the developed countries health facilities require some process of licensing or accreditation or both. These procedures call for examination of the facilities and reports on their structure and services. In less-developed countries detailed information is often not available and if one wishes to plan, it is essential to make special surveys of existing facilities to determine whether they are usable or not.

Surveys should include structural reviews of the condition of the building; its ability to withstand structural stresses such as snow loads, earth tremors, and so on; and its fire resistance.

Mechanical devices should be surveyed to determine condition and safety. The services such as water, sewage, electricity, and gas should be reviewed to determine their adequacy and safety.

Access to the facility should be reviewed to determine any barriers to utilization of the structure by the public. Information should also be gathered on types of services the health unit is prepared to offer, as well as the number of services actually performed in relation to capacity.

COST ANALYSIS AND ACCOUNTING

Estimation of Costs of Construction or Renovation

The estimation of cost of construction is extremely difficult. Hospital costs vary greatly depending on locality, availability of capital, and interest rates charged. There are two good sources of current information on hospital construction: the *Dodge Building Cost Calculator and Evaluation Guide*[7] and Means' *Building Construction Costs Data*.[8] These manuals give costs of the different elements of construction for hospitals built in the past year in different parts of the United States. They enable one to make comparisons and approximate the cost of hospital construction closely enough for planning purposes. Less-developed countries have less information and a greater spread of construction costs. Some figures are given for comparative purposes in Table 11.1.

The cost of renovation is even more difficult to estimate. Contractors have great difficulty in knowing what problems will be encountered in modernizing a facility. The costs of relocating service lines for electricity, water, gas, and sewage make up a major part of the price of renovations.

One of the major elements driving up the cost of health facilities construction is construction codes that lag behind the state of the art in the building trades. Frequently strong labor unions are able to delay the introduction of technological change for several years.

Conversion of Capital Costs to an Annual Basis

In many developing countries the government pays for the cost of all construction, which is budgeted as a one-time capital cost. However, there is an increasing trend

Table 11.1

ILLUSTRATIVE CONSTRUCTION COSTS ($)

	Cost	Year	Location - Type
General Hospitals (Cost per Bed)	50,000	1975	U.S. 100-bed unit
	65,000	1975	U.S. 400-bed unit
	250,000	1975	U.S. teaching hospital
	105,000	1980	U.S. 200-bed unit
	25,000	1975	Singapore
	375,000	1975	Abu Dhabi
	290,000	1981	Saudi Arabia
	19,000	1986	Malawi
Nursing Home (Cost per Bed)	25,000	1985	U.S.
Health Center (Cost per sq. meter*)	300	1975	Ethiopia - brick
	100	1975	Ethiopia - mud, thatch
	250	1975	Turkey - brick, concrete
	200	1975	Bolivia - avg. for mud, brick
	170	1975	Indonesia - concrete
	330	1986	Malawi - brick, concrete

*Costs are estimated to have increased by at least ten percent per year since the survey was done in 1975.

toward use of nongovernmental funds for hospital construction and for a realistic allocation of the governmental funds on an annual cost basis. This is particularly true as the use of government loans or bonds to finance construction of government hospitals increases.

To convert the cost of construction to an annual basis, one should use the concept of *debt servicing* charge: Such a charge includes the payback of principal, plus the interest on the remaining principal. For example, one may have a twenty-year loan in which one-twentieth of the principal is paid back each year, along with annually decreasing payments of interest. A more common method of allocation of debt servicing charges is to make equal payments each year for the twenty-year period of the loan. In this case the payments for the earlier years have a much higher component of interest and the overall interest charges over the twenty-year period are larger. However, in the real world, where inflation is a fact of life, it is probably advantageous to defer payback as long as possible, even if the overall interest charges are higher, as the payback in later years will be with deflated money. A practical tip for health facilities planners is to learn to use one of the inexpensive financial calculators to estimate the impact of different systems of allocation of the debt servicing charges for hospital construction.

Comparison of New Facilities Cost with Old

In estimating the costs of operating new facilities, one starts with the debt servicing charges, unless one is operating in a system in which the capital costs are maintained in a completely separate budget. Even in this case an estimation of "shadow pricing" of debt servicing costs is important for reaching rational decisions on whether or not to construct a new facility.

In addition to the cost of debt servicing, one must estimate the cost of maintenance of the facility. Maintenance cost for a new facility may be substantially less than that for an existing one. Figures should be available from the hospital budgetary department on the costs of maintaining the old facility, though those should be judged according to whether the upkeep has been adequate. Estimates of future costs of maintaining the proposed facility should be appraised as realistically as possible, of course, rather than relying on optimistic hopes or contractor promises.

Apart from these directly comparable costs, less-measurable benefits of the new facility may have to be considered. Professional opinions on ease and reliability of operation, convenience for workers and/or patients, and other intangible factors can be meaningful and should be carefully weighed.

Sources of Funding for Construction

Estimation of the availability of funds for health facilities construction is a difficult and complex art. Essentially all funding is financed by loans which depend on current interest rates and the existing money market. In developing countries where the government finances hospital construction, the interest rates are often hidden, as construction costs become a part of the national debt. International agencies provide funds on varying terms. For some purposes, for example, the World Bank can be a source of substantial funds at low interest. Numerous other possibilities include fund-raising within the community; short-term debt financing; issuance of bonds, both tax-exempt and taxable; convertible mortgages; and other sources of private funding. Frequently funds gathered from the community or from individuals or through loans are matched by state and local authorities; often the local funds are augmented by central-level matching grants or loans. The terms of the financial arrangements are sometimes dictated by the nature of the institution that will operate the health facility.

These complex elements come together to give rise to the debt servicing cost (interest plus payback of loan), which must be counted as part of the ongoing operating expenses of the health facility.

Operating Costs

The decreased cost of operating new facilities compared to old includes efficiencies that can be built into new facilities through such techniques as automation, spoke construction of facilities, and progressive patient care (intensive, intermediate, minimal). Hospital administrators and systems analysts should be called on to make estimates of the saving in personnel and materials through the use of new systems in comparison to old systems before reaching decisions as to whether to continue with the old system, to renovate, or to build anew.

Operating costs vary by size of hospital, by ownership, by type of hospital and, of course, by country. There is no consensus as to the most cost-efficient size of hospitals in the broad range of one hundred to one thousand beds. In 1983 the average in-patient cost in U.S. short-term nonfederal hospitals was $368. In 1977 nursing home costs averaged $689 per month depending on the type of nursing home and source of payment.[9] (Of course, charges are now higher and costs are increasing each year.) In developing countries operating costs may be as low as 10 percent of U.S. costs because of their large, low-paid personnel component.

FOCUS ON IMPLEMENTATION

Alternatives and Constraints

The tug between elegance and economy is ever-present, and much of the pressure generated in society favors construction of expensive health facilities. Builders, insurers, as well as health providers exert pressures on governing bodies, boards of trustees of nonprofit organizations, and other decision-making groups to opt for new construction. There is an almost instinctive drive toward extravagant facilities. Monument building seems to have been a human trait since the days of the pyramids.

The need to economize can also be carried too far. The dilemma was best expressed by a dean of a medical school on undertaking construction of new teaching facilities. He said somewhat sadly, "Today, everyone curses me for spending too much; ten years from now they will curse me for not spending enough."

Another likely trade-off concerns site selection of the cheaper peripheral location which is less convenient to the bulk of potential users versus a more expensive central site. As mentioned earlier, efficiency in operation must be balanced against construction costs. Similarly, less flexibility in construction might lead to decreased construction costs, but must be balanced against the problem of early obsolescence.[10]

Furthermore, particularly in the developing countries of the world, the cost of building hospitals must be balanced against the cost of building health centers and health posts.[11] This, in effect, is a decision on how to divide resources between urban and rural populations.

Planners should be familiar with the new techniques in hospital architecture such as (1) the computer design for similar health facilities, (2) the "fast tract" system[12] for initiating construction before design is complete (to prevent increased construction costs from inflation), (3) the use of interstitial floors to provide easier access for the various services such as water and electricity, (4) the use of traffic models for hospital design, and (5) the use of flexible designs with open options for expansion or change of facilities.

Master Planning

While it is essential for health planners to be knowledgeable of the basic elements of individual facility construction, it is also important for them to have a grasp of overall planning of facilities to serve regions, provinces, and entire nations. As is the case in essentially all health planning, the starting place for master planning is the population, its distribution, and its demographic attributes, such as age distribution, birth rate (for calculating maternity services), economic levels, and current patterns of utilization of facilities.

After basic information is collected on the current parameters, changes should be predicted for the future: increases in population and increases in per capita utilization. The increased per capita utilization will arise from increased economic levels and social changes such as preference for modern medical facilities instead of traditional medicine. Also migration patterns and changes in birth rates should be projected. In general the same factors determining the need for additional health personnel (detailed in Chapter 10) dictate the need for facilities in which the additional personnel will work.

Besides projections of objective need, current and anticipated government policies and priorities should be realistically considered. Attitudes toward primary health care in comparison to high-technology specialized services should be appraised, along with regional preferences and attempts to overcome existing inequities. One must always contend with the winds of political change, of course, and facilities master plans may be in jeopardy as a result. The facilities planner should not, as a rule, attempt to prejudge the political factors, however, but should force any alterations on political grounds to be made in the best professional and technical master plan that can be developed.

In summary, master planners must take a comprehensive view of the rapid changes that are occurring in most developing nations. They must build for the future, not the past, anticipating worldwide trends, such as urbanization, and plan for facilities to meet these major trends.

Use of Consultants

Once the decision to build a facility has been made, specialized architectural firms dealing primarily in health facilities should be consulted. Health facilities construction is a very special field in which many architectural firms have no competence at all.

In planning the actual design of a facility the basic team should include architects, engineers, physicians, hospital administrators, nursing supervisors, and informed representatives of the patient population. Frequently architectural firms have numerous planning sessions, involving community and health professionals, before any design is initiated.

SUMMARY

A broad range of potentially complex topics in facilities planning has been covered briefly and simply. As a result, planners without sophistication in the intricacies of construction should be started on the path toward learning some of the important basic facts dealing with demand for facilities and their cost, changes in demand and cost, possible sources of funding, and other factors of practical importance for rational planning of health facilities in developing countries.

REFERENCES

1. Mein, Philip, and Thomas Jorgensen, *Design for Medical Building: Manual for the Planning and Building of Health Care Facilities Under Conditions of Limited Resources*, Housing Research and Development Unit, Nairobi: University of Nairobi, 1975.

2. Smythe, C. M., "New Resources for Medical Education: Start-up Expenditures in 22 New U.S. Medical Schools," *Journal of Medical Education*, 47:690–701, 1972.

3. Cheesbrough, M., and J. McArthur, *A Laboratory Manual for Rural Tropical Hospitals*, Edinburgh: Churchill Livingstone, 1976.

4. *Appropriate Industrial Technology for Drugs and Pharmaceuticals*, Vienna: United Nations Industrial Development Organization, 1980.

5. Wells, Mark, *A Model Health Center*, London: Conference of Missionary Society, 1976.

6. Bridgman, R. F., and M. I. Roemer, *Hospital Legislation and Hospital Systems*, Public Health Papers No. 50, Geneva: World Health Organization, 1973.

7. *Dodge Building Cost Calculator and Evaluation Guide*, New York: McGraw-Hill Information System Co., revised annually.

8. Godfrey, R. S. (ed.), *Building Construction Costs Data*, Kingston, MA: R. S. Means Co., Inc., revised annually.

9. *Health: United States 1985*, U.S. Department of Health and Human Services, Public Health Service Publication No. PHS 86-1232, Hyattsville, MD: National Center for Health Statistics, December 1985.

10. Weeks, J., and G. Best, "Design Strategy for Flexible Health Science Facilities," *Health Services Research*, 5,3:263–284, 1970.

11. Shastri, J. B., "Physical Planning and Primary Care: The Problems of Developing Countries," *World Hospitals*, 14,3:156, 1978.

12. Price, D. L., "Fast Tract and New Methodology in Hospital Planning and Construction," *Hospital Progress*, 53,6:50–57, 1972.

PRIMARY READINGS

Appropriate Industrial Technology for Drugs and Pharmaceuticals, Vienna: United Nations Industrial Development Organization, 1980. Discusses principles involved in establishing domestic pharmaceutical production, with reference to several country studies.

Berki, S. E., *Hospital Economics*, Lexington, MA: Lexington Books, 1971. Covers costs of operations, demand utilization, productivity and efficiency, pricing and reimbursement.

Cheesbrough, M., and J. McArthur, *A Laboratory Manual for Rural Tropical Hospitals*, Edinburgh: Churchill Livingstone, 1976. Discusses essential laboratory equipment related to microscopy, hematology, blood transfusions, bacteriology, and parasitology, as well as examination of stools, urine, and other body fluids.

Kleczkowski, B. M., and R. F. Pibouleau (eds.), *Approaches to Planning and Design of Health Care Facilities in Developing Areas*, Vols. 1–4, WHO Offset Publications Nos. 29, 37, 45, and 72, Geneva: World Health Organization, 1976, 1977, 1979, 1983. Thorough documentation for designing health care facilities and taking into account special disease problems and unusual climatic conditions.

Llewelyn-Davies, R., "Planning Health Facilities in Developing Countries: Case Studies and Their Lessons," *World Hospitals*, 12,3:159–163, 1976. A leader in the field presents philosophies derived mainly from experiences in Thailand and Bahrain.

Pacey, A., *Sanitation in Developing Countries*, New York: John Wiley & Sons, 1978. Examines unconventional techniques of sanitation including thirty latrine models.

The Selection of Essential Drugs, WHO Technical Report Series No. 641, Geneva: World Health Organization, 1979. Presents criteria for application in individual countries to identify priorities in establishing drug lists.

SECONDARY READINGS

Alford, T. W., *Facility Planning: Design and Construction of Rural Health Centers*, Health Services Research Center, Chapel Hill: University of North Carolina, 1976.

Bridgman, R. F., B. M. Kleczkowski, R. F. Pibouleau and M. E. F. Torfs, "Health Care Facilities in Developing Countries: Prevailing Concerns and Possible Solutions," *World Hospitals*, 16,1:38–43, 1980.

Gish, O., and L. Feller, *Planning Pharmaceuticals for Primary Health Care: The Supply and Utilization of Drugs in the Third World*, International Health Programs Monograph Series No. 2, Washington: American Public Health Association, 1979.

Kleczkowski, B. M., and N. O. Nilsson, *Health Care Facility Projects in Developing Areas: Planning, Implementation, and Operations*, Geneva: World Health Organization, 1984.

Quick, J., et al. (eds.), *Managing Drug Supply: The Selection, Procurement, Distribution and Use of Pharmaceuticals in Primary Health Care*, Boston: Management Sciences for Health, 1981.

Rosenfield, E. D., "Limitations on Planning for Health Facilities in the Various Developing National Situations," *World Hospitals*, 13,3:126–129, 1977.

Segall, M., *Pharmaceuticals and Health Planning in Developing Countries*, IDS Communication 119, Brighton: Institute of Development Studies, 1975.

Simmonds, S. P., "Essential Drugs for Primary Health Care Standard Packages," *Lancet*, 1,8269:435–436, 1982.

12

Financial Analysis

WILLIAM A. REINKE

The ultimate test of an agency's priorities is in its budget. Resources can be actually utilized in the provision of services only to the extent that funds are made available. Thus, financial considerations are at the heart of the planning process.

SCOPE AND PURPOSES

Those considerations can range from mechanisms for tracking petty cash expenditures on pencils and paper clips to comprehensive and sophisticated cost-benefit analyses for establishing rational program priorities. Table 12.1 establishes four categories of financial analysis that conform to the planning, budgeting, implementation, and evaluation stages of the programming cycle. First, the fiscal implications of program options are assessed for the purpose of establishing an action strategy. A schedule of funding, that is, a budget, is then prepared for the program option chosen. In the course of implementation funds are disbursed, ideally according to procedures of adequate accountability. Each of the four categories of financial analysis is further elucidated in the following paragraphs in order to provide the structure and understanding necessary for subsequent discussion.

Strategy Formulation

Sometimes the purpose of financial analysis in strategy formulation is simply to enable predetermined services to be offered. If the decision has been made, for example, to establish five mobile vasectomy units, the financial planner must calculate the associated costs of personnel, fuel, supplies, and other resources so that the units can, in fact, become operative. More often comparative costing will be necessary. The incremental cost of including family planning services with antenatal care may be determined for comparison with the vasectomy camp alternative. Perhaps the financial feasibility of mounting both approaches to family planning simultaneously is at issue. Finally comparative costs may be related to expected results. Thus cost per acceptor or cost per birth averted through a vasectomy program might be compared with the corresponding ratio for a postpartum program. Methods for conducting such cost-effectiveness studies[1] are described in detail in Chapter 20.

Table 12.1

PRINCIPAL CATEGORIES OF FINANCIAL ANALYSIS

1. Cost Analysis for Strategy Formulation	PLANNING
2. Scheduling of Financial Needs: Tactics for Implementation	BUDGETING
3. Management of Disbursements: Expenditures	IMPLEMENTATION
4. Accountability and Control	EVALUATION

To summarize, financial planning may consist of straightforward cost analyses or more complex cost-effectiveness studies. That is, the intent may be to select a program of services that is merely feasible, or the intent may be to achieve the optimum. In principle the latter is more desirable in economic terms. Since noneconomic factors often enter into planning decisions, optimality may not be a practical possibility; nevertheless, the financial planner should at least determine realistic financial needs for the programmatic strategy selected.

Tactics for Implementation: Budgeting

The budgeting process translates those needs into a schedule of financial outlays.[2] The link between the medium-term plan (frequently five years) and the annual work plan and budget is crucial. Indeed, successful plan implementation is largely dependent upon arrangements made for personnel deployment and for expenditures. As Waterston notes, "for less developed countries, annual plans and budgets, and their coordination, are virtually sine qua non for putting medium-term plans into effect. The task of implementing a medium-term plan, without first phasing it into annual plans appears to be well beyond the capacity of most developing countries."[3]

The financial arrangements made should be organized around specific cost centers that serve as the locus of management activity. With the recognition that budget preparation and monitoring of actual expenditures are essential management functions, sound management practice demands that financial authority and responsibility be clearly placed at appropriate levels and that carefully formulated procedures for accountability be established.

Less obvious, but equally important tactical considerations relate to levels of utilization of services and their equitable distribution. A legitimate aim of planning is rationalization of the process of service delivery in order to direct supply and demand in accordance with genuine need and in a manner that minimizes financial and other hardships on clients as well as providers. This is a tall order requiring careful analysis of costs and mechanisms for meeting them.[4] Services that are free to clients may encourage overutilization. On the other hand, charges may be burdensome, especially to the needy poor, and may therefore form a barrier to needed utilization. Depending upon the methods employed in raising revenues, services might be rationed in desirable or undesirable ways. Because providers often induce demand, methods used to reimburse them can also affect services use, as well as productivity, efficiency, and quality.

Management of Disbursements: Expenditures

Health budgets in developing countries are notoriously low, frequently amounting to no more than a dollar or two per capita annually. It might be expected, therefore, that any funds budgeted would be quickly spent. Such is not the case, however; it is not uncommon for ministries of health to reach the end of the fiscal year with one-fourth to one-half of their budgets unexpended. Three principal factors account for the shortfall.

First, cumbersome disbursement procedures may block expenditures, even those fully authorized in advance. Before actually purchasing a budgeted piece of equipment, for example, a refrigerator at a peripheral health unit, a host of approvals from district to central levels of the ministry may be necessary.

Second, shortfalls in expenditure may also occur because planned resources are not, in fact, made available. Staff vacancies or drug shortages obviously have a direct impact on expenditures, and in addition the resulting curtailment of activities may limit the use of other resources. Thus, actual expenditures must be examined in relation to both budget and performance. Expenditures at 80 percent of planned levels could give evidence of exceptional efficiency. If at the same time, however, only half of the intended services were provided, the program might actually be inefficient, as well as ineffective.

A third difficulty frequently arises from the fact that poorly trained personnel are employed to carry out ill-defined procedures of financial accounting. As a result, the current status of expenditures may not be known. When information on total disbursements does not become available until after a budget audit is conducted at the end of a fiscal year, financial planners are forced to rely upon educated guesses and probabilities instead of hard data in making budgetary decisions. Expenditure reports a year or more behind schedule are commonplace.

Accountability and Control

Timely recording and reporting of expenditures are necessary but not sufficient to ensure appropriate management action. Effective control requires, in addition, the compilation of useful indicators of financial performance at relevant decision points. If staffing assignments and salary determinations are made at district headquarters, local health center managers can hardly be held accountable for personnel costs incurred at their units. They should account, however, for the way in which existing personnel are being utilized. For example, indicators depicting trends in the center's cost per home visit would be useful.

ORGANIZATIONAL IMPLICATIONS

We have stressed the importance of attributing achievements and associated resources expenditures by cost centers in accordance with the locus of management decision making and control responsibility. This has organizational implications, particularly with regard to issues of centralization and decentralization.

Centralization connotes detailed advance planning leading to uniform local action. In contrast, decentralization permits local decisions to be made flexibly "as needed," coupled with post facto accounting for the appropriateness of the decisions made under prevailing circumstances. The notion of flexibility is attractive, and accordingly decentralization is frequently cited as an ideal state toward which health systems should move.

The issue is not so simple, however. Under certain circumstances uniformity is desirable and centralization is clearly more efficient. If the essential conditions for action are unvarying from place to place, why should multiple decision makers repeat the same tedious process to arrive at similar conclusions? Even if decisions themselves are appropriately individualized, a uniform set of decision rules may be applicable. To illustrate, well-defined procedures have been formulated for ensuring that adequate stocks of drugs and supplies are maintained at minimum cost. While the exact quantity ordered varies from item to item, time to time, and place to place, cost minimization requires that a single objective decision algorithm be applied uniformly. Results are bound to be superior to those obtained from decentralized subjective assessments.

In the event that recognized advantages are to be gained from decentralization, certain requirements must be met in order to realize the advantages. First, locally competent staff must be available. In effect centralized competence must be replicated. Second, clearly defined procedures of accountability must be applied from a carefully structured information system through a highly developed network of timely communication. The increased availability of microcomputers should provide a substantial stimulus to the decentralization movement.

ORGANIZATIONAL ARRANGEMENTS

Exposition of the multiple factors that impinge on specific organizational arrangements is beyond the scope of present discussion. Rather, our attention is limited to arrangements directly associated with financing mechanisms and to factors of services delivery that have a major bearing on financing alternatives. For example, the handling of insurance claims is likely to be different for private providers of care than for public services. In addition, the following discussion focuses on the public role in these organizational arrangements. In particular, arrangements whereby services are provided by public agencies lead directly to government planning and activation. In other cases the government role is indirect and regulatory, as when limits are placed upon levels of reimbursement for specified private services. In this regard one should not underestimate the influence that accrues to government through its authority to grant and withhold funds for private institutions that act or fail to act "voluntarily" according to specified guidelines.

Arrangements Regarding Services Delivery

Three categories of services provision are worth distinguishing: (1) the individual practitioner as private entrepreneur, (2) private corporate medicine, and (3) public agencies directly engaged in the provision of services.

Because private physicians are relatively scarce, especially in rural areas of developing countries, planners sometimes act as though these populations are unserved except by the few existing government health centers. In fact, however, many local healers are likely to be active, offering a variety of folk remedies not recognized by Western medicine. Qualified or not, these private entrepreneurs are important for planning purposes inasmuch as expenditures to them, in money and in kind, are usually several times higher than either health center budgets or payments to private physicians.[5] Questions being raised about the feasibility of schemes for the community financing of primary health care have heightened concern for the full accounting of local expenditures on health care from all sources.[6]

In the private corporate category we include philanthropic nonprofit hospitals and other enterprises, as well as proprietary hospitals and clinics. Industrial clinics and other health units of large employers are also included. A few of these organizations have been notable in offering comprehensive health care to employees, their dependents, and in some cases the community at large. Such endeavors are likely to expand in importance with trends toward urbanization and industrialization.

Public service agencies fall into four categories reflecting the special need they seek to meet and/or the clientele they serve. The first group includes those disadvantaged in some respect. Because the disadvantaged are likely to be poor and unable to pay for needed services, they represent a group of special interest in financial planning. The second category is made up of population groups considered dangerous and therefore isolated from the rest of the community. Mental hospitals, leprosy hospitals, and prison services exemplify this category. The third category relates to problems that are professionally recognized but that generate little felt need among clients. Nutrition education programs are a case in point. Finally there are programs providing community services that may be of recognized importance but that cannot be carried out readily by individuals. Water and sanitation projects are obvious examples.

Arrangements Regarding Financing

Financial planners should be alert to three patterns in the flow of funds for health services. The client might pay the provider directly; payment might be through a third party intermediary between client and provider; or the provider agency may offer "free" services from a pool of funds supplied independently of the services provided. A number of variations on the three themes are possible. For example, the client's direct payment to the provider might be made as a fee for service at the time care is provided, or a prepayment might be made periodically to cover all eventualities during a subsequent time period.

Table 12.2 shows the combinations of service delivery and funding arrangements that emerge from the foregoing classifications. All combinations are feasible, but the ones more commonly employed (X) relate mainly to the public or private nature of the system. Where public funds are used to reimburse private providers, at least two agencies are necessarily involved in the transactions. In totally private or totally public systems a single agency might be both provider and funder, or separate organizations might be involved.

Unfortunately, fragmentation of care and financing is too often the norm. A financial report from Indonesia[7] voiced a common complaint that there is no direct correspondence among functions, budgets, and administrative hierarchies. Virtually every health system function is financed from more than one budget deriving from more than one level of government. This makes meaningful cost analysis difficult and violates the already cited management dictum that decision-making authority, control, and accountability should be exercised through clearly defined cost centers.

The many ramifications of possible arrangements within the framework of Table 12.2 are illustrated by circumstances in Indonesia. Government health centers treat government workers free of charge through an insurance scheme that is government-sponsored but supported through employee premiums based upon income. The health center also treats private citizens. Preventive services are offered without charge through general tax revenues. Curative services are government-subsidized but require payment of a patient fee which is channeled back to local and higher levels of government. Plans are under way to bring all residents of specified catchment areas into an insurance scheme financed by client premiums. Thus the intent is for public employees of government facilities to offer preventive services supported by government revenues and curative services paid for privately by the community of clients served.

Table 12.2

SERVICE DELIVERY-FINANCING ALTERNATIVES

Flow of Funds for Service	Category of Provider		
	Private Individual	Private Corporate	Public Agency
Direct from Client	X	X	
Through Private Intermediary	X	X	
Through Public Intermediary	X	X	X
Free Service			X

X - More common arrangements

FINANCING MECHANISMS

Service organizations and programs require financial support to enable them to become going concerns, able to deliver the intended services. In addition financial transactions may occur in connection with the provision of individual services. Financing mechanisms operative at each of these levels are considered separately later. In either case the mechanisms are to be distinguished by whether the burden of financing is borne on the basis of ability to pay or according to level of need or use. Mechanisms for financing individual services may also be distinguished by the timing of payment in relation to receipt of services.

General Agency or Program Support

Private Savings/Investment

The profit motive has stimulated the formation of private hospitals, clinics, pharmacies, and other health enterprises. Such endeavors require that those with savings to invest have entrepreneurial interests in health care and/or they anticipate a favorable return on health sector investment in relation to other options. These considerations have sometimes deterred, but have by no means precluded, private enterprise in the field of curative health services.

Public Taxing/Investment

Government taxing is in essence forced saving and raises the fundamental question, Who must "save" how much for what purpose, and is the purpose in line with the "saver's" needs and interests? In principle, taxes could be levied according to expected use of services, but the need for services may not match ability to pay.

More equitable arrangements can be made for raising revenues, for example, through a progressive income tax, but difficulties remain if the revenues are earmarked for specific services. Consider the typical case in which a specified proportion of one's income is taxed in support of health services. In the short run, demand for services is likely to be fairly constant, whereas the amount of revenue generated varies with the state of the economy. Deficits may accrue in times of recession when they are most troublesome. The arrangements tend to produce even greater problems in the long run because of demographic changes. As populations age, the presence of fewer workers of productive age causes a decline in the revenue base at the same time that the number of older persons with greater service needs is increasing.

To avoid these dilemmas governments sometimes budget health services out of general revenues. This tends to foster stability in the level of health services support, but the level can be quite low, depending upon the priority accorded the health sector. The ministry of health is forced to compete with other ministries for a "fair slice" of the revenue pie. Health and other social service agencies can be at a disadvantage in this competition if criteria of economic growth are stressed at the sacrifice of less tangible concerns for social welfare and quality of life.

Deficit Financing/Inflation

Public service needs typically outrun the taxing capabilities of government, especially in rural subsistence economies. As a result, services are frequently provided through deficit financing. The effect is that of an indirect tax, but the specific impact is less clear. A direct tax measurably reduces disposable income available for the purchase of goods and services. The deficit financing alternative leads to the creation of additional money to pay for the same limited volume of goods and services, thus driving up their prices. How the indirect effects of inflation are distributed is problematic, but the total effect is certainly equivalent to that of a direct tax.

Foreign Investment

Faced with revenues that are inadequate, even to meet minimal service needs, governments often view external grants or loans as attractive alternatives to deficit financing. Foreign assistance is usually limited, however, to building construction, procurement of equipment, training of personnel, or other start-up activities. Large as these initial outlays may be, they invariably represent only a small fraction of costs incurred over the life of the facility or project. One-time costs of preservice training are likely to be less than the resulting *annual* commitment for salaries, supervision, and other support of the personnel trained. Careful calculation of the annual recurrent cost implications of development projects is an extremely important, but frequently neglected, aspect of program planning. The result is facilities left idle or, worse yet, ineffective and understaffed programs that are wasteful and inefficient in their utilization of whatever limited resources are made available.

Financing at Point of Service Delivery

Considerations of adequacy and equity in funding have dominated the discussion of general program support. These issues are also important in relation to payment for specific services. In addition, financing mechanisms, including matters of timing, in connection with services delivery must be judged by their effect on demand relative to genuine need.

Private fee-for-service arrangements provide the closest link between service delivery and payment and therefore offer the greatest possibility for inhibiting demand in that need must be matched by ability and willingness to pay. The effect on demand is considerably dampened if services are supported through periodic prepayment of a fixed premium set independently of actual service use. This sharing of risks and costs succeeds in spreading the burdens of health care, but because of differences in income and ability to pay, equal sharing of costs does not translate into equitable sharing of burden. Differential premiums based upon ability to pay obviously produce the least burdensome arrangements, assuming that "ability" can be determined objectively in practice. The equity dilemma is largely avoided, of course, if premiums are paid by groups, for example, employers, other than the clients themselves.

Despite the obvious advantage of equitable cost sharing, it has the disadvantage of failing to discourage unnecessary utilization. To offset this disadvantage, arrangements are sometimes made to couple prepayment with a modest charge to the client at the time each unit of service is provided. Obviously, if the service fee is too small, it will be ineffective in controlling utilization. On the other hand an unduly large fee can have the same undesirable effect as a straight fee-for-service arrangement. Achievement of an equitable balance between need and demand remains one of the principal challenges to the financial planner and the health services researcher.[8]

General acceptance of the principle that health care is a fundamental human right has led many governments to pursue a policy of free care, thereby skirting the issue of payment mechanisms altogether. The fact that removal of economic barriers to service has seldom led to obvious overutilization is more an indication of failure of government policy than success. Three principal reasons for failure have been cited. First, many governments simply have not had the will or means to implement the policy meaningfully. As a result, the majority of rural residents do not have access to the government services within the three to five miles they are willing to travel for care. Long-accepted local healers are more conveniently available and continue to be used as in the past. Second, even if accessible, the government service may be perceived to be of poor quality. Patients have come to realize that a trip to the health center offers no guarantee that staff will be present who understand the patient's complaint or, if the illness is successfully diagnosed, medicines to treat it will be available. Patient "perceptions" noted earlier are the third source of difficulty. Experience has shown that people tend to value more highly commodities and services that require sacrifice, that is, payment. If something is being given away, ipso facto it must not be worth very much.

The net result is that even with the expansion of free services, communities continue to receive the bulk of their care from local healers deemed unqualified by the health professionals. We return to the point that payments to these healers represent a significant expenditure of community resources that financial planners should take cognizance of and seek to channel more effectively.

The technical nature of health care has meant that demand is stimulated by providers, as well as consumers. Indeed the medical profession has fostered a dependence upon providers for making treatment decisions. For this reason mechanisms for provider reimbursement can conceivably affect demand as much as mechanisms for client payment. Especially when provider income accrues directly from the volume of services given, the temptation to encourage use of services exists. Thus, fee-for-service arrangements, which can inhibit consumer demand, can work in the opposite way regarding provider-induced demand.

To counter the effects of this direct link between service and payment, capitation arrangements have been proposed for providers, much as prepayment arrangements have been put forward for consumers. Under capitation, providers are paid according to the number of clients they serve regardless of the number of services provided to them. Hence there is an incentive to limit the number of costly services performed. If this is accomplished through activities intended to keep the client healthy, the incentive is in the interest of both parties. To the extent that the system fosters the postponement of needed services, however, it produces undesirable results.

Despite certain attractions of capitation schemes, salary arrangements have been more common in practice. Because salaries are based neither on volume of services performed nor on number of clients served, they offer no particular stimulus to overutilization but likewise do not encourage improvements in quality of care or productivity. Experience seems to indicate, however, that the latter are more influenced by organizational and practice arrangements than by form of remuneration.

TIMING OF PROGRAM EXPENDITURES

The health sector is notoriously labor-intensive, meaning that the largest single element of cost is that associated with the ongoing support of personnel. Nevertheless health programs, like most other major endeavors, do usually require that substantial start-up costs be incurred initially in contrast to the intended benefits, which accrue more slowly over a period of time as clients are served. Capital costs amortized over several years become a relatively small item of annual cost but are an important budgetary concern at the time they are incurred. For this reason the distinction is made between *capital budgets* and *budgets of recurrent costs*.[9] Moreover, new programs frequently require special support in early stages of growth until they become routinely operational. Apart from provision for one-time expenditures for such items as equipment and training, special arrangements may be necessary for a period of time to cover operating expenses, such as salaries, until they can be accommodated in the regular budget. Thus, the further distinction is made between development budgets and routine budgets. *Development budgets* are usually formulated in support of medium-term (usually five-year) plans, whereas *routine budgets* are prepared in connection with annual work plans.

International donor agencies typically support capital expenditures and items included in development budgets. Reference has already been made to the importance of fully enumerating all routine internal budgetary commitments arising from external capital assistance. External development assistance for noncapital items of expenditure requires caution as well in a couple of regards.

First, in order to attract highly qualified personnel into a new program, higher-than-normal salaries and/or fringe benefits may be offered. Development budgets often permit such special provisions, especially if the costs are borne by external donors. The donors themselves are likely to support the arrangements; indeed by donor standards the salaries may be very modest. In the course of implementation, however, resentments harbored by similarly trained, but less-favored personnel in other programs could be devastating. Equally important, civil service regulations or budgetary constraints may make it impossible to carry over the initial arrangements into the routine budget, but it may be equally difficult to do otherwise.

Inclusion of drug purchases in the externally aided development budget may also create difficulties. After withdrawal of aid, the flow of supplies that the program had come to depend upon may be disrupted because of foreign exchange restrictions, budgetary limitations, or inadequacies in the logistics system.

BUDGET PREPARATION AND ANALYSIS

Concepts enunciated in preceding sections are put into practice through the budgetary process. This concluding section, therefore, is a practical summary of the principal forms of budgeting. Numerical examples are introduced within a context of financial analysis that ranges from planning to evaluation and accountability.

Line-Item Budgets

The planning of inputs requires determination of personnel requirements, anticipated expenditures on supplies, types of equipment needed, and so forth. The line-item budget organizes planned costs along lines of such input categories, as shown for an illustrative health unit in Table 12.3. In practice, more detailed subcategories of expense would usually be identified, but the gross breakdowns of the table are adequate for our purposes in distinguishing among budget formats and in describing methods of financial analysis.

Program Budgets

Let us suppose that the health unit illustrated in Table 12.3 is a pediatric unit engaged in two basic programs: well-child care and treatment of sick children. (Although a more complex array of activities might be distinguished in practice, this simple breakdown is adequate for discussion purposes.) In fiscal terms, programs should be set up as cost centers that are foci of accountability.

Means must be established for allocating line-item costs among programs. Personnel costs are usually the largest single component and and can normally be related to specific programs without difficulty. Where persons distribute their time among programs, the proportional allocation can be determined in advance, estimated, or ascertained by the methods of work sampling microanalysis described in Chapter 19. Allocation of the cost of expendables is made according to purpose. Antibiotics would obviously be charged to the illness-care program, whereas vaccines would be charged to well-child care.

Other costs are likely to be minor and can be allocated in any reasonable manner without distorting analysis. Building costs provide a good example. While large initially, when amortized over the life of the facility, they contribute less than 10 percent of the annual operating cost in most cases. One method for allocating space costs is discussed on the following page.

Table 12.3
ILLUSTRATIVE LINE-ITEM BUDGET

Line Item	Amount
Professional Staff	$300,000
Non-Professional Staff	240,000
Total Personnel	540,000
Expendables	150,000
Fixed Capital and Equipment	60,000
Total	$750,000

A facility of 1,000 square feet, costing $300,000 and expected to last 30 years might simply be budgeted at $10,000 per year, or $10 per square foot. The space within the building would then be charged according to its use. Suppose, for example, that an office of 200 square feet is used by physicians who devote 80 percent of their time to curative services. Of the total budgeted space charge of $2,000, $1,600 would be allocated to the curative program and $400 to the well-child program.

The allocation process results in a program budget as illustrated in Table 12.4. The data apply to the same health unit depicted in Table 12.3 but are organized programmatically, rather than strictly in line-item terms.

Performance Budgets

In spite of the programmatic orientation of program budgets, they still focus on resource inputs. Relating these inputs to intended outputs converts the presentation to a performance budget. Suppose, for example, that the curative budget of Table 12.4 is based upon the expectation of 90,000 patient visits, whereas 75,000 well-child visits are anticipated. Thus, the budgeted cost per unit of service is

$$\frac{516,000}{90,000} = \$5.73$$

for illness care and

$$\frac{234,000}{75,000} = \$3.12$$

for well-child care. Addition of this information concerning output and budgeted cost per unit of output transforms the program budget into a performance budget.

Comparison of Actual Experience with Budget

We now turn to a review of experience at the end of the budget period in comparison with planned expenditure and performance. For evaluative purposes it is most useful to judge actual expenditures against achieved outputs. That is, the performance budget

Table 12.4

ILLUSTRATIVE PROGRAM BUDGET

Item	Illness Care	Well-Child Care
Professional Staff	$225,000	$ 75,000
Non-Professional Staff	144,000	96,000
Total Personnel	369,000	171,000
Expendables	105,000	45,000
Fixed Capital and Equipment	42,000	18,000
Total	$516,000	$234,000

is the point of departure, as in Table 12.5. A comprehensive evaluation would, of course, include consideration of the effectiveness of services rendered as well.

Costs of fixed capital and equipment have been excluded from Table 12.5 on the assumption that these are beyond the control of the managers of the program cost centers being evaluated. The pattern of variable costs that emerges from the table reveals overexpenditures for curative care and savings in well-child care. The significance of the pattern is unclear, however, inasmuch as the performance of curative services exceeded expectation, while the number of well-child visits, like expenditures, fell considerably short of planned levels. We recognize that actual expenditures are a function of two factors: actual levels of performance and the efficiency with which those levels were achieved. The influence of these two factors must be separated in any fiscal analysis.

To do this, the principle of standard costing is introduced. Accepting for the moment any deviations in service performance from budget, we derive an adjusted budget as if the achieved level of output had been planned in the first place. In the case of curative care, the originally budgeted 90,000 services were associated with a budgeted, or standard, cost per unit of service. In fact, the number of services rendered, 93,214, was 3.6 percent above budget. If each of the rendered services had been provided at standard cost, then each line-item expenditure under curative care should have been 3.6 percent above that originally planned. Differences between the resulting adjusted budget levels and actual expenditures (Table 12.6) are due strictly to variances in efficiency, since variances in output have already been accounted for. Such comparisons assume constant marginal costs of shifts from planned outputs, an assumption that must be examined critically.

Unlike in Table 12.5, the main feature of Table 12.6 is overexpenditure in both programs on professional staff in contrast to slight underexpenditures on nonprofessional staff. In relation to services provided both programs were overspent on expendables, but the variance in both cases was well under 1 percent of adjusted budget.

Overall the evaluation in performance budget terms produces two major findings

Table 12.5

COMPARISON OF EXPENDITURES WITH BUDGET

Item	Expenditures		Variance	
	Illness Care	Well-Child Care	Illness Care	Well-Child Care
Professional Staff	239,716	64,111	-14,716	+10,889
Non-Professional Staff	148,029	76,848	- 4,029	+19,152
Total Personnel	387,745	140,959	-18,745	+30,041
Expendables	109,337	37,046	- 4,337	+ 7,954
Total Variable Cost	497,082	178,005	-23,082	+37,995
Service Units	93,214	61,543	+ 3,214	-13,457
Var. Cost per Service Unit	$5.33	$2.89	$-0.06	$-0.01

Table 12.6

COMPARISON OF EXPENDITURES WITH BUDGET ADJUSTED FOR SERVICES PROVIDED

Item	Adjusted Budget		Adjusted Variance	
	Illness Care	Well-Child Care	Illness Care	Well-Child Care
Professional Staff	233,035	61,543	-6,681	-2,568
Non-Professional Staff	149,142	78,775	+1,113	+1,927
Total Personnel	382,177	140,318	-5,568	- 641
Expendables	108,750	36,926	- 587	- 120
Total Variable Cost	490,927	177,244	-6,155	- 761

worthy of further investigation. First, performance in the well-child program fell far short of expectation. Second, adjusting for this shortfall, both programs made unexpectedly heavy use of professional staff. Is the relatively "rich" personnel mix being employed an error in need of correction, or is it a practical necessity that should be acknowledged in next year's budget?

Conclusions

Budget formats vary according to the nature of decisions to be made and controls to be exercised. Of the three types of budgeting discussed in the present chapter, however, we have found the performance budget to be the most useful throughout the process of planning, implementation, monitoring, and evaluation. In the evaluative mode, it is worth reemphasizing that fiscal analysis must be tied realistically to conditions of accountability and control. If evaluation is to be forward-looking in seeking better decisions for the future, the evaluative analyses must focus on decision makers and viable options available to them.

REFERENCES

1. Reynolds, Jack, and K. Celeste Gaspari, *Cost-Effectiveness Analysis*, Pricor Monograph Series: Methods Paper 2, Chevy Chase, MD: Center for Human Services, 1985.

2. Mach, E. P., and B. Abel-Smith, *Planning the Finances of the Health Sector: A Manual for Developing Countries*, Geneva: World Health Organization, 1983.

3. Waterston, A., *Development Planning: Lessons from Experience*, Baltimore: The Johns Hopkins University Press, 1965, p. 203.

4. deFerranti, D., "Paying for Health Services in Developing Countries: A Call for Realism," *World Health Forum*, 6,2:99–105, 1985.

5. Ahmed, Paul, *Guidelines for Analysis of Indigenous and Private Health Care Planning in Developing Countries*, Office of International Health, Rockville, MD: U.S. Public Health Service, 1979.

6. Stinson, W., *Community Financing of Primary Health Care*, Primary Health Care Issues Paper No. 4, Washington: American Public Health Association, 1982.

7. Wheeler, Mark, *Financing of Health Services in Indonesia*, Sectoral Study No. 2, Institute of Government Studies, Birmingham, England: University of Birmingham, 1983.

8. Zschock, Dieter K., *Health Care Financing in Developing Countries*, International Health Programs Monograph Series No. 1, Washington: American Public Health Association, 1979.

9. Waterston, A., "An Operational Approach to Development Planning," *International Journal of Health Services*, 1,3:247, 1971.

PRIMARY READINGS

Caiden, Naomi, and A. Wildavsky, *Planning and Budgeting in Poor Countries*, New York: John Wiley & Sons, 1974. An early, comprehensive treatment of the fiscal aspects of health planning.

deFerranti, D., "Strategies for Paying for Health Services in Developing Countries," *World Health Statistics Quarterly*, 37,4:428–442, 1984. A comprehensive and thoughtful review of past national trends, as well as current options and issues in health care financing.

Howard, L., *A New Look at Development Cooperation for Health: A Study of Official Donor Policies, Programmes and Perspectives in Support of Health for All by the Year 2000*, Geneva: World Health Organization, 1981. A thorough review of donor policies in health matters reveals that there is room for expansion in the number of health programs in developing countries receiving help from international agencies.

Mach, E. P., and B. Abel-Smith, *Planning the Finances of the Health Sector: A Manual for Developing Countries*, Geneva: World Health Organization, 1983. The manual presents a methodology for collecting, organizing, and using data on health expenditures and sources of finance.

Stinson, W., *Community Financing of Primary Health Care*, Primary Health Care Issues Paper No. 4, Washington: American Public Health Association, 1982. A review of community resources generation methods in one hundred projects.

Zschock, Dieter K., *Health Care Financing in Developing Countries*, International Health Programs Monograph Series No. 1, Washington: American Public Health Association, 1979. An appraisal of health financing practice and sources of funding with reference to case studies in Bolivia, Botswana, Colombia, the Dominican Republic, and South Korea.

SECONDARY READINGS

Ahmed, Paul, *Guidelines for Analysis of Indigenous and Private Health Care Planning in Developing Countries*, Office of International Health, Rockville, MD: U.S. Public Health Service, 1979.

Financing of Health Services, WHO Technical Report Series No. 625, Geneva: World Health Organization, 1978.

Maxwell, R. J., *Health and Wealth: An International Study of Health-Care Spending*, Lexington, MA: Lexington Books, 1981.

Parker, D. A., "The Use of Indicators of Financial Resources in the Health Sector," *World Health Statistics Quarterly*, 37,4:451–462, 1984.

Robertson, R. L., D. K. Zschock and J. A. Daly, *Guidelines for Analysis of Health Sector Financing in Developing Countries*, Office of International Health, Rockville, MD: U.S. Public Health Service, 1979.

Rodwin, Victor G., *The Health Planning Predicament*, Berkeley: University of California Press, 1984.

13

Community Involvement

CARL E. TAYLOR

Community involvement is one of the main pillars of primary health care as defined at the Alma Ata Conference on Primary Health Care in 1978.[1] Although everyone seems to agree that it is important, there is no consensus about what it is or how to achieve it. Yet it is not surprising that problems of implementation remain, because systematic efforts to promote community involvement in health care have only recently received serious attention.

A spectrum of definitions of community involvement includes at one extreme those who put great effort into finding ways by which people can be persuaded to do what health personnel want. At the opposite end of the spectrum are those who feel that the community should make the decisions and the health system should have a purely supportive role. Between these extremes, notions of community participation range from inducing communities to help promote utilization of services, to having communities provide some labor and financial support and letting people have some say in what they find acceptable.

In recent years there has been a trend toward shifting more responsibility for planning and decision making about primary health care and all development activities to the community. A major international effort to improve understanding of community participation as part of general social development has been conducted since 1979 by the United Nations Research Institute for Social Development in Geneva.[2] A report on fifty-two primary health care projects supported by the U.S. government during the 1970s identified community participation as an area particularly needing study and discussed those elements of primary health care that will benefit most from community involvement.[3] Similarly, a WHO review of seventy country programs in primary health care showed the tremendous diversity in approaches that are emerging.[4]

HISTORICAL BACKGROUND

Social Change Theory and Practice Generally

Growing recognition of the need for social change to maintain the momentum of any development has led to systematic efforts to understand the dynamics of how community involvement can be promoted. In the 1950s intensive efforts to promote large-scale community development programs, starting in India and eventually extending to twenty-five countries,[5,6] focused on improving both agricultural production and rural living conditions. After considerable success in pilot projects,[7] national programs failed to produce equivalent results because of the tendency to substitute a burden of top-down bureaucratic compulsion and national targets for the flexible, adaptive approaches by which local projects promoted community initiative.

A more fundamental problem was the failure to recognize as constraints the competing interests of factions at village level, as well as larger-scale intergroup rivalries among local and national power structures. Egalitarian initiatives alarmed community leaders and regional power structures. This condition changed only when local elites found that through community participation they could benefit from the unpaid labor of the poor. In spite of these problems community development had the long-term benefit that in some places it began to show people that change was possible. It also provided training to community members in technical skills and ways of mobilizing community effort.

Much research has been done on problems of social change, with the findings relating to diffusion theory being of special relevance.[8] In the 1960s and 1970s, in Latin America, the theology of liberation movement developed an extensive literature[9] and experiential background. Commitment to changing oppressive political and social structures produced both an intense ideological orientation[10] and examples of successful change. The underlying principle of conscientization stresses the need to empower the people with an understanding of their own capacity so that they will stand up for their rights and change the way they live. The change agent stimulates but never tells the community what to do.

The Professionalization of Medicine

In health similar patterns can be traced. In ancient times in most cultures health activities involved much community involvement. An example is a quotation from Herodotus[11] describing medical care in ancient Babylon:

> Having no use for physicians they carry the sick into the market place; then those who have been afflicted themselves by the same illness as the sick man, or seen others in like case come near and advise him by what means they have themselves recovered of it or seen others so recover. None may pass by the sick man without speaking and asking what is his sickness.

As medicine became professionalized, people seemed relieved to be able to turn their cares and worries over to doctors. The family physician as described in folklore used family members in the home to provide routine care. Even this minimal involvement has tended to disappear as medical care moved from homes to institutions.

In public health especially there has been a continuing tendency for professionals to assume responsibility for decisions and implementation of health programs with less and less consultation with the people. When dealing with environmental problems the tendency was to proceed directly to implement what professional judgment suggested would be best unless embarrassing public protests emerged. The presumed good of society took precedence over individual wishes, and there was no hesitation in passing laws and regulations. Health education was considered mainly a means of convincing the people to do what the health professionals thought was best. Most health education messages ended with the injunction "see your doctor" rather than "take care of yourself." As the focus of health activities shifted from communicable to noncommunicable conditions, this approach was also applied to the many activities in which prevention depended on personal changes in life-style more than mass implementation of societal and environmental interventions. In many doctor-dominated health systems a strong tradition of limiting community participation to inducing people to do what they are told has evolved. The common term *compliance* carries that connotation.

A dramatic shift in thinking reached its most general articulation in the Alma Ata definition of primary health care. It was realized that many health programs were achieving less than had been anticipated. Problems of utilization and compliance had been identified and studied extensively. When well-intentioned efforts to work with communities were only marginally successful, health workers tended to blame the people for not cooperating.

When field studies began to show the dramatic effectiveness of projects in which communities took responsibility for their own health care,[12,13] some health workers reacted by wanting to dump responsibility for primary health care back on the community so that they could return with relief to their institution-based activities. These health workers had been uncomfortable when they were expected to do community work because they found it difficult to accept the notion that the people must ultimately be in control. In their institutions health workers were accustomed to being clearly in charge.

Since Alma Ata a beginning in resolving these ambivalent feelings has come from better clarification of relative roles of health workers and communities. Primary health care depends on a new partnership between the community and the health system. Functional responsibilities on both sides of this interface should be complementary. Specific allocation of responsibility, however, must be different, depending on local traditions of administration, culture, and political and social authority. We need means of defining what the right balance should be in each individual situation.

JUSTIFICATIONS FOR NEW CONCEPTS OF COMMUNITY INVOLVEMENT

Many justifications have been mobilized to support community involvement.[14,15] Advantages can be summarized under the following headings, which are obviously not mutually exclusive.

Effectiveness

In situations in which formal health services provide inadequate coverage the only care possible is from people helping themselves. Even where health services are well developed, there are many activities that can be carried out best when the people understand the problem and help work out solutions. This is true not only of developing countries but has become most obvious in the long-term changes in life-style which are essential to the prevention of the chronic diseases that have become the greatest health problems of affluent societies.

Efficiency

Direct community support for health programs is often more cost-effective than raising money through taxation or other sources of public funding. The basic principle is that the government should pay only for those activities that no one else will pay for. By making use of local expertise and understanding of what works, many costly mistakes can be avoided. People tend to value and use services more when they know they have helped pay for them directly. The quality of commitment in voluntary work is particularly valuable for short-term intensive activities.

Response to Felt Needs of Community

One of the principal functions of community involvement is to give people an opportunity to express their desires in health care. All programs can benefit from indigenous knowledge to become more relevant. When communities also assume responsibility for supporting them directly, assurance is gained that effective demand will be a reflection of true local priorities.

Development of Community Cohesion and Capacity to Act Together

Most communities are so split into factions that it is sometimes necessary to treat each faction as a separate community. Mobilizing community organization for action is difficult except when it is done around specific activities for which there is overt demand. Successful action on such issues develops community cohesion and a new awareness of what people can do together.[16] As enlarged communities take on a real identity, they grow less dependent on professionals and become self-reliant, fulfilling a specific objective of the primary health care movement. Bureaucracies typically are an impediment to such a process, and ways must be found to involve them in a learning partnership with the people.[17] Possible new responsibilities for the community include participating directly in planning and decision making, carrying out specific tasks, serving as communication channels to specific groups, mobilizing support of all kinds, supervising health workers, collecting data, and participating in evaluation.

Conscientization

A further stage in the process of developing community awareness occurs when underlying changes in values and attitudes begin to appear. The fundamental importance of value change is epitomized in the term *conscientization*, which has become important in the philosophy of the theology of liberation movement.[9] Empowering the people so that they can stand up for their rights represents a tremendous change from centuries of social and economic oppression. Practical mechanisms to encourage conscientization are being adapted to local social and political situations.[18] The hazard should be recognized that when change agents are being most successful they may get into political trouble with repressive regimes.

Promoting Equity

One of the dilemmas in community involvement is the constant tension produced by the tendency of elite or special groups to try to take over the benefits of the change process for themselves and their families. A strong advantage of health programs as contrasted to programs which have high economic demand, such as the package of agricultural technologies that produced the "green revolution," is that the compulsion to monopolize inputs for personal profit is somewhat less. A limitation of the green revolution was the lag period before economic benefits began to trickle down to the poor. Health programs have the great advantage of being able to get communities involved in surveillance to gather or interpret information on whether those in greatest need receive care. If the community leaders are aware that people know that high child mortality is concentrated in certain areas and groups, there is much greater community compulsion to ensure that equitable coverage is being achieved.

THE MAJOR COMPONENTS OF COMMUNITY INVOLVEMENT

Experience thus far indicates that for community involvement to become self-sustaining it is important first to get a clear definition of what the local community is. In general the definition should be functional and based on local perceptions of the best local grouping that can be mobilized to promote action. The units may be based on geographical contiguity, on cultural tradition, economic production, or political association. The indicator of community in any case is a local group that can be characterized as sharing the same values.

Some specific organizational components of community involvement have to be considered and an appropriate balance worked out. Choices about how to organize each component vary, but something should be done in each of the following areas.

Official Commitment

Community involvement for systematic program development is unlikely to start in traditional societies unless it is stimulated from outside and perceived as being in accordance with government policy. Clear statements of national or regional policy are therefore necessary as a starting point. Continuing support and commitment by those in authority is equally essential. In the negotiations between government officials and communities, high officials often make promises which local personnel then have trouble implementing. Those who promise should be committed to carrying out their promises. It helps if communities have the stimulus of knowing that other communities are moving in the same direction.

Community Committees or Other Organized Groups

Several mechanisms have been used to promote community organization, but most of them involve some kind of local committee. A formal arrangement helps to provide some continuity and gives the group standing and recognition so that they can carry out activities in the name of and for the good of the people. Committee members almost always are volunteers. They function best in intermittent activities which do not require day-to-day commitment that would interfere with personal responsibilities for work or family. They can carry out well-organized routine or continuing tasks if sufficiently large numbers are involved so that each individual only occasionally has to take responsibility. Committees are best at organizing activities which may take a great deal of effort over a short period, but not if it is necessary to make such an effort frequently. Community committees are, therefore, excellent for starting projects and giving them a periodic stimulus, but they are not the best way of maintaining routine activities. Committee members should receive special training.

Community Health Workers (CHWs)

The most visible component of most community involvement efforts has been the community health worker. Tremendous diversity of experience is evident in programs and projects around the world. In most places the only way equitable coverage can be ensured is through an appropriate distribution of CHWs. Many documents and manuals describing successful approaches which fit specific situations are being produced. Comparative analyses are synthesizing experience from many countries.[19] The following general classification is based on a WHO study[20] of experience from forty-six countries.

Tasks and Functions

The tremendous variation in what CHWs do has been decided usually by the health system with little involvement of the community. This has not worked as well as when the people were involved in defining roles. Usually CHWs are supposed to carry out a combination of simple curative care and preventive activities. In their training great stress is placed on teamwork and on their relations with peripheral health workers. A problem is frequently encountered when workers coopt CHWs as their assistants.[21] Various studies suggest that by working at least thirty hours a week they should be able to cover five hundred to one thousand population in providing a relatively focused package of services. In general it has been found that coverage is better when a multipurpose worker is responsible for a package of half a dozen services in a small population than if several workers provide only one or two services for considerably larger populations.

Selection and Recruitment

Generalizations that apply in most places are that CHWs should be mature and respected in the community, at least half should be women because of the importance of services to mothers and children, and literacy is desirable for maintaining records, though outstanding successes have been achieved with illiterate women.[22] Selection processes should include both the community and the health system. In an outstanding project in Kenya,[23] a useful compromise evolved with the community selecting three candidates and the health team then making the final selection by objective testing. It may also be desirable to keep the final selection open until after the basic training is completed and course performance evaluated.

Training

Duration ranges from a few days to two years. Often arrangements can be worked out for part-time training so that CHWs are away from their homes and work for limited blocks of time. An important educational consideration is to alternate periods of theoretical training and practical field experience.[24] Content and teaching methods should be determined by precise job definition and task analysis to focus on developing the knowledge, skills, and attitudes needed to provide a limited range of specific tasks. Continuing education should relate directly to supportive supervision. CHWs should have regular opportunities to get together with other CHWs to discuss mutual problems and prevent a feeling of isolation. Trainers should include experienced CHWs.

Remuneration

To maintain continuity and to increase competence, CHWs should be compensated for their time, either by money or by other culturally appropriate rewards. It is not realistic to expect volunteers to maintain regular services. Three types of incentives are possible. First, in some successful programs government allocates money to the community to cover basic salaries. It is not advisable to have CHWs paid directly by the health services because their loyalty then shifts to their official supervisor rather than to the community. Second, the community may pay the CHW either in money or in kind. In some instances increased social status and recognition are considered sufficient compensation, but this is not usual. Incentives should be sustainable and paid regularly; otherwise there will be loss of interest and a high turnover. The third possibility is fee for service, or payment for drugs, but this requires careful control and definition of relations with existing traditional practitioners.

Career Prospects and Attrition

Job security and a sense of career achievement are important in maintaining continuity of service among CHWs. A powerful motivational support is opportunities for career advancement, as when CHWs know that a few of their colleagues are being selected for training as health professionals. More commonly it should be possible for the best CHWs to be chosen as supervisors. In some programs there has been concern about attrition and turnover, but this is not necessarily negative because former CHWs can still have great influence in their communities. Where such turnover occurs it is essential to have a continuing program for training new CHWs. Turnover rates seem to be much higher for men than women, and this may be a reason for giving preference to women in selection.

Support Services

Extension of coverage using CHWs necessarily increases demands for drugs, supplies, and logistic support. It is counterproductive to select and train CHWs and then fail to provide this needed support. Management systems must be devised to control the usual tendency of health centers and hospitals to drain off into their activities materials that are supposed to go to peripheral workers. Highest priority should be given to peripheral workers in distributing drugs and supplies, for centrally located institutions have more options and alternative sources than people in remote areas. Private sector distribution manages to get drugs and supplies to remote areas, but at prohibitive cost to the poor, who then may have to depend on erratic supplies to formal health facilities. CHWs tend to be scattered in villages. An effective communication system is needed so that they can reach out and get appropriate help when they need it. This includes referral and the chance to call for consultation when a clinical or community problem arises. Without such support the CHWs' credibility will be problematic.

Supervision

Continuous, educative, supportive supervision is the single most important characteristic that distinguishes effective community programs. Two types of supervision should be recognized. The first is technical supervision by peripheral health workers who can provide consultation and referral. If distances are great, ingenuity is needed in using two-way radios, records, pigeons, or other locally appropriate means. If health center doctors have competing clinical demands that interfere with the regularity of their visits, then other supervisors have to be identified. Where multiple categorical programs are trying to work through CHWs, a strong mechanism is needed to make local workers coordinate their peripheral activities. The representatives of special programs should work through supervisors rather than directly with CHWs. Supervision is often most meaningful when provided by people who have previously done the same job themselves and have received appropriate additional training. An effective working relationship between CHWs and communities requires reorientation of all members of the health team. Experience in the Indian CHW program is instructive.[25] At first health center personnel opposed the idea of CHWs, but evaluation one year later showed them to be enthusiastic because CHWs had proved useful in carrying out programs they had been trying to implement. The danger emerged that CHWs were being coopted by the health system.

The second type of supervision is of routine operations and administration. This can be done by community representatives. The CHW should usually be responsible to the community health committee, which will typically control remuneration. A dynamic two-way interaction is needed with the CHW's providing stimulation and focus for the activities of the committee.

Cooperation with Other Sectors

CHWs can be an important link between health activities and other development programs at the community level. Intersectoral cooperation has been difficult to implement in government hierarchies. At village level there is more tendency to get together because separate sectoral distinctions mean little to village people. Their everyday problems cannot be artificially divided to fit government sectors. In promoting intersectoral cooperation it is necessary to develop better ways of identifying and articulating community priorities. As they develop awareness of their needs, community representatives learn how to draw on resources from the government and elsewhere.

Information Systems and Evaluation

Health information systems are often among the least satisfactory components of health systems. Basic data on health status and health care must be collected by peripheral workers, and the information system is usually too complicated to match field realities. If the raw data are not good then no amount of sophisticated handling can improve their validity. CHWs can provide good information if data collecting and recording are simple and if they understand that these activities serve a useful function. Data should be rapidly analyzed for local, regional, and central use. Evaluation should be fed back promptly to improve services. If the purpose of evaluation is perceived to be punitive and a means for superiors to demonstrate their authority, then workers find ingenious methods of covering up the facts. Some of the most effective new approaches in improving health information involve the community in gathering and analyzing data as part of making their own evaluations.[26]

Patterns of Funding

Community involvement is most clearly demonstrated when people contribute to the financial support of primary health care. A major obstacle in many countries is that politicians have been promising free care with no recognition of the fact that health care is never really free, since the people eventually pay. The recurrent question is, How can the costs of care be equitably distributed? Health services are increasingly expensive. The limited free care available benefits urban populations in close proximity to health facilities. As a result of the new rhetoric of community involvement the people who are most remote and deprived are sometimes being asked to finance their own care. The social injustice of this process cannot be rationalized away. If rural people are asked to pay for their own care, the same requirement should apply in urban areas. The hard fact is that tax-supported care cannot be provided equitably for everyone unless the government gives high priority to health.

Patterns of funding primary health care other than by direct support from tax revenues may follow many different channels. Government planners should reserve public funds for high-priority activities of largely unrecognized importance such as preventive services and family planning. For other services they should follow the axiom that "any planner is a fool to pay for anything that someone else will pay for."

Some of the most successful community-based payment schemes are those associated with cooperatives or in which a health maintenance organization has negotiated a group contract to provide care. An extensive review of community financing in one hundred projects[27] showed that people were most commonly contributing to drug costs, payment of community workers, and provision of facilities and labor. The major inducement to participate was always curative services, with preventive activities being added at the insistence of health workers. A period of education was needed to help people to understand the insurance concept of spreading costs among a large number of people and over time. A generalization that seems valid is that prepayment schemes work best if there is a continuing money flow from which premiums can be deducted. For example, in the dairy cooperatives in India, arrangements for health services developed when people realized that their buffaloes were getting better health care than their children. It is often difficult to induce people to pay premiums directly for health care, even if the program is called a cooperative. In spite of this, the aforementioned review showed that there were twice as many projects using direct payment into a fund compared with those drawing funds from productive enterprises. The success of any payment mechanism depends eventually on whether people are satisfied with the care they receive.

PRACTICAL PROCESS OF IMPLEMENTATION

The major problem in planning for community involvement is that we have not yet learned how to apply lessons from special projects to promoting national programs. The theory seems reasonably well developed, but practical questions remain about why the implementation of some programs succeeds remarkably while others have no impact. Officials tend to take patterns evolved in flexible local programs and make them rigid and locally irrelevant by taking decision making away from communities. Paperwork becomes so massive that the community cannot cope.

The first need is for a clear national policy supporting the concept of community-based decision making related to health. Too much centralized planning is contrary to the fundamental principle of encouraging community decisions. On the other hand leaving everything entirely to the communities is little more than romantic idealism because usually nothing will happen. If communities could generate their own process of change using modern knowledge and technology, they would do so on their own.

A recurring source of disagreement between proponents of centralized direction and advocates of community control revolves around who should select the priority components of the primary health care package. Everyone agrees that selectivity based on priority setting is needed. The reality is that the only way of ensuring that all eight components of primary health care are implemented is to work first on a few interventions, with others' being phased in over time. Multipurpose peripheral health workers should only be expected to manage a half a dozen tasks at a time. This means that choices have to be made that will:

- focus on the greatest problems
- be effective enough to make a difference
- use appropriate technology that is within the limited resources and competence available in the community
- be cost-effective, implementable, and acceptable to the people
- have characteristics that make equitable coverage possible
- initiate a systematic process in places and activities where cooperation is easiest in order to demonstrate success and justify to the people the benefit they will receive when they show the necessary initiative and cooperation

A great deal of energy is wasted in arguments between proponents of top-down and bottom-up programs. Centralized programs are said to have the advantage that they can achieve a quick impact within a two- or three-year period, but they tend to show less concern about continuity once the initial impact has been made. Any such program should eventually fit into the health infrastructure. On the other hand, proponents of community control sometimes seem to be more interested in promoting sociopolitical change than in saving the lives of babies.

Obviously the optimum approach is not either-or but both. Developing the infra-structure should be complementary to implementing practical interventions. Ways must be found to persuade health services and communities to work together in a partnership. Health planning should concentrate on devising facilitating mechanisms so that health personnel can recognize and act on their responsibility to help people solve their own problems. In the series of steps that follow some suggestions are made for achieving this difficult reorientation in interactions between the health system and community.

Situation Analysis

Two sources of information have to be brought together in the situation analysis. First, locally appropriate ways for the community to articulate its own perceptions of needs should be developed. Efforts should be made to develop community capacity to do much of this analysis. This should be followed naturally by a review of what is being done to solve the problems identified and what might be done. To ensure adequate objective attention to the needs of the poor it may be necessary to include health personnel from outside the community to define where the health problems are concentrated.

The second source of information is professional determination of health needs using appropriate scientific analysis. These epidemiologically defined problems should be compared with community perceptions. Dialogue with the community should lead to priority ranking. Joint review of what the health services and community are doing about priority health problems should lead to joint planning. It is often desirable first to work on problems considered important by the people and to use joint activities as a means of creating awareness of problems not recognized earlier. When efforts were made to compare community and professional perceptions in Nepal,[28] it was found that half of identified problems were recognized as a need by both, one-fifth only by the community, and 15 percent only by health professionals. National and international agencies sometimes provide funding only for specific priorities, and in this case care should be taken to permit communities to decide whether to go along with those priorities with full awareness of the continuing costs they will have to bear.

Interventions to Be Selected for Primary Health Care Package

A systematic analysis of alternative interventions which might be applied to the prior-ity problems is the next step. At the local level this mainly involves helping commu-nity leaders understand technical methods and approaches that have been successful in national or international programs. Community involvement can help greatly in adapting procedures to the ecologic, cultural, economic, and administrative condi-tions of the area that will influence implementation. For instance, oral rehydration is usually accepted most readily if it is based on locally prepared liquids such as carrot juice or rice flour.

Mobilization and Reallocation of Resources and Personnel

Health personnel and community representatives should together review the resources available or needed to carry out the interventions which are selected. These range from material supplies to the time of community members. The process of reallocating roles among health personnel and community workers is especially important and delicate. All activities should be simplified and routines established so that they can be brought as close to the village home as is technically safe. Appropriate technology should be used. The general experience is that about 90 percent of primary health care can be provided by peripheral workers under supervision.

Management, Supervision, and Logistics

Most community programs encounter their greatest obstacles in being unable to establish appropriately simple arrangements for management, supervision, and logistics. Ensuring technical quality should be the particular responsibility of the health system. The fact that community-based activities are often poorly performed may be due to the less than total commitment to community involvement by health workers. Community members may test the commitment of health workers by raising irrelevant obstacles and constraints. Past experiences tend to make many communities skeptical about the sincerity of people who come from outside saying they want to help. These attitudes can be changed only through patient persistence.

Training and Retraining

A considerable educational effort is needed to train CHWs and members of community committees. This should be followed by repetitive continuing education. It will be necessary to reorient all health personnel in how to work with the community. This may be difficult since doctors and other health workers often do not take community activities seriously. They resist showing the respect and cooperation which are needed for a new collaborative style of work and try to keep peripheral workers "in their place" by exerting professional dominance as they reiterate concerns that CHWs will become quacks. This lack of trust interferes with the educational objectives of developing competence and confidence.

Information, Evaluation, and Feedback

A partnership between a health system and communities cannot be expected to succeed spontaneously when first tried. A learning process of flexible change and progressive modification is needed as problems are identified and improved solutions discovered. More than with almost any other type of planning, therefore, community-based programs need systematic means of gathering simple data for decision making about the adaptive changes that are inevitably needed. Decentralized control and management are essential.

Surveillance for Equity

Health for all is more than anything else a call for equity. It will not evolve easily or automatically. A major responsibility of the health system should be to establish surveillance for key health indicators, implementation of selected priority services, and coverage of high-risk groups. When it is shown that particular needs are concentrated in certain groups, then community leaders will be more likely to ensure appropriate distribution of benefits. Systematic use of the high-risk approach for surveillance of women and children will lead to focusing services where needs are greatest.

To summarize, community involvement is recognized to be an important part of primary health care, but we have a great deal to learn about how it should be implemented. Approaches must be adapted to local conditions. A general process has been described that provides a starting point in working out a locally appropriate balance in responsibility between the health system and the community.

REFERENCES

1. *Primary Health Care: Report of International Conference on Primary Health Care, Alma Ata, USSR*, Geneva: World Health Organization, 1979.

2. Stiefel, M., and A. Pearse, "UNRISD's Popular Participation Programme," *Assignment Children*, 59 and 60:145–162, 1982.

3. *Primary Health Care: Progress and Problems*, Washington: American Public Health Association, 1982, p. 101.

4. "Review of Primary Health Care Development," SHS/82.3, Geneva: World Health Organization, 1982, p. 357.

5. Council of Social Development, *Action for Rural Change*, New Delhi: Munshiram Manoharlal Publishing Co., 1970, p. 495.

6. Holdcroft, L. E., "Community Development: Rise and Fall," *Journal of Community Action*, I,6:41–46, 1983.

7. Wiser, C. M., and W. H. Wiser, *Behind Mud Walls*, Berkeley: University of California Press, 1983.

8. Rogers, E. M., *Communication and Development*, Beverly Hills: Sage Publications, 1976.

9. Gibellini, R., *Frontiers of Theology in Latin America*, trans. by John Drury, New York: Orbis, 1979, p. 321.

10. Freire, P., *Pedagogy of the Oppressed*, St. Louis: The Herder Book Co., 1970.

11. *Herodotus* (English trans.), Loeb Classical Library Edition B1, 1976, p. 25.

12. Djukanovic, V., and E. P. Mach, *Alternative Approaches to Meeting Basic Health Needs in Developing Countries*, Geneva: World Health Organization, 1975, p. 116.

13. Newell, K., *Health by the People*, Geneva: World Health Organization, 1975, p. 206.

14. Korten, F. J., "Community Participation: A Management Perspective on Obstacles and Options," in Korten, D. C., and F. B. Alonso (eds.), *Bureaucracy and the Poor: Closing the Gap*, Singapore: McGraw-Hill International Book Co., 1981, pp. 181–200.

15. White, A. T., "Why Community Participation?" in *Community Participation: Current Issues and Lessons Learned, Assignment Children*, 59 and 60:17–34, 1982.

16. Banerji, D., *Poverty, Class and Health Culture in India*, New Delhi: Prachi Prakastan Publishing Co., 1982, p. 309.

17. Korten, D. C., and F. B. Alonso (eds.), *Bureaucracy and the Poor: Closing the Gap*, Singapore: McGraw-Hill International Book Co., 1981, p. 258.

18. Goulet, D., *The Cruel Choice: A New Concept in the Theory of Development*, New York: Atheneum, 1973, p. 360.

19. *The Community Health Worker, A WHO/UNICEF Workshop in Jamaica*, PHC 80.2, Geneva: World Health Organization, 1980, p. 69.

20. Ofosu-Amah, V., *National Experience in the Use of Community Health Workers*, No. 71, Geneva: World Health Organization, 1983, p. 49.

21. Maru, R., "Organizing for Rural Health," in Korten, D. C., and F. B. Alonso (eds.), *Bureaucracy and the Poor: Closing the Gap*, Singapore: McGraw-Hill International Book Co., 1981, pp. 35–43.

22. Arole, R., and M. Jamkhed, "A Comprehensive Rural Health Project in Jamkhed (India)," in Newell, K., *Health by the People*, Geneva: World Health Organization, 1975, pp. 70–90.

23. Were, M., *Organization and Management of Community-Based Health Care*, Nairobi: UNICEF Regional Office, 1982, p. 149.

24. Taylor, C. E., D. G. Carlson and A. S. Golden, "Education of Primary Health Care Workers," *UNICEF News*, 100:3–13, 1979.

25. National Institute of Health and Family Welfare, *An Evaluation of Community Health Workers Scheme in India, A Collaborative Study*, Technical Report No. 4, New Delhi: National Institute of Health and Family Welfare, 1978, p. 134.

26. "Use of Epidemiology in Primary Health Care," *WHO Chronicle*, 34:16–19, 1980.

27. Stinson, W., *Community Financing of Primary Health Care*, Primary Health Care Issues Paper No. 4, Washington: American Public Health Association, 1982, p. 90.

28. DeSweemer, C., R. L. Parker, C. E. Taylor and W. A. Reinke, "Unresolved Issues in Primary Care in the Developing World," in White, K. L., and P. J. Bullock (eds.), *The Health of Populations: A Report of Two Rockefeller Foundation Conferences*, New York: Rockefeller Foundation, 1979.

PRIMARY READINGS

Cohen, J., and N. Uphoff, *Rural Development Participation: Concepts and Measures for Project Design, Implementation and Evaluation*, Rural Development Committee, Center for International Studies Monograph Series No. 2, Ithaca, NY: Cornell University Press, 1977. Presents a framework, including graphs and charts, for analyzing community participation, then describes application to a specific project.

Coombs, P. (ed.), *Meeting the Basic Needs of the Rural Poor: The Integrated Community-Based Approach*, Elmsford, NY: Pergamon Press, 1980. A useful commentary on community participation in major projects in Bangladesh, Sri Lanka, and Thailand.

Kark, L., *The Practice of Community-Oriented Primary Health Care*, New York: Appleton-Century-Crofts, 1981. Based upon extensive experience, this text is useful for both developed and developing countries.

Korten, David C., "Community Organization and Rural Development: A Learning Process Approach," *Public Administration Review*, 480–511, September 1980. Describes a systematic three-phase approach to learn from experience in carrying out community programs.

Newell, K., *Health by the People*, Geneva: World Health Organization, 1975. The case studies presented in this volume provided basic background for the deliberations on primary health care at Alma Ata.

Rifkin, Susan B. (ed.), *Health, The Human Factor: Readings in Health, Development, and Community Participation*, Geneva: Christian Medical Commission, 1980. Difficulties in gaining community participation are cited through position papers and accounts of field experience.

Were, Miriam K., *Organization and Management of Community-Based Health Care*, New York: UNICEF, 1980. An important community health program in Kenya was subjected to extensive analysis as reported in this document.

SECONDARY READINGS

Connor, Eileen, and Fitzhugh Mullan (eds.), *Community Oriented Primary Care: New Directions for Health Services Delivery* Washington: National Academy Press, 1983.

Metsch, Jonathan, and James Veney, "Measuring the Outcome of Consumer Participation," *Journal of Health and Social Behavior*, 14:368–374, 1973.

Ofosu-Amah, V., *National Experience in the Use of Community Health Workers: A Review of Current Issues and Problems*. Geneva: World Health Organization, 1983.

Rifkin, Susan B., *Health Planning and Community Participation: Case Studies in South East Asia*, London: Croon Helm, 1985.

Silver, G. A., "Community Participation and Health Resource Allocation," *International Journal of Health Services*, 3,2:117–131, 1973.

Twumasi, P. W., "Community Involvement in Solving Local Health Problems," *Social Science in Medicine*, 15A,2:169–174, 1981.

Uphoff, N., et al., *Feasibility and Application of Rural Development Participation: A State of the Art Paper*, Rural Development Committee, Center for International Studies Monograph Series No. 3, Ithaca, NY: Cornell University Press, 1979.

Vaughan, J. P., "Barefoot or Professional? Community Health Workers in the Third World," *Journal of Tropical Medicine and Hygiene*, 83,1:3–10, 1980.

Werner, D., *Where There Is No Doctor: A Village Health Care Handbook*, Palo Alto, CA: The Hesperian Foundation, 1977.

14

Organizational Structure and Process

WILLIAM A. REINKE

Individual words by themselves are quite useless until they have been molded into a language through which ideas are communicated. Likewise the organization, through which decisions are communicated and actions taken, is an entity worthy of study in its own right apart from the individuals whom it comprises. We hardly need to be reminded that the organization has a mission and character quite separate from, though necessarily compatible with, the goals of its members. Planners and policymakers have argued with good reason over the ramifications of placing environmental control matters under the jurisdiction of health departments, recreational agencies, or natural resources development bodies.

Organizations are essentially channels for the flow of information, ideas, and influence for the purpose of making decisions and taking action. To begin with, organizational analysis deals with structural matters of responsibility, authority, and coordination of decisions and actions. Structural issues regarding the anatomy of organizations are discussed in the next section.

Individuals cannot act in a coordinated, organized fashion in the absence of a communications network that both stimulates and controls the flow of information needed to make and disseminate decisions. This network is the organization's circulatory system that deserves attention, along with specification of relevant features of the information to be communicated.

Continuing the human analogy, we next deal with the organization's physiology, that is, the process by which decisions are made. Elements of the decision process have already been outlined in Chapter 4. The present chapter offers concrete examples of the application of that process and its functional attributes.

While this chapter focuses on the organizational entity with regard to structure, communication, and decision making, we can never disregard the individuals making up the organization. Likert[1,p.207] has observed that organized effort is ideally a dynamic process whereby individual and organizational goals are examined and modified, and methods are devised for rewarding their achievement.

> A. The relevant goals of persons in the organization, or related to it, develop so that these goals achieve a satisfactory level of compatibility between them;
>
> B. The objectives of the entire organization and of its component parts are in satisfactory harmony with the relevant goals and needs of the great majority, if not all, of the members of the organization and of the persons served by it;

C. Each member of the organization has objectives and goals which have been established in such a way that he is highly motivated to achieve them and which, when carried out, will result in his doing his part in enabling the organization to achieve its over-all objectives;

D. The methods and procedures used by the organization and its subunits to achieve the agreed upon objectives are developed and adopted in such a way that the members of the organization are highly motivated to use these methods to their maximum potentiality; and

E. The reward system of the organization is such that the members of the organization and the persons related to it feel that the organization yields them equitable rewards for their efforts in assisting the organization to achieve its objectives.

STRUCTURAL CONSIDERATIONS

Organizations are formal structures. Yet they exhibit nearly lifelike emotional qualities, as well as patterns of growth, development, and decay. Since they are made up of individuals, consideration must be given to interpersonal relationships and motivations. Each of these features of the organization deserves comment.

Formal Structure

The formal structure is first of all characterized by specialization because of the limited capacity of single individuals to perform the wide range of activities required in an organization. Although compartmentalized to some extent, the individuals must interact, and frictions inevitably arise as a result. Some stem from the functional interdependence among officials, whereas others are allocational conflicts. Problems of a functional nature arise whenever the actions of one individual or segment of the organization have repercussions upon the effectiveness of others, regardless of the type or amount of resources used. For example, decisions regarding the nature of a family planning program may have a substantial impact upon child-care programs under the direction of entirely different members of the organization. In contrast, allocational conflicts arise when two or more activities must be supported by a single pool of scarce resources, so that an increase in the money and/or personnel allotted to one reduces the amounts available to support the other.

Administrators have generally felt that arbitration of these conflicts is best resolved by a hierarchical type of organization structure. Embedded in the hierarchy is a system of formal rules designed to reduce to a minimum the cumbersome communication required in the appeals process. The formal rules are likely to cover a fairly wide range of behavior in recurrent situations for which precedents have been established. Beyond this range are, on the one hand, decisions deemed too important to make without prior review by higher authorities and, on the other hand, matters that are sufficiently inconsequential to permit lower level discretionary action.

Granted the general use of hierarchical structure, organizations differ markedly according to whether they employ a relatively "steep" structure or a "flat" one. In the former case we have a long chain of command with many layers, so that administrators at the top receive only a limited amount of thoroughly screened information.

Presumably, they are then able to give adequate attention to a small number of critical decisions that are made in the light of a broad overview of organizational activities, undistracted by petty details. The difficulty with a steep structure is that movement of information up and down the line may be accompanied by distortion or improper selection. Important information may reach a dead end, and relatively inconsequential data may be unnecessarily passed on.

The obvious way to reduce this difficulty is to flatten the structure so that higher-level administrators have direct contact with more subordinates. This can lead, however, to a deluge of information that cannot be assimilated and to an unwieldy "span of control." Flat hierarchies, therefore, tend to be useful only where decision making and control can be largely decentralized.

Our discussion of organizational hierarchies has led us to consider chains of command. Earlier we spoke of the need for specialization within an organization. We must bring these two notions together and remark that not all the individual specialists have authority and responsibility in the chain of command, at least not in the strict sense. Thinking more broadly, individuals' status within an organization can come from the confidence they command through their special knowledge or education as well as through their official position in the chain of command. Thus, there are "staff" personnel and "line" personnel who differ formally in three ways[2,p.143]:

> staff members perform purely advisory functions, whereas line personnel have operational responsibility; each staff reports directly to its top-level boss, whereas most line officials report to their ultimate boss through hierarchical superiors; staff members are technical specialists, whereas line members are generalists.

It follows that "staff work influencing future action of organizations is based upon an ability to persuade,"[3,p.718] whereas line officials can rely upon formal authority. We must not overemphasize this distinction, however, for the effectiveness of all officials is determined informally in large part through their ability to influence, rather than to command.

Lifelike Characteristics of Organizations

Organizational entities are far more than inanimate structures. Their observed rise and decline and their need for viability in the face of destructive forces cause them to have a dynamic, if not entirely animate, character. In the long run they face extinction unless they can change and innovate. In the short run, however, they demand stability, causing them to seek a comfortable routine. As a result organizations are continually in a state of tension. In some the forces of energy and movement are dominant, while others have a clearly sluggish nature. In short, organizations have metabolic levels much as individuals do. While the biochemistry of the former is not as well understood as it is for individuals, two "laws" are worth noting. The first is the *law of countervailing goal pressures*, which states, "The need for variety and innovation creates a strain toward greater goal diversity in every organization, but the need for control and coordination creates a strain toward greater goal consensus."[2,p.150]

Much lip service is given to rewarding innovation, but unfortunately control and compliance are the more dominant characteristics of many organizations. To illustrate, Argyris has performed an extensive analysis of 265 corporation decision-making meetings at the board or presidential levels. Among the nearly 12,500 units of behavior identified from tape recordings, "there were almost no instances in which executives took risks, experimented with new ideas, or helped others to experiment with new ideas."[4]

> Second, we have the so-called <u>Law of Increasing Conservatism</u>: All organizations tend to become more conservative as they get older, unless they experience periods of very rapid growth or internal turnover. . . . They formulate more extensive rules, learn to perform their tasks more efficiently, broaden the scope of their activities, develop more rigid procedures, shift their attention from task-performance to organizational survival, and devote a higher proportion of their activities to internal administration.[2,p.31]

No doubt other "laws" could be formulated and instances could be found which would tend to invalidate the ones presented here. The point is, however, that organizations as entities possess rather predictable characteristics that extend beyond but are not entirely independent of those of the individuals in them.

Informal Nature of Organizations

The individuals themselves deserve attention, of course. In studying ways in which relationships among various health services and structures were modified in six different communities, Morris found that the major impetus to change could usually be traced back to one or two key leaders.[5] Moreover, within a total agency there was often one guiding subgroup with religious or ethnic similarities.

Downs has postulated and discussed in some detail five different types of officials who fall into two broad classes.[2,pp.8-9] Each type is motivated differently by such factors as power, income, prestige, security, creativity, loyalty to an ideal or institution, and desire to serve the public interest.

A. Purely self-interested officials are motivated almost entirely by goals that benefit themselves rather than their bureaus or society as a whole. There are two types of such officials:
   1. Climbers consider power, income, and prestige as nearly all-important in their value structures.
   2. Conservers consider convenience and security as nearly all-important. In contrast to climbers conservers seek merely to retain power, income, and prestige they already have, rather than to maximize them.
B. Mixed-motive officials have goals that combine self-interest and altruistic loyalty to larger values. The main difference among the three types of mixed-motive officials is the breadth of the larger values to which they are loyal. Thus:
   3. Zealots are loyal to relatively narrow policies or concepts, such as the development of nuclear submarines. They seek power for its own sake and for the purpose of effecting the policies to which they are loyal. We shall call these their sacred policies.
   4. Advocates are loyal to a broader set of functions or to a broader organization than zealots. They also seek power because they want to have a significant influence upon policies and actions concerning those functions or organizations.

5. Statesmen are motivated by loyalty to society as a whole and a desire to obtain the power necessary to have a significant influence upon national policies and actions. They are altruistic to an important degree because their loyalty is to the "general welfare" as they see it. Therefore statesmen closely resemble the theoretical bureaucrats of public administration textbooks.

Relating these categories of individuals to the law of increasing conservatism, Downs observes that almost every organization goes through a period of rapid growth before reaching what he calls "its initial survival threshold." During the growth period the organization contains a high proportion of zealots who helped to establish it and climbers who have been attracted by its fast growth. Ultimately a high proportion of the organization's membership tends to be converted into conservers because of increasing age and frustration of ambitions for promotion. The squeeze on promotions also tends to drive many climbers out of the organization into faster-growing agencies if alternatives are available. From this point of view, then, the nature of individuals, with their private goals, combined with the more or less natural course of events, results in the organizational patterns of growth and decline, energy and stagnation that we have come to recognize.

COMMUNICATIONS NETWORKS

Information received by any organizational unit can be a prescription for a defined course of action, a mandate to decide upon appropriate action, or a passive acknowledgment of activity undertaken elsewhere. As a decision point the organizational unit must utilize or acquire relevant information from multiple sources, must process the information to arrive at decisions, and must disseminate the results of decisions to other units whose actions or reactions are needed.

The organization's information network is an important determinant of how this process works. How is it determined whether information received is to be filed or acted upon? What determines the information to be sought in support of decision making? How is it determined who needs to know about decisions made? These questions cause us, first, to seek better understanding of the networks through which bits of information move and, second, to identify effective systems into which the bits can be assembled.

Information coming to a given individual can be forgotten or destroyed, retained for personal use, or passed on. If it is passed on, it can be forwarded in total, in part, or in some distorted manner. The individuals deciding what to do with the information are affected by their own self-interest, their understanding of the organization's interests and goals, their perception of the real world, and their interpretation of those specific data on hand. Even a piece of concrete information may have a great deal of uncertainty attached to it. For example, one may learn that 112 cases of pertussis have been reported during a certain period in an adjacent district and still be unsure when, where, how, or whether there will be a local impact. The greater the inherent uncertainty the more latitude officials have in interpretation. They tend to emphasize one ramification of the data as being most probable, not because it really is, but because the occurrence of that result would benefit them more than other possible outcomes.

We shall discuss these communications problems in three respects: the effect of information screening, the impact of distortion, and the nature of redundancy. As an integral part of the exposition we shall employ a model which, although artificial and oversimplified, will contribute to the understanding of the phenomena of interest.

In the model we postulate a hierarchy of authority containing seven levels. We will assume that the officials on the lowest (G) level are in the field. The information that they collect is sent to their F level superiors who screen it and relay the most salient parts to their superiors on the E level. The screening continues in this way until eventually the information reaches the top person in the hierarchy after being screened six times in the process.

Carrying the model a step further, we assume that each official on the G level collects one unit of data in a single time period. We further suppose that the average span of control in the organization is four, that is, that each individual above the G level has four subordinates on the average. This means that there are 4^6, or 4,096, units of data gathered at the G level during each time period.

Screening of Information

In order to appreciate the effect of screening, let us see what would happen if the average official forwarded only one-half of the information received. Then 2,048 units of data per time period would be received at the F level, 1,024 at the E level, and so on, until A would receive only 64 bits of information. The winnowing process would have removed 98.4 percent of the data originally generated. By comparison, if the average official screened out only one-fourth of the data received, Official A would ultimately receive 729 units per time period, more than 11 times the amount previously calculated.

The screening process is obviously essential if higher-level officials are not to be inundated with communications. The process will be successful, however, only to the extent that unimportant information is screened out and useful data are forwarded for use in higher-level decision making. Let us suppose, initially, that only one-half of the information received at any level of the hierarchy is worthy of being forwarded and that one decision results from each item of information that passes through the organization. We assume further that officials tend to usurp authority, in that at each organizational level 20 percent of the information that should be passed on for action at a higher level is held for action at the lower level.

The flow of information and decision making is then as shown in Figure 14.1. At the bottom of the hierarchy (Level G) only 1,638 of the 2,048 items of information deserving the attention of superiors is forwarded. If Level G personnel are ineffective in acting upon this information, 410 inadequate decisions are made at that level. In following the information screening upward to Level A, we find that the top executive receives only 17 of 64 units, or 27 percent of the vital information needed. Furthermore, the accumulation of ineffective decisions, indicated by the "held" entries, reveals that 680 of the 4,096 organization decisions (17 percent) are ineffective.

On the contrary some organizations are plagued by officials who are reluctant

Organizational Level	Status of Information*	Items of Information Meriting Upward Transmittal	Action
A	Received		17
	Forwarded	17	
B	Held	4	21
	Received	21	21
	Forwarded	42	
C	Held	10	52
	Received	52	52
	Forwarded	104	
D	Held	26	131
	Received	130	131
	Forwarded	261	
E	Held	66	328
	Received	327	328
	Forwarded	655	
F	Held	164	819
	Received	819	819
	Forwarded	1638	
G	Held	410	2048
	Received	2048	2048

*20 Percent of Information Meriting Upward Transmittal is Retained.

Figure 14.1   Hypothetical flow of information

to take certain actions of which they are fully capable. Let us suppose that at each hierarchic level, 20 percent of the information that should be acted upon is instead forwarded to superiors. Thus in our illustration 410 of the 2,048 decisions that should be made at Level G are passed upward, along with all of the 2,048 decisions that truly merit higher action. In this case, an information flow diagram analogous to Figure 14.1 would reveal that Level A receives the 64 units of information essential to effective action at that level and 22 additional items of data as well. The top-level executive is forced, therefore, to make 86 decisions (64 + 22), of which 22 could be made equally well at a lower level in the organization. The ratio 22/86, or 26 percent, might be considered an index of inefficiency for Level A. In all, 807 of the 4,096 decisions are taken at an unnecessarily high level under these circumstances, so that overall organizational inefficiency is at a 20 percent level.

In practice the screening of information may be imperfect in a manner which produces both ineffectiveness and inefficiency. Suppose we combine the two foregoing sets of circumstances to postulate a situation in which 20 percent of the information deserving upward transmittal is instead retained, while 20 percent of the information that could be retained for action is instead forwarded. The information flow diagram in this case reveals that 17 percent of the 4,096 decisions are handled inefficiently and a similar percentage are ineffective. Level A receives only 17 of the 64 vital items of information but receives 8 units of unnecessary information.

With calculations such as these, we begin to gain some appreciation for the practical implications of such factors as steep and flat hierarchical structures, principles of management by exception, and advantages of clear-cut, formal decision rules.

Quality of Informational Flow

This screening process is likely to affect not only the quantity and type of information received at each decision point but its quality, that is, its substantive content as well. The selection principles and interpretations applied by officials at the various levels may well be different. Hence the information that finally reaches A will have passed through six filters of different quality, and the "facts" reported to A will be quite different in content and implication from those gathered at the lowest level.

To illustrate the potential magnitude of the resulting distortion, let us simply assume that each screening destroys a certain fraction of the true meaning of the information from A's point of view. If this fraction is 10 percent, then by the time the information passes through all six filters, only about 53 percent of it will express the true state of the environment as A would have observed it. In particular if individuals at Level G were to initiate budget requests which were then reduced by 10 percent at each level, the final amount determined at A would be 53 percent of the original request.

Redundancy

Recognizing that incoming information is incomplete or distorted, A may try to establish more than one channel of communication to report the same events and topics. From one point of view this redundancy approach is wasteful, yet under the circumstances it may be quite productive.

Let us suppose that an administrator receives from one source only six-tenths of the necessary information. A second, independent source of the same kind would likewise report 60 percent of the total, although a certain amount of duplication would be expected. The two sources combined could be expected to report to him 84 percent of the total information needed, from the *additivity law of probability*:

$$(.6) + (.6) - (.6)^2 = .84$$

The second channel of communication, therefore, would increase the administrator's knowledge by 24/60, or 40 percent.

While our assumption of independence between the two channels of communication has been convenient, in practice the lack of independence may be by design, in order that competition may stimulate each of the two sources to become more productive of useful information.

THE DECISION PROCESS

Information is communicated in an organization in order to make decisions and to disseminate knowledge of the consequent actions taken. As outlined in Chapter 4, the decision process begins with the statement of objectives and specification of alternative strategies for achieving them.[6,7] Even when available information is fully utilized in the appraisal of alternatives, a degree of uncertainty concerning possible outcomes from specific strategies usually remains. Some or all of the uncertainty might be removed through acquisition of additional information, but only at a cost. Thus, rational decision making involves mobilization of as much information as can be economically justified, followed by objective appraisal of alternatives in the face of remaining uncertainties. The concrete example employed in the following discussion to illustrate the process was chosen to keep the arithmetic simple in order to focus attention on principles and methods.

Decision Analysis

We suppose that a certain Under-Fives Clinic conducts morning and afternoon sessions daily. The need for pediatric specialist services occurs randomly and arises at 70 percent of the sessions on average. To cope with this uncertainty, specialists can be employed *on call* at $30 each or *on demand* at $50 each. If they are *on call*, they must be paid whether utilized or not. Because of other duties they cannot be utilized in more than one session per day. Hence, an on call specialist needed in the morning cannot be employed again in the afternoon. Specialists *on demand* are employed only as needed for a particular session.

The circumstances give rise to the three possible strategies indicated in Figure 14.2 to place zero, one, or two specialists on call and to fill any further need through services "on demand."

In any case three possible (uncertain) results must be considered, along with their cost implications. To illustrate, if one specialist is on call, the cost will be $30, unless a second is needed at an additional on demand cost of $50. This will happen 49 percent of the time because 70 percent of the time the on call specialist will be needed in the morning, and on 70 percent of those occasions another need will arise in the afternoon (i.e., .7 × .7 = .49). The possible costs of $30 and $80 might be evaluated in any of several ways, but the most common approach is to weight them

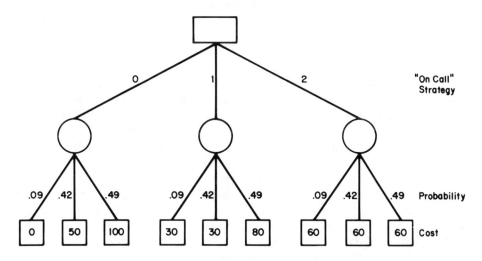

Figure 14.2   Illustrative decision tree

according to their likelihood of occurrence. The thinking is that if a cost of $30 is to be incurred 51 percent of the time and that of $80 is applicable the remaining 49 percent of the time, then the average cost of the strategy of concern is

$$(.51)(30) + (.49)(80) = \$54.50.$$

Similar appraisal of each of the three strategies yields the following.

None on call: $(.9)(0) + (.42)(50) + (.49)(100)$ $= \$70.00$
One on call: $(.51)(30) + (.49)(80)$ $= \$54.50$
Two on call: $= \$60.00$

The optimal strategy is that in which one specialist is placed on call each day and a second is summoned only if needed; this will occur less than half the time.

Any other strategy would be irrational because of its excessive cost. Even the rational strategy suffers a cost of uncertainty, however. If need could be foreseen in advance and specialists placed on call accordingly, the cost would be:

$$(.9)(0) + (.42)(30) + (.49)(60) = \$42.$$

The $12.50 difference between the cost of the most rational protection against uncertainty ($54.50) and that incurred if uncertainty were removed ($42) is the *cost of uncertainty*. If any further strategies that involve elimination of uncertainty at a cost of under $12.50 per day can be formulated, they should be evaluated. For example, an appointment system might be introduced so that patients and their needs could be determined in advance.

The circumstances surrounding most practical decisions are considerably more complex than in the foregoing example. As a result the number of possible options for action is tremendous, and the amount of information required for full appraisal of all of them is overwhelming. Determination of truly optimum strategies is simply not feasible. Rather than seeking elusive optima, decision making in practice usually is restricted to consideration of a modest number of attractive alternatives leading to choices expected to produce outcomes that are considered generally satisfactory, though possibly not the best possible.[8]

Sensitivity Analysis

This approach makes limited demands for precision of data. Using best estimates that are currently available, decision makers ascertain the range of conditions over which a specified strategy can be expected to yield satisfactory results. If the range is broad enough to encompass all realistic expectations, the strategy is chosen with confidence in spite of existing imprecision. If such confidence cannot be exhibited, decision makers seek additional, more precise data that will allow them to be more sensitive to small differences between strategies.

Consider a health unit that provides care 250 days (D) per year to a target population (T) of 50,000 whose utilization (U) of the health unit is expected to average between two and three visits annually. In choosing among staffing alternatives for handling the anticipated service volume, consideration is given to the employment of medical assistants (A) whose qualifications permit them to handle a proportion (P) of patients roughly estimated to be 20 to 40 percent. The issue for decision is whether to employ assistants, and if so how many, assuming a desirable service load (S) for each to be 30 patients per day. The issue is resolved in a three-stage process.

First, the needed items of information are established along with their interrelationship. Interest mainly centers on the number of assistants, which depends on the relationship

$$A = \frac{TUP}{DS}.$$

The numerator describes the total volume of patients to be seen by assistants annually, and the denominator defines the number to be seen per worker. Once the number of workers is fixed, the number of patients per worker per day can be calculated as

$$S = \frac{TUP}{DA}.$$

At the second stage of analysis, existing information, including uncertainties, is applied to the preceding models of relationships in order to establish the range of possible solutions. In the illustrative case uncertainty regarding per capita utilization and the ability of assistants to handle individual cases leads to

$$\text{Minimum } TUP = (50,000)(2)(.2) = 20,000;$$
$$\text{Maximum } TUP = (50,000)(3)(.4) = 60,000.$$

If the intent is for each assistant to treat

$$DS = (250)(30) = 7,500$$

patients annually,

$$\text{Minimum } A = \frac{20,000}{7,500} = 2.7;$$
$$\text{Maximum } A = \frac{60,000}{7,500} = 8.0.$$

We find that with existing information, the estimation of personnel needs is exceedingly imprecise; yet a specific decision must be made. Suppose the planner settles on 5 assistants per health unit, a reasonable compromise between the extremes of 2.7 and 8. As a result the effects of uncertainty inherent in the decision are transferred to the daily work load (S) of each assistant. In particular, with $A = 5$:

$$\text{Minimum } S = \frac{(50,000)(2)(.2)}{(250)(5)} = 16;$$
$$\text{Maximum } S = \frac{(50,000)(3)(.4)}{(250)(5)} = 48.$$

These second-stage calculations provide a sensitivity analysis that reveals the effects of imprecise information on the quality of impending decisions. In the present case the possibility of a threefold difference (48/16) in worker productivity is due to uncertainty regarding per capita utilization (U) and case mix (P). The separate effects of each factor can be calculated. For example, holding P fixed at .3, the separate effect of U is found to be

$$\text{Minimum } S = \frac{(50,000)(2)(.3)}{(250)(5)} = 24;$$

$$\text{Maximum } S = \frac{(50,000)(3)(.3)}{(250)(5)} = 36.$$

The magnitude of each effect can then be judged in relation to the feasibility and cost of reducing the effect through acquisition of more precise information.

In the present case, the staffing decision is less sensitive to utilization uncertainties than to considerations of case mix. Let us suppose, further, that experience elsewhere is readily available to reduce utilization uncertainties, whereas experience with medical assistants is not yet adequate to permit sharper estimates of their degree of effectiveness. In particular suppose that review of programs in other areas with service accessibility similar to that contemplated in the present case suggests that utilization is very likely to reach the higher level considered; that is, $U = 3$. Then we are left with

$$\text{Minimum } S = \frac{(50,000)(3)(.2)}{(250)(5)} = 24;$$

$$\text{Maximum } S = \frac{(50,000)(3)(.4)}{(250)(5)} = 48.$$

The remaining twofold difference in possible levels of productivity arises from the twofold difference in possible values of P. In effect P is estimated to be $.3 \pm .1$. If the level of imprecision (L), .1 is excessive, it can be reduced through acquisition of additional information in a survey designed to test the ability of medical assistants to treat a random sample of patient complaints.

Determination of sample size to be used in the survey forms the third stage of analysis. The sample should yield the desired improvements in precision but should not be larger and most costly than necessary. It can be shown that the level of imprecision associated with a sample of size N does not exceed $1/L^2$. (This point is considered more fully in Chapter 16. For the present the relationship $N = 1/L^2$ can be accepted as a useful rule of thumb.) Thus the planner who seeks an estimate of P that is within 5 percent (not 10 percent as at present) of the level that will be confirmed ultimately in practice is advised to mount a survey such that

$$\begin{aligned} N &= 1/L^2 \\ &= 1/(.5)^2 \\ &= 400. \end{aligned}$$

SUMMARY

Planning is necessarily shrouded in uncertainty. It is equally unrealistic to expect that management of the present can be based solely on "hard" data. Decision objectives and alternatives must be formulated carefully with information requirements and tolerable levels of uncertainty in mind. The resulting information system should then be applied through a communications network within an organization structure that promotes the organization's unity of purpose, ensures decision making at appropriate organizational levels, controls the flow and quality of information flow to those decision points, and effectively communicates the results of decisions to other organizational units as necessary.

REFERENCES

1. Likert R., "A Motivational Approach to a Modified Theory of Organization and Management," in Haire, Mason (ed.), *Modern Organization Theory*, New York: John Wiley & Sons, 1959.

2. Downs, A., *Bureaucratic Structure and Decision Making*, Memorandum RM-4646-1-PR, Santa Monica, CA: Rand Corporation, 1966.

3. Fleck, A. C., Jr., "Evaluation of Research Programs in Public Health Practice," *Annals of the New York Academy of Science*, 107:717–724, 1963.

4. Argyris, C., "How Tomorrow's Executives Will Make Decisions," *Think*, 18–23, November–December 1967.

5. Morris, R., "Basic Factors in Planning for the Coordination of Health Services," *American Journal of Public Health*, 53:248–259 and 462–472, 1963.

6. Raiffa, Howard, *Decision Analysis: Introductory Lectures on Choices under Uncertainty*, Reading, MA: Addison-Wesley, 1968.

7. Keeney, Ralph L., and Howard Raiffa, *Decisions with Multiple Objectives: Preferences and Value Tradeoffs*, New York: John Wiley & Sons, 1976.

8. Simon, Herbert A., *Administrative Behavior: A Study of Decision-Making Processes in Administrative Organization*, 3rd ed., New York: The Free Press, 1976.

PRIMARY READINGS

Downs, A., *Bureaucratic Structure and Decision Making*, Memorandum RM-4646-1-PR, Santa Monica, CA: Rand Corporation, 1966. Contains many practical insights on organizational behavior.

Leonard, David K., and Dale Rogers Marshall (eds.), *Institutions of Rural Development for the Poor: Decentralization and Organizational Linkages*, Institute of International Studies Research Series No. 49, Berkeley: University of California, 1982. Dealing with development generally, this volume gives particular attention to organizational requirements for serving the rural poor.

Raiffa, Howard, *Decision Analysis: Introductory Lectures on Choices Under Uncertainty*, Reading MA: Addison-Wesley, 1968. This remains the clearest description of decision analysis based upon probability considerations.

Walsh, J. A., and K. S. Warren, "Selective Primary Health Care: An Interim Strategy for Disease Control in Developing Countries," *Social Science in Medicine*, 14,2:145–163, 1980. A provocative approach to the organization of basic health services that has stimulated much discussion.

SECONDARY READINGS

Brolly, E. H., "Health Care Data Recording System for Developing Countries," *Tropical Doctor*, 12,3:105–109, 1982.

Keeney, Ralph L., and Howard Raiffa, *Decisions with Multiple Objectives: Preferences and Value Tradeoffs*, New York: John Wiley & Sons, 1976.

Simon, Herbert A., *Administrative Behavior: A Study of Decision-Making Processes in Administrative Organization*, 3rd ed., New York: The Free Press, 1976.

Toward Plan Implementation: Analytic Techniques and Tactical Considerations

The preceding series of chapters has established the conceptual basis and defined the scope of health planning, described the essential content and presented relevant methodology, and raised a number of important strategic issues. In short, Part II was an exposition of the planning process.

We now turn to specific analytic techniques that have proved useful in carrying out that process. Whereas the relevance of demography and the role of demographic methods were discussed in Part II, we describe in Part III techniques for making population projections. To take another example, we have already reviewed the main principles of economic analysis from the planning perspective; we now present the techniques of cost-effectiveness analysis for choosing among program options.

Taking another perspective, the preceding discussions have had an essentially strategic orientation, whereas henceforth we focus on the tactics of plan implementation. To illustrate, having earlier considered the overall assessment of need for additional facilities of various types, we turn in Part III to specific techniques for scheduling construction, so that implementation proceeds within a realistic time frame.

The underlying theme in the chapters that follow is that planning does not end with the preparation of a plan. Because planning can be considered effective only if it leads to successful implementation, it must be a practical guide to managers. This means that elements of the plan should be readily translated into a realistic budget and set of feasible time-phased activities capable of achieving clearly defined objectives. Although Part III is not meant to be a compendium of management techniques as such, it is written more for those charged with implementation, in contrast to Part II, which was mainly directed to policymakers and planning strategists.

15

Tools for Improving the Process of Planning

WILLIAM A. REINKE

Planning techniques usually relate to specific aspects of the process of clarifying health needs and allocating resources to meet those needs. Thus, for the most part, the discussion of techniques in Part III parallels the topical structure of Part II. For example, methods for deriving estimates of current population distributions and future projections are described in Chapter 17 in accordance with demographic principles enunciated in Chapter 8. Similarly, specific procedures for the measurement of health problems (Chapter 18) build upon the epidemiologic base of Chapter 9.

Additionally, certain analytic procedures are broadly applicable to the entire planning process. For example, because planning at all stages is a group effort, methods for establishing group consensus are highly valued tools of planning. Further the measurable goals and priorities on which consensus has been achieved must be translated into similarly explicit actions for achieving them. Practical techniques for defining clearly and appraising objectively the relationships between actions and results, that is, between inputs and outputs, are also among the tools needed by planners. The logical framework for program development and evaluation is one such technique commonly employed. Finally, the actual carrying out of plans of action requires detailed attention to the scheduling of a host of interrelated activities. Knowledge of scheduling techniques is therefore crucial for operational planning. The present chapter covers these generic issues in planning.

PROCEDURES FOR OBTAINING GROUP CONSENSUS

Health planners play an important mediating role among health professionals, their associations, and service agencies; the public at large and community organizations; and public officials and government administrators. Planners must recognize mutuality of interests among groups, be sensitive to potential areas of conflict, and be adept at resolving differences. To illustrate, consider the assignment given by one state governor[1] to a health planning task force.

> I will instruct the Task Force to ascertain the health needs of our citizens and to design a comprehensive system which will provide the services health consumers require. The Task Force will work to develop realistic health and health service goals. I will also ask it to

compile a health plan, designate health priorities, recommend a legislative program and suggest any necessary administrative reorganization.

In order to fulfill this charge it was clearly necessary to obtain the constructive participation of a large and varied representation of the affected citizens of the state. In carrying out its assignment the task force benefited markedly from the use of the two group process techniques described later. Although their exposition is given in a more limited setting for purposes of clarity, it is helpful to bear in mind this broader, realistic framework in considering their value in practice.

Nominal Group Technique

Andre Delbecq[2] and his colleagues at the University of Wisconsin have developed a systematic five-phase group process model for problem identification and program planning. The elements encompassed by the model include (1) listing of specific problems to be attacked, (2) listing of possible approaches to solutions, (3) establishment of program priorities, (4) program development, and (5) program evaluation. Thus the model is comprehensive in scope and thereby involves a host of interested parties representing both the community with its defined needs and the providers of service programs addressed to these needs. It is to be expected that clients will find difficulty in listing, not to mention ranking, their principle problems; professionals will not be unanimous in their judgment regarding the appropriateness of alternative means of attacking these problems; and the two groups will have difficulty in establishing consequent priorities. Therefore Delbecq relies heavily upon the *nominal group technique* (NGT) for resolving these conflicts.

Silent Generation of Ideas

For our purposes the use of this technique is perhaps most appropriately illustrated with respect to the specification of alternative strategies (Phase 2). Suppose that a major problem that has been identified in a particular locale is the lack of convenient access to primary health care. A group of from six to nine persons with knowledge and understanding in these matters from several perspectives is convened to explore possible solutions. During an introductory period of approximately ten minutes the convener, serving as moderator, outlines the problem, explains the nominal group technique, and distributes to each participant a stack of three-by-five-inch cards. During the next fifteen to twenty minutes each group member independently considers specific actions that might be taken to alleviate the problem and writes each of the possibilities on a separate card.

Assembly of Ideas

After a short rest break the group comes together again and one member is asked to read one item from a card. This is transcribed by the moderator without discussion onto a flip chart, and the next person is asked to identify a different item from the list. After each group member has contributed an item, the first member is asked to present a second item, and the process continues until all items on all lists have been recorded on the flip chart. Typically a group of six people generates a total of twenty or more items of varying merit. Since no discussion has been allowed, the contribution of everyone is assured, in contrast to unstructured group discussions in which certain individuals would be reluctant to express themselves for fear that they would be put down by articulate colleagues.

Discussion for Clarification and Editing

After all items have been recorded, a thirty-minute structured interactive group discussion is held for purposes of clarification of meaning, rewording and combining of related items, and elimination of duplication.

Priority Setting

After this discussion participants independently review the final list of items and identify the five which they consider to be most important. They establish a score of five for the item they consider to have top priority, four for the second-priority item, and so on. After all members have made their own judgments, the votes are tallied to determine the items with the highest combined totals of votes. After this exercise the group discusses the results in order to be assured that they do indeed reflect group consensus.

The nominal group technique draws upon multiple sources of judgment and experience to the extent that varied insights can be beneficial, but it succeeds in avoiding interactive conflict that tends to be counterproductive. The net result, of course, can be no better than the composite knowledge and insight of the group members, so that group composition is an important consideration. Lay-persons, notably consumers, should dominate groups attempting to identify problems, whereas considerable technical expertise is important for solution-oriented groups.

Delphi Technique

The second approach to group decision making, the *Delphi technique*,[3] is useful in achieving consensus on the utility of a specified course of action and in assessing the likelihood that the action will produce the desired result. The technique permits the participation of large numbers of individuals and does not require the physical presence of all persons in one place. The technique, developed at the Rand Corporation, grew out of the recognition that knowledge is seldom absolute, but can be placed upon a continuum, with factual data at the one extreme and sheer speculation at the other. The vast area in between is represented by opinion, or experienced judgment. Consider, for example, the probability that a truly effective vaccine against malaria will be developed within the next five years. Conclusive factual information is obviously unavailable for making this assessment, but it is not entirely speculative either. Considerable knowledge concerning the present state of the art and what is yet needed to achieve a breakthrough exists. The required probability is therefore a matter of opinion based upon experienced judgment, although we must recognize that the level of knowledge varies among individuals, along with the way in which different individuals may process their knowledge to form opinions, that is, probability judgments. The question is, How can the opinions of several reasonably knowledgeable persons be appropriately combined to form the best composite judgment?

Initial Estimates

The Delphi technique, which has been developed and tested in response to this question, works as follows. Each of a group of individuals, say five for purposes of illustration, is asked to provide an independent numerical response to a question of concern. In the case of the malaria vaccine probability, for example, the group members may independently respond with estimates: .2, .7, .6, .9, .4. Each response is given to a moderator, taking care that no individual knows the judgment expressed by any colleague. The moderator notes the median response, .6 in this case, and reports this result to the entire group.

Repeated Revisions and Movement Toward Consensus

Now all participants have two pieces of information: their own initial judgment and the nonpersonalized average of the group. Taking both factors into consideration all individuals form a revised judgment and secretly report their response to the moderator. A new median is calculated, and the process is repeated for as many rounds as are necessary to achieve stability in the individual assessments. Seldom are more than three or four rounds required in practice.

Comparison with Nominal Group Technique

As in the case of the nominal group technique the Delphi technique takes advantage of multiple viewpoints while avoiding damaging interactions and the dominance of one or two intimidating or prestigious individuals. Experience has shown that the more truly knowledgeable individuals tend to follow their own convictions rather than the group average, so that the average tends to move toward their level, and consensus is thereby established in an automatic, impersonal way.

Although we have described two distinct approaches to the establishment of group consensus, they are sometimes applied in combination. The priority health problems in a specified region might be determined by the nominal group technique, for example; then a quantification of the relative importance of each, using the Delphi approach, could be achieved.

LOGICAL FRAMEWORK FOR PLANNING AND EVALUATION

Broad programs are often made up of several interrelated projects, each of which must be planned to contribute to the overall effort. While anticipated project results must conform with broader program goals, they must also be clearly related internally to the resources and activities necessary to achieve project intentions.

Moreover, if the hierarchic relationships among inputs, outputs, purposes, and goals are to be more than conceptual, concrete measures of progress must be established, along with an information base for providing the data necessary for project monitoring and evaluation.

The hierarchical relationships and the basis for quantification have been incorporated into a matrix known as the *logical framework*[4] shown in Figure 15.1. The hierarchic vertical logic of the framework clarifies why and how a project is to be undertaken. The horizontal informational logic depicts the evidence to be used to signal project success and to make explicit important assumptions, some of which may be so shaky that they deserve to be tested before the project starts. A project to immunize preschool children against measles is used to illustrate these features of the matrix.

Vertical Framework

The project purpose must first be placed within the context of broader organizational aims. The immunization project, for example, may be part of a maternal and child health effort designed to reduce mortality and morbidity among infants and preschool children. The direct purpose of the project itself might be the elimination of measles from the target community. Achievement of this result is presumably contingent upon the mobilization of certain resources to produce a targeted level of service coverage (assumption). Specifically, the output should be immunization of 80 percent of the target population of 10,000 preschool children. This level of coverage is expected to require inputs of two person-months of physician effort, five person-months of nurse time, and ten person-months of input from health auxiliaries. Other input requirements for vaccines, transport, and so on, should also be specified.

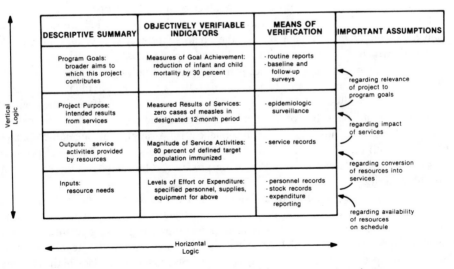

Figure 15.1   Logical framework for summarizing project design

Horizontal Framework

To make the preceding hierarchy of relationships operational, it is necessary to specify performance indicators that can be measured objectively so that performance can be reliably monitored. The matrix also indicates how the specified measures are to be obtained and verified. This ensures the practicability of the designated indicators and outlines the required system of data collection, including the need for special surveys. The matrix format requires that (frequently ignored) quality control procedures be incorporated explicitly into the data collection system.

Important Assumptions

The rationale behind the logical framework depends upon the validity of certain assumptions that underlie the linkages elaborated in the matrix. To further enhance the realism of the logical framework, the most important of these assumptions are recorded. Project objectives can thus be pursued with due caution, and in the event that expectations are not realized, the original assumptions can be examined.

In the course of project implementation some assumptions are inevitably invalidated, factors initially overlooked turn out to be severely constraining, certain planned inputs prove to be unattainable for well-documented reasons, and numerous other changes take place. The logical framework, therefore, cannot be an inflexible blueprint for action. Moreover, it must be supplemented by information systems that fully encompass the dynamics of monitoring and evaluation. Nevertheless, subject to appropriate modification as necessary, the logical framework can be a most useful tool for planning and evaluation.

SCHEDULING: NETWORK ANALYSIS

Any project of consequence invariably involves a multiplicity of discrete activities, each of which contributes in some way to overall project success. Failure to complete even a seemingly insignificant link in the chain of project events may produce a bottleneck which ultimately jeopardizes the entire project.

To cite a rather mundane example, many separate activities go into the preparation of a meal. These activities must be scheduled so that all of the individual components of the meal are ready when the guests are to be served. Some of the activities can be undertaken simultaneously; for example, the salad can be prepared while the meat is roasting. Other activities must occur in sequence; for example, the vegetables cannot be cooked until they have been washed, peeled, sliced, and so on. Failure to peel the potatoes on schedule can delay the cooking process, in turn delaying the serving of the entire meal.

The systematic scheduling of activities is at least as important in the conduct of a health project as it is in the preparation of a meal. Similarly, it is an essential element in the planning process. Adequate preparation for planning requires explicit specification of activities which must be undertaken to ensure the development of planning competence. Meaningful project formulation cannot take place in the absence of planning authorization and budget, competent planning staff, an adequate data base, and other components of the process. In any event, the large number of activities to be tracked requires their organization into a systematic framework.

Basic Considerations

Whatever the scheduling problem the program of interest can be divided into a series of discrete activities, each with a time requirement and a well-defined end point. For example, the development of a multiphasic screening program might include such activities as the installation of an x-ray unit and provision of a supply of Pap kits. The end point of such activities, called *events*, might be identified by such statements as "x-ray unit in place" and "Pap kits on hand." Another general feature of programs, as already noted, is that the individual activities are ordered to some extent. The installation of the x-ray unit cannot begin, for instance, until blueprints have been drawn up, specifying locations for the various pieces of equipment. These features of systematic scheduling are brought together in various techniques which come under the general heading of network analysis. Although specific techniques vary in purpose and sophistication, they all begin with a listing of relevant events, along with associated activity times and sequencing constraints.[5]

Network Construction—CPM

The general scheduling procedure is described with the aid of a hypothetical, over-simplified illustration. We suppose that a crisis has arisen which requires the construction, staffing, and outfitting of an emergency health center. Ideally, this is to be accomplished within a fifteen-day period.

The planning begins with the identification of individual jobs to be performed. Table 15.1 lists the associated events and arbitrarily assigns reference numbers to them. The order of listing is unimportant; events are simply noted as they come to mind until all requisite tasks have been enumerated. The expected time required to perform each of the tasks is also specified. Table 15.1 lists these times in days, but other time units can be used according to individual circumstances. Finally, considering the problem of sequencing, one must identify for each task the last job that must be completed before the one in question can start. For example, job number 5, which involves the laying of brick to form the exterior wall of the building, cannot begin until the basic framework, identified with job number 1, is in place.

Once the information of Table 15.1 is compiled, the network of Figure 15.2 can be diagramed to display graphically the required sequence of events and time commitments. The network analysis can then proceed either from the diagram itself or, in more complicated cases, from a computerized analog of the network.

Critical Path

The first point to note from the diagram is that there are many paths leading from start to finish of the project. Presumably one of these requires more time to traverse than any of the others, and thus is of special concern. In the present illustration this so-called critical path is the sequence 0–1–6–14 and is denoted by a double line. Only by finding ways to shorten jobs along the critical path can the overall project time be

Table 15.1

HYPOTHETICAL EMERGENCY HEALTH CENTER ACTIVATION PROBLEM

Event Number	Event Description	Estimated Time (Days)	Predecessor Event
0	Start	-	-
1	Building framework in place	4	0
2	Electrical wiring installed	2	1
3	Plumbing installed	3	0
4	Cement floor ready for use	2	3
5	Brick outer wall completed	6	1
6	Inside walls plastered and dry	10	1
7	Roof installed	2	1
8	Drug list authorized	4	0
9	Drugs ordered	1	8
10	Drugs received	7	9
11	Personnel authorized	2	0
12	Personnel recruited	3	11
13	Personnel trained	5	12
14	Health center finished	2	2, 4, 5, 6, 7, 10, 13

reduced. In our case the estimated time required to traverse this path is sixteen days, one more than the number tentatively allotted to the project.

Slack Time

Each path other than the critical one has *slack time*, which is the difference between the critical path time and that associated with the particular path of interest. As an example, the estimated time required for path 0–11–12–13–14 is twelve days, indicating that this path has four days slack time.

Such calculations are useful for two reasons. In the first place the noncritical path with the least slack time gives evidence of the maximum reduction in total project time that can accrue from modifications on the critical path. Suppose, for example, that the project director in our illustration, recognizing job number 6 to be critical, decides to consider the use of a more costly, prefabricated substitute for plaster. If this substitution reduces job number 6 time from ten days to six, the time of the

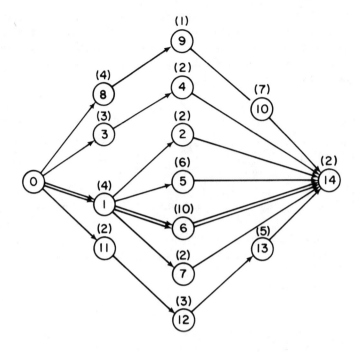

PATH	TIME	SLACK
0-8-9-10-14	14	2
0-3-4-14	7	9
0-1-2-14	8	8
0-1-5-14	12	4
0-1-6-14	16	0
0-1-7-14	8	8
0-11-12-13-14	12	4

KEY

(6) TIME (DAYS)

(5) EVENT NUMBER

Figure 15.2   Activity network based upon Table 15.1

formerly critical path is reduced by four days, but the total project time is reduced by only two days. This is because path 0–8–9–10–14 will become critical, so that the only saving in project time will be the two days of slack formerly associated with this path.

The second use of slack time is to provide flexibility in the conduct of the project. Consider, for instance, the fact that path 0–11–12–13–14 has two days more slack than path 0–8–9–10–14. Both paths entail administrative action in the form of personnel authorization in the one case and drug authorization in the other. Recognizing the difference in urgency between these two administrative tasks, the project officer might choose to take early, perhaps costly, action to expedite the drug authorization, even at the expense of a slight increase in personnel authorization time. In order to visualize opportunities in this direction better, the project officer will probably compile a list of late start and late finish times for each job. These will indicate the maximum delay that can be tolerated in the initiation or completion of any activity without affecting the total project time. Recognizing, for example, that conditions on the critical path make it impossible to initiate job number 14 before day 15 without special action, we observe that accomplishment of job 4 can be postponed until days 13 and 14 without causing project delay.

Gantt Charts

Network analysis as diagramed in Figure 15.2 is a relatively recent innovation. However, it is an outgrowth of Gantt charting procedures long employed in the industrial engineering field. In fact, Gantt charts can be used operationally in conjunction with network analysis in the actual scheduling of project activities. This is shown in Figure 15.3, which assumes that the activities of Figure 15.2 are to be scheduled during the period April 1 through 16. Again using job number 4 for purposes of illustration, the chart tentatively schedules this activity for April 4 to 5 but indicates (by dotted lines) that completion could be delayed until April 14 without adverse repercussions.

PERT

The approach to network analysis described previously is called the *critical path method* (CPM), which is among the earliest and simplest forms. Perhaps the most important factor which it fails to recognize is the possibility of error in the time estimates. The *program evaluation and review technique* (PERT) is the best known

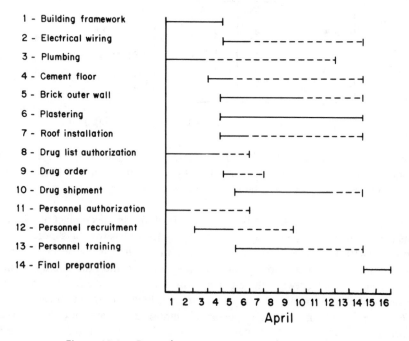

Figure 15.3   Gantt chart representation of Figure 15.2

approach that includes the error feature.[6] In PERT applications, the estimator provides not only an expected time requirement for each activity but "most pessimistic" and "most optimistic" estimates as well. The calculated required time is then a weighted average in which the best estimate is given four times as much weight as either of the other two. The range of possible error incorporated into the estimates is further used to calculate such probabilistic aspects as the likelihood of completion by the target date and most probable completion date.

Further Refinements

PERT/COST adds the consideration of resource costs to the activity schedule produced by the PERT procedure. As we have seen in our simple illustration of plastering, time can often be purchased at a price. Thus PERT/COST determines the most inexpensive way to meet a specified project deadline. It also relates project progress to budget expenditures. To illustrate, suppose that a two-year project has expended only one-third of its total budget during the first year of operation. On the face of it, financial control appears adequate. However if delays have caused only one-fourth of total project to be completed during the first year, the project is actually in financial, as well as scheduling, difficulty.

While CPM or PERT in principle permits certain activities to be scheduled simultaneously, this may become impossible in practice if the same personnel are required to perform multiple tasks. A more refined PERT/MANPOWER analysis includes constraints on personnel availability as well as activity sequencing constraints, thereby highlighting the importance of worker allocation and utilization.

In view of the fact that a plan usually includes several projects, a technique known as *resource allocation and multiproject scheduling* (RAMPS) has been developed.[7] Finally, for cases in which results can be achieved in a variety of ways, the alternative sets of activities can be analyzed by means of *decision CPM*.[8]

Greater sophistication in approach may produce more meaningful results, but it also requires more and better information and greater analytical effort. Even in its simplest form, however, network analysis is useful in providing a framework for the orderly consideration of complex problems. It is not enough to produce an initial schedule of activities, though. That schedule must be constantly monitored to identify impending bottlenecks and to adjust project targets as necessary.

REFERENCES

1. Lucey, Patrick, address delivered May 18, 1971.
2. Delbecq, Andre L., and Andrew H. Van de Ven, "A Group Process Model for Problem Indentification and Program Planning," *The Journal of Applied Behavioral Science*, 7, 4:466–492, 1971.
3. Dalkey, Norman C., *The Delphi Method: An Experimental Study of Group Opinion*, Memorandum RM-5888-PR, Santa Monica, CA: Rand Corporation, 1969.
4. Office of Program Evaluation, *Evaluation Handbook*, 2nd ed., Washington: Agency for International Development, 1974.
5. Levy, F. K., G. L. Thompson and J. D. Wiest, "The ABCs of the Critical Path Method," *Harvard Business Review*, 41:98–108, 1963.

6. Merton, W., "PERT and Planning for Health Programs," *Public Health Reports*, 81:449–454, 1966.

7. Lambourn, S., "Resource Allocation and Multiproject Scheduling (RAMPS): A New Tool in Planning and Control," *The Computer Journal*, 5:300–304, 1963.

8. Crowston, W., and G. L. Thompson, "Decision CPM: A Method for Simultaneous Planning, Scheduling and Control of Projects," *Operations Research*, 15:407–426, 1967.

PRIMARY READINGS

Department of Industrial Engineering, *Delphi Summary: Health Planning Barriers*, Madison: University of Wisconsin, 1973. A report on applications of the Delphi technique to health planning.

Fink, Arlene, et al. "Consensus Methods: Characteristics and Guidelines for Use," *American Journal of Public Health*, 74, 9:979–983, 1984. Reviews and provides guidelines for the use of Delphi, nominal group, and other consensus techniques.

Levy, F. K., G. L. Thompson and J. D. Wiest, "The ABCs of the Critical Path Method," *Harvard Business Review*, 41:98–108, 1963. A very readable description of the essentials of network analysis.

Merton, W., "PERT and Planning for Health Programs," *Public Health Reports*, 81:449–454, 1966. Presents a somewhat more sophisticated, but very practical, approach to activities scheduling.

Office of Program Evaluation, *Evaluation Handbook*, 2nd ed., Washington: Agency for International Development, 1974. A general review of evaluation that includes a description of the logical framework.

SECONDARY READINGS

Dalkey, Norman C., *The Delphi Method: An Experimental Study of Group Opinion*, Memorandum RM-5888-PR, Santa Monica, CA: Rand Corporation, 1969.

Delbecq, Andre L., and Andrew H. Van de Ven, "A Group Process Model for Problem Indentification and Program Planning," *The Journal of Applied Behavioral Science*, 7, 4:466–492, 1971.

16

Sample Surveys

WILLIAM A. REINKE

Perhaps the fondest dream of the planner is to have ready access to a data base that accurately documents all current conditions of interest and places them within the context of important time trends. The reality is, however, that certain critical information is invariably out of date, inaccurate, incomplete, or lacking altogether. As a result the sample survey can be an invaluable planning tool, but it can also be costly and time-consuming. The planner must know enough about the principles of sampling to use them effectively.

Indeed, carefully controlled sampling can produce more accurate results than complete enumerations that suffer from underreporting, inability to obtain data of uniformly high quality from a vast army of data gatherers, and errors, as well as delays, in processing masses of data. In principle complete enumerations can achieve absolute precision, whereas samples inevitably risk the possibility of being less than perfect representations of the universe sampled. In practice, however, the potential precision of censuses is seldom attained and the imprecision associated with sampling is measurable and controllable.

THE STANDARD ERROR AS A MEASURE OF IMPRECISION

Suppose that interest centers on the prevalence (p) of a particular condition, for example, hearing impairment, in a defined population. A random sample of size n will yield a more or less precise estimate of p. The degree of imprecision is measured by the standard error (SEp), which is defined as

$$SE_P = \sqrt{\frac{p(1 - p)}{n}}$$

Thus, a sample of 100 taken from a population with prevalence 20 percent gives a result with standard error

$$SE_P = \sqrt{\frac{(.2)(.8)}{100}}$$
$$= .4.$$

According to probability theory, amply demonstrated in practice, there are roughly two chances in three that sample findings will be within one standard error of the true population prevalence. Of more practical importance, sample results are nearly always (95 times in 100) within two standard errors of the true population prevalence.[1] If the prevalence of hearing impairment is, indeed, 20 percent, a random sample of 100 individuals is quite likely (2 chances in 3) to identify from 16 to 24 with hearing impairment. The sample will almost certainly (95 chances in 100) contain between 12 and 28 hearing-impaired persons ($20 \pm 2 \times 4$ percent).

In practice, of course, the true prevalence is not known, but the preceding reasoning is still applicable. For example, what if a random sample of 100 persons yielded 18 with hearing impairment? It is extremely doubtful that this finding is in error by more than 8 percent, and most likely the error is considerably smaller. Therefore, the population prevalence can be conservatively estimated at 18 ± 8 percent, that is, between 10 and 26 percent.

The calculation of sampling error is made somewhat more complex when variables are measured on a continuous scale, not simply classified according to the presence or absence of a condition. Suppose, for example, that hearing loss were measured on a scale from 0 to 100. If loss in excess of 30 were considered impairment and persons were classified only according to whether they scored above or below 30, we would be dealing with the prevalence situation previously described. Often, however, the average is of greater interest for planning. For example, the average number of antenatal cases among a sample of health centers could be useful in estimating the total volume of antenatal care being provided.

The standard error of an average is a function of the variation among individuals included in the average. If substantial variation exists, then selection of a few exceptional individuals in the sample would affect the sample mean $(\bar{x})$ markedly, causing imprecision. In particular, variation among individual measurements (x) is depicted by the standard deviation (s), where

$$s = \sqrt{\frac{\Sigma (x - \bar{x})^2}{n - 1}}.$$

The standard error $(SE_{\bar{x}})$ is, in turn

$$SE_{\bar{x}} = \frac{s}{\sqrt{n}}.$$

If hearing loss in a sample of 100 individuals averages 25 and has a standard deviation of 15, then

$$SE_{\bar{x}} = \frac{15}{\sqrt{100}}$$
$$= 1.5.$$

Hence the sample mean of 25 is most likely within ± 3 (2×1.5) of the population mean.

Regardless of which standard error formula is applicable, SE_p or $SE_{\bar{x}}$, the extent of imprecision can be reduced to any level desired by appropriate increase in the denominator, that is, increase in sample size. There is a rapidly diminishing benefit from increased sampling, however. In the preceding prevalence example we saw that a sample of 100 would produce an estimate accurate within ±8 percent. The next 100 observations, that is, $n = 200$, would reduce the level of imprecision to ± 5.7 percent (a 2.3 percent reduction), the third 100 observations would bring it down to ±4.6 percent (a further 1.1 percent reduction), and so on. To double the level of precision from ±8 to ±4 percent requires a quadrupling of the sample size from 100 to 400. Then a further halving of the sampling error to ±2 percent would again require a quadrupling of the sample size to 1,600. It is important to make explicit in advance the level of accuracy that is acceptable for planning purposes, for a relatively small sample can usually produce satisfactory results in a fraction of the time and at a fraction of the cost of complete enumeration.

METHODS AND TIMING OF DATA COLLECTION

The universe to be sampled may consist of persons (e.g., all residents of a defined district) or of inanimate objects (e.g., all of the country's general hospitals with 200 beds or fewer). Records of individuals (e.g., records of all patients admitted to Hospital X in March 1983) can also define a universe, recognizing that the records contain limited information, perhaps of questionable validity, about individuals not likely to be representative of the larger community from which they were drawn. In any event, unambiguous, prior definition of the universe of interest is essential in order that an adequately representative sample may be identified for data gathering.

Types of Survey Instruments

Once sample respondents have been identified, the required information about them can be obtained from a review of existing records, direct questioning, observation, or physical examination. The direct questioning approach is the most common and is accomplished verbally through interview or in writing via questionnaire. Since all approaches have been used successfully and none is without certain disadvantages, a brief commentary on the pros and cons of each is in order.

Records review is relatively quick, inexpensive, and unobtrusive. If the purpose of the survey is not the same as that which motivated the compilation of records in the first place, however, the information may be misleading in unknown ways. For example, client reports on cost of seeking care may be of little value unless it had been made clear in advance whether interest was limited to expenditures on direct services or whether costs for transportation and child care were to be included. Moreover, recording errors made some time earlier at the time of recording may now be hidden or impossible to trace.

Questionnaires can provide an inexpensive means of securing broad geographical coverage in a survey, provided that literacy can be assumed and that an effective postal service or other means of questionnaire dissemination exists. Even when the assumptions hold, problems of nonresponse can be serious.

Interviews guarantee, or at least maximize, the likelihood of response and, in addition, permit face-to-face clarification of misunderstanding of the intent of questions being asked. On the other hand, the personal contact may inhibit honesty and objectivity in response. This approach requires well-trained interviewers capable of producing reproducible responses. Health professionals tend to make poor interviewers in morbidity surveys, for example, because they tend to apply their own diagnostic interpretations, rather than simply accepting respondents' accounts of reported illness.

Medical examinations can go to the heart of biologic need for health care, identifying asymptomatic conditions, but examinations are extremely costly and time-consuming and cannot hope to cover more than a small portion of those reached in a household interview survey. The use of morbidity information in planning is also at issue. A strong case can be made for the overwhelming importance of client perceptions of illness in triggering the demand for medical care. Since such perceptions are most readily identified through a household survey, the value of this approach for planning purposes is evident, quite apart from cost considerations.

Observation is an attractive means of identifying actual behavior. Is it better to observe how workers actually spend their time or to ask them what their perceptions are? Is it better to observe mothers' feeding practices or to ask them to report them? The answers clearly favor the observational approach provided that the respondent maintains "typical" patterns of behavior while being observed. Behavior modification is a genuine concern, but work sampling procedures adapted from the industrial engineering field can minimize the risk.

The recording of activity in a *diary* or *log* is an alternative to observation. Instead of engaging a nonparticipant observer in the time-consuming task of observing and recording, the respondent does the recording as part of a daily routine. There is the danger, of course, that the respondent will not give the same undivided attention to completeness and accuracy of recording as an observer would. On the other hand, if the respondent does take the recording seriously, the recording activity itself is likely to distort normal behavior patterns, thereby invalidating the record.

Survey Timing

Associated with the question of how to gather information is the matter of when to obtain it: at a point in time or over a period of time.

Cross-sectional studies are conducted at a point in time and are used to characterize a population in certain respects at that time. For example, cross-sectional surveys would be appropriate for determining the prevalence of specified morbid conditions or for depicting current patterns of health services utilization.

Longitudinal studies, in contrast, employ procedures for repeated sampling of a population in order to assess changes over time. A group of toddlers, for example, might be measured periodically after introduction of a nutrition intervention program in order to evaluate gains in height and weight.

Longitudinal designs can be cohort studies or panel studies. In either case a specified population is sampled repeatedly. In the *cohort* approach a new sample of individuals is selected randomly for each set of measurements. The *panel* approach selects a sample initially and follows the same individuals over time. Cohort studies of given age groups are commonly used by demographers.

While panel studies are highly sophisticated, allowing maximum explanation of change over time, they are expensive and time-consuming and can produce serious problems of nonresponse through attrition. They also require complex statistical analysis. In order to avoid these problems and still capture many of the benefits of panel studies, surveyors frequently attempt in a single respondent contact to reconstruct retrospectively the history of interest, for example, through a pregnancy history. Obviously one must be alert to the danger of faulty recall in employing this approach.

CONSIDERATIONS OF SAMPLE SIZE

Having established the items of information needed, how they will be obtained, and within what time frame, the question of magnitude of information, that is, sample size, comes into focus. This returns us to consideration of the formulas for sampling error.

Based on Tolerable Level of Imprecision

Recall, in the case of discrete data,

$$SE_P = \sqrt{\frac{p(1-p)}{n}}.$$

We observed, further, that seldom does sampling error exceed two standard errors, and, of course,

$$2SE_p = 2\sqrt{\frac{p(1-p)}{n}}.$$

In particular, we found that with $p = .2$ and $n = 100$, sample estimates are likely to be in error by no more than ± 8 percent, meaning that

$$2SE_p = .8.$$

Rather than accept the level of precision dictated by a fixed sample size, the planner would prefer to specify a tolerable level, L, of imprecision, and let the sample size be determined accordingly. In effect, the relationship

$$L = 2SE_p = 2\sqrt{\frac{p(1-p)}{n}}$$

is to be restated with n as the unknown. This yields

$$n = \frac{4p(1-p)}{L^2}.$$

In the illustrative case suppose that an estimate within ± 8 percent is unsatisfactory, but precision of ± 5 percent is acceptable. Then

$$n = \frac{(4)(.2)(.8)}{(.5)^2}$$
$$= 256.$$

Determination of L in a specific situation is a matter of judgment by the planner. The value of p, on the other hand, is beyond the planner's control and is not known prior to the conduct of the survey. Realistically, moreover, surveys elicit several items of information, so that several values of p and associated levels of precision are of interest.

The derivation of sample size ultimately depends upon the limiting case; that is, the sample must be large enough to accommodate that variable which demands greatest precision. In this connection we observe that the quantity $p(1 - p)$ is largest when $p = .5$. Thus a sample size large enough to gain the required precision when prevalence is 50 percent yields even greater precision when p is anything other than .5. With p unknown, therefore, the most conservative approach is to assume it is .5, in which case

$$n = \frac{1}{L^2}.$$

This becomes a useful rule of thumb for sample size, based solely on the maximum tolerable error in estimation.

Stratification

It is important to recognize that the size of the universe is of no consequence in the preceding formula for sample size determination. The common practice of sampling a fixed percentage of the population, therefore, has no rational basis. A 10 percent sampling of a large population may be unnecessarily costly, whereas a 10 percent sampling of a small population could be inadequate. The absolute size of the sample is the important factor.

Sample size determination is applicable to each population group subject to analysis. If health care–seeking behaviors of females in and out of the work force were to be examined separately, for example, an adequate sampling of each group must be assured. Because "adequate" is expressed in absolute, rather than percentage, terms, a simple random sample of an entire population may give inadequate representation to a rare component of interest. In the present case, for instance, suppose that only 10 percent of women are in the work force, yet for purposes of analysis equal samples of three hundred are needed from both participants and nonparticipants in the work force. A simple random sample of six hundred would yield only about sixty work force participants and would provide an excess of nonparticipants. In order to achieve appropriate representation of each population component of interest, subgrouping or stratification procedures are employed. In the present example the universe of employed women would somehow be identified separately from all others and independent random samples would be selected from each group.

Multistage Cluster Sampling

The selection of a genuinely representative sample from a large, geographically dispersed population is seemingly difficult. If five hundred households are to be selected from an entire province of ten million population, for example, it is clearly infeasible to construct a list of all households in the province and then to select a simple random sample from the list. Equally absurd would be the administrative nightmare experienced in trying to reach all of the scattered individual households selected in the sample. Yet it is important that sufficiently varied district, subdistrict, and village conditions be represented in the sample, along with household variability.

Such circumstances suggest the use of a sequential approach. First, all districts are listed and a specified number are selected at random. Subdistricts are then listed only in the districts selected, and a second stage of random selection takes place. Similarly, a third-stage selection of villages is undertaken. Only in those villages selected for sampling is it necessary to follow the laborious mapping procedures necessary for the random selection and contact of households. To further ease the burden of sampling, households are sometimes selected in clusters. When one household is selected at random, for example, it might be understood that two adjacent households are also to be included. Under some circumstances clustering of villages might be appropriate. Guidance of a survey statistician is advised when setting up a complex multistage sampling procedure, but with such guidance the advantages of purely chance selection can be achieved feasibly at modest cost.

The decision on how many districts, subdistricts, and villages to select at each stage of the process can be rather tricky. Referring to the formulas for standard errors, we recall, first, that sampling error is a function of individual variation, noted in the numerator of the formula. The surveyor then seeks to make n in the denominator large enough to effectively iron out this individual variability in the averaging process.

The presence of several sources of variability at district, subdistrict, village, and household levels complicates the procedure but does not alter the principle involved. If differences between districts are large, for example, confining the sample to a single district would cause sampling error to be large, regardless of the number of households chosen because the n in relation to district variability is only one. On the other hand if the magnitude of variation between districts is no greater than that observed between adjacent households, then sampling might as well be confined to a single village for reasons of economy. The choice of multistage sampling procedure in a specific case thus involves a trade-off between statistical efficiency and administrative simplicity.

Sampling Unit Versus Unit of Analysis

The presence of multiple layers of variation must be considered at the time of analysis as well as in sample selection. To illustrate, morbidity surveys are obviously designed to investigate differences among individuals. Yet the household is usually the unit sampled, and then information is collected on all household members. During analysis individual morbidity experience is likely to be related to household characteristics, such as family income, or to village variables, such as proximity to an urban center or to a government health facility. The household characteristics of large families and the village features of heavily represented villages therefore tend to dominate the analysis.

The statistical implications are beyond the scope of present discussion. Two points of concern in survey design and analysis are worth highlighting, however. First, basic plans for analysis should already be formulated at the time the survey is being designed in order that sampling units may be as compatible with units of analysis as possible.

Second, even though the sample size may be considered large for most purposes of analysis, one must be alert to the presence of important factors, for example, village features, whose variability is not represented to the extent suggested by the overall sample size.

SURVEYS FOR COMPARATIVE ANALYSIS

Two Sources of Error

The sample-size formula developed previously has important, but rather restricted, uses. It defines the quantity of information needed to estimate current conditions in one population at levels of precision deemed adequate to make reasonable plans for the future. Frequently, however, surveys are conducted in order to compare two or more sets of conditions as a basis for choice among future alternatives. To illustrate, consider an investigation of DPT immunization protection achieved in two sets of communities, one with a particular prepaid insurance scheme and one without. The statistical question is whether there is a significant association between a specific preventive activity and the system of care and payment. Sample surveys of the two types of communities would serve to answer the question.

Either one of the areas could be surveyed with a designated level of precision, applying the sample-size formula

$$n = \frac{4p(1 - p)}{L^2}.$$

The issue now is not the precision of each estimate, however, but rather the magnitude of difference between them. In calculating the difference between two imprecise estimates the two errors are compounded. Thus, for example, if one sample produces an estimated coverage of 60 ± 10 percent and the other sample gives an estimate of 40 ± 10 percent, then the estimated difference between the two populations is 20 percent and the possible error in this estimate is something more than ± 10 percent. In short, because the difference of interest has two sources of error, the preceding formula applicable to each source separately is inadequate.

Two Possible Types of Error

Two kinds of analytical risk must also be taken into consideration. First, the sampling procedure may produce apparent differences between the two populations that are, in fact, only due to sampling error. Such an erroneous judgment is known as *Type I*, or *false-positive*, *error*. On the other hand, sample differences may, by chance, be so small that genuine population differences remain undetected. The result is *Type II*, or *false-negative*, *error*.

The risk of Type II error is associated with the magnitude of real population difference. A small difference, say 1 percent, would have a high risk of going undetected. If results in the insured and uninsured communities differed by as much as 30 percent, however, one would expect the risk of failing to detect a significant difference would be low. In practice one must specify the minimum magnitude of difference *(D)* that is of practical significance and then must choose a sample size large enough to limit the risk of Type II error under such conditions to a tolerable level. Suppose, in the present illustration, the planner determined that if the insurance scheme produced immunization levels at least 10 percent higher on the average than those found in noninsured communities, then this factor definitely should be recognized in future planning. In effect, the planner has specified that *D* is .1 and *n* should be established accordingly.

Our discussion of risk leads to the need to specify three factors: (1) the tolerable risk of Type I error, (2) the value of *D* to be used, and (3) the tolerable risk of Type II error associated with *D*. The first risk is conventionally taken to be 5 percent. Let us assume that a 5 percent risk of Type II error can be similarly tolerated. Then we can derive a simple sample-size formula based upon *D* analogous to that obtained earlier for *L*:

$$n = \frac{6.5}{D^2}.$$

The calculated value of *n* is applicable to *each* of the two groups sampled.

Recalling the earlier formula,

$$n = \frac{1}{L^2},$$

we note that estimates of immunization level in either set of communities, accurate to within ±10 percent, can be obtained with a sample of 100. If we wish to compare the two groups and seek assurance that a real difference as large as 10 percent is detected, then a sample of 650 must be taken from each group, 1,300 in all.

In the present chapter we have barely touched upon the many features of survey methodology; yet the importance of statistical considerations has become apparent. In more realistically complex circumstances the counsel of a survey statistician is essential. Nevertheless the importance of survey information for planning dictates that every planner have a firm grasp on the statistical concepts and principles elucidated here.

REFERENCES

1. Snedecor, George, and William Cochrane, *Statistical Methods*, 7th ed., Ames: Iowa State University Press, 1980.

PRIMARY READINGS

Cartwright, Ann, *Health Surveys in Practice and in Potential: A Critical Review of Their Scope and Methods*, London: Oxford University Press, 1983. Provides a detailed and wide-ranging review of methodology and subject matter for application of survey procedures.

Kish, Leslie, *Survey Sampling*, New York: John Wiley & Sons, 1965. A complete technical presentation of survey methods.

Ross, David, and J. Patrick Vaughan, *Health Interview Surveys in Developing Countries*, London: Evaluation and Planning Centre, London School of Hygiene and Tropical Medicine, 1984. Concise presentation of one of the most useful forms of health survey.

SECONDARY READINGS

Daza, C. H., and M. S. Read, "Health Related Components of a Nutritional Surveillance System," *Bulletin of the Pan American Health Organization*, 14,4:327–336, 1980.

Ghana Health Assessment Project Team, "A Quantitative Method of Assessing the Health Impact of Different Diseases in Less Developed Countries," *International Journal of Epidemiology*, 10,1:73–80, 1981.

Griffiths, M., *Growth Monitoring of Preschool Children: Practical Considerations for Primary Health Care*, Primary Health Care Issues Paper No. 3, Washington: American Public Health Association, 1981.

Improving Social Statistics in Developing Countries: Conceptual Framework and Methods, U.N. Statistical Office, New York: United Nations, 1979.

17

Population Estimates
and Projections

WILLIAM A. REINKE

Health planning seeks to direct services according to the distribution of need among members of the target population. In order to accomplish this, planners must be able to make reasonable estimates of the current population size, composition, and characteristics, along with anticipated trends. Although planners are not expected to be professional demographers, they should be able to apply certain fundamental demographic techniques to population data, and they should be sufficiently knowledgeable of demographic concepts to be able to utilize demographers effectively.

PREPARING FORECASTS

Population data tend to be among the more accurate sets of information available to health planners. We usually know more about population denominators than about health status numerators that provide the basis for calculating morbidity, mortality, fertility, and services utilization rates. Regardless of the accuracy of our knowledge of current conditions, however, future projections are inevitably subject to uncertainty and imprecision. Moreover, highly detailed projections are not only technically complex; they are especially subject to error. Armed with the information that the most recent census identified 5,260,000 residents in the subject population, which has been growing steadily at a rate of 2 percent annually, we have a solid basis for projecting the population over the next ten years. It is quite another matter, however, to judge what proportion of the total will be made up of employed, married female secondary school graduates residing in urban areas.

Level of Detail Required

The principle underlying the discussion of this chapter is that population projections should be no more detailed than is truly necessary for planning purposes. In particular, disaggregated projections are needed only to the extent that: (1) population composition is expected to change, and (2) service needs or demands differ by population subgroup. The point is of sufficient importance to merit careful illustration.

Suppose that a defined population of one thousand made five thousand out-patient visits, or five per capita, during the most recent year. If the population is expected to increase by 50 percent over the next ten years and there is no reason to question the existing rate of use of out-patient services, the first approximation plan would presumably aim to accommodate 50 percent more visits, that is, seventy-five hundred in all.

Individuals in the population differ in a number of ways, by education attainment, for example. If health services use is unrelated to education, that is, each educational category has an average of five visits per capita, then the planner can disregard both current educational status and changing patterns.

Consider the more likely circumstances of Table 17.1, however, in which services use increases with education. Then the planner must examine educational trends. Case A in the table depicts the situation in which the proportional change in all subgroup sizes is expected to be the same (50 percent in the present case). Thus, the highly educated currently account for one-fifth of the total, and under Case A they will continue to constitute 20 percent of the larger total after ten years. Case B, in contrast, shows the highly educated growing more rapidly in numbers than other groups, so that after ten years they are expected to represent one-third of the total.

In Case A the different rates of services use among educational groups have no effect on future per capita use. Current per capita use is a weighted average of use rates in the three educational groups. Because of the anticipated uniformity in population growth by educational category, the weighting factors are not expected to change and the values of the individual components to be weighted, that is, use rates, are therefore immaterial.

In Case B, however, the disproportionate growth in size of the highly educated class means that this group will exert a greater future influence on overall per capita service use. It is important to know this group's per capita use rate that is to be given greater future weight in order that the new overall per capita rate can be determined. Only under Case B conditions is it necessary to project the population by educational attainment, for only in that case is the population composition changing with respect to a factor that correlates with services use.

Table 17.1

ILLUSTRATION OF EDUCATION EFFECT ON SERVICES USE

Education	Current Pop.	Current Services	Per Capita	Case A Pop.	Case A Services	Case B Pop.	Case B Services
Low	500	1,800	3.6	750	2,700	550	1,980
Moderate	300	1,800	6.0	450	2,700	450	2,700
High	200	1,400	7.0	300	2,100	500	3,500
Total	1,000	5,000		1,500	7,500	1,500	8,180
Per Capita			5.0		5.0		5.45

Consider a second factor, residence location. If services use rates for urban and rural residents differ and the proportion of the population that is urban is changing, then separate urban/rural population breakdowns are necessary.

If Case B also prevails with respect to education, does this mean that the urban/rural breakdown must be further disaggregated by educational attainment? Only if the two factors interact. If urban residents average, say, one more visit per year per capita than rural residents, regardless of education, then the two factors can be considered independently and separate population projections can be made by education and by residence (provided they both yield the same total). If, however, urban/rural differences in services use vary by education, then a combined population breakdown by education and residence is needed. A numeric example of this type of interaction analysis is given later in the chapter.

Obtaining Baseline Estimates and Trend Information

Censuses, vital registration systems, surveys, national social insurance records, or other specialized data sources may be used singly, or in combination, for obtaining estimates of current population conditions as baselines for judging anticipated growth or decline.[1]

When the same information is available, directly or indirectly, from two sources, it is generally advisable to use both sources for purposes of confirmation and thereby to gain greater confidence in the estimates. To illustrate, population distributions by age from two consecutive censuses give evidence of population change through birth and death during the interval between censuses. The evidence should be compatible with data available from the routine vital registration system or from special surveys. The several sources are not expected to yield identical results, of course, since errors are undoubtedly present in each. If findings are similar, however, composite indicators can be derived that should be superior in quality to each of the individual estimates.

Data sources can be complementary as well as redundant. Underenumeration, for example, is a problem that plagues all national censuses. Unfortunately, the magnitude of underenumeration usually differs by ethnic groups, age, residence location, or other characteristics. Other data bases such as employment or school enrollment statistics, social insurance records, or special surveys may provide clues regarding the true proportional distribution of certain population subgroups and therefore permit appropriate adjustment factors to be applied to the census data.

Because of the central role of forecasting in planning, estimates of population changes are at least as important as estimates of current conditions. Although reference is frequently made to *population projections*, the term *forecasts* is used here advisedly. Projections connote extrapolation from past trends; forecasts interpret past trends critically and make adjustments, often qualitative, as necessary. Recent changes in national policy regarding health insurance, for example, undoubtedly disrupt services utilization patterns in ways that are not yet clearly discernible. Nevertheless the planner must make forecasts, combining qualitative judgment with whatever quantitative data remain relevant. Regardless of terms employed, the planner should be aware of existing trends and patterns and should in addition be prepared to judge their future relevance.

The three major demographic components of change—births, deaths, and migration—are influenced by different forces and are frequently investigated separately. Urbanization and population movement between geographical regions often represent the largest component of change, yet the least predictable because of the shifting dynamics referred to previously. For this reason the planner may have to look beyond past migration trends to an appraisal of the likely impact of government multisector development policy, plans for the development of roads and other infrastructure, and private sector strategies of significance.

Planners sometimes work directly from crude birth and death rates, estimating population growth simply as the difference between the two rates. This is sometimes acceptable, especially at the national level, where net migration is likely to be near zero. Even in the absence of migration, however, changes in population composition that require more detailed examination of vital events by age may be occurring. On the basis of birth and child mortality rates twenty years ago, a large cohort of females may now be entering the age of high fertility and causing the crude birth rate to rise without any change in age-specific fertility rates. Thus it becomes necessary to determine the number and age distribution of young females, move them conceptually through various age brackets over time, and apply appropriate fertility rates to those in each age group at each point in time.

Similarly, the age distribution of the population, coupled with mortality rates applicable at each age, dictates the overall death rate. Equally as important, the age distribution of survivors determines the quantities of specific age-related services needed in, for example, school health or geriatric care. Along with current population estimates by age, planners need to employ life tables that depict survival rates for each age group. They can then develop a model that moves survivors through successive age groups over time and thereby determine the age composition of the population to be anticipated at a designated point in the future for which services are being planned.

Factors other than age and sex are usually of interest for planning. This condition can lead the health planner to a variety of agencies and data sources other than demographic institutes or government statistical bureaus. Departments of education usually maintain detailed information about school-age children, including numbers entering, remaining in school, and leaving at each educational level. Analyses of industrial, commercial, agricultural, and overall economic growth are made by a number of government, international, and private agencies. The health planner needs to examine and compare the various economic reports and to make judgments concerning the realism of each.

Overall Annual Growth Rates Compounded

We now turn to a series of specific techniques of increasing complexity for estimating the future size and/or composition of specified populations. The simplest approach, of course, is to project the impact of a constant annual growth rate over a period of years. The impact is compounded year by year. Thus a population of 1,000 that is growing by 10 percent annually will have 1,100 inhabitants at the end of the first year, 110 percent of 1,100, or 1,210 at the end of the second year, and so on until the tenth year, when the population will reach 2,594. Noting that a constant *absolute* increase of 100 per year would total 1,000 after ten years, we observe that the impact of a constant *percentage* increase is, in the illustrative case, nearly 60 percent higher after ten years and continuing to accelerate.

The required calculation is essentially that used in determining the value (V_n) of an investment (V_0) after n years, when the annual yield (r) is fixed and compounded annually:

$$V_n = V_0(1 + r)^n.$$

Thus, for example, $1,000 invested at an interest rate of 2 percent will grow to

$$V_n = \$1,000(1.02)^{20} = \$1,486.$$

at the end of twenty years. More to the point, a population of 1,000 increasing by 2 percent annually will total 1,486 after twenty years. This and other numerical results selected to cover a realistic range of conditions are summarized in Table 17.2.

The effect of compound growth is especially noteworthy when improvements in service coverage are planned at the same time. To illustrate, consider a population of 2 million served by 1,000 paramedical workers, or one per 2,000 population. Suppose further that the national goal is to have one worker per 1,000 population within twenty years. If current staffing standards were maintained, the projected population would call for 1,486 workers, an increase of 48.6 percent (see Table 17.2). Improved staffing standards applied to the present population would require a 100 percent increase in the size of the work force. The combined influences of population growth and higher staffing ratios lead to the need for 2,972 workers, an increase of 197.2 percent, which is considerably greater than the sum of the two effects separately.

CHANGING POPULATION CHARACTERISTICS

Aging

Reference has been made to the use of fertility and survival rates to model the aging of a population in order to derive the size and composition expected at a specified time in the future. In illustrating the procedures employed we consider a hypothetical population of nursing personnel, rather than a general population, in order to emphasize the versatility of the model. The work force of nurses is subject to phenomena of recruitment and retirement that are mathematically comparable to births and deaths in the general population. Moreover temporary departures and reentry for child rearing and other activities are simply special cases of migration.

It is necessary to estimate attrition rates for cohorts of graduates during each period (usually five years) following training. This is done for the illustrative case in Table 17.3A. The table indicates that of 1,000 recent (within the past five years) graduates who are currently employed, 30 percent, or 300, can be expected to leave the work force permanently within the next five years and another 300 will leave temporarily for child rearing. During the next five years the 400 continuing employees are subject to a 40 percent attrition rate, and the 300 temporary dropouts of the previous period are expected to return. The resulting work force is subject to a 50 percent attrition rate during the next five years, the "survivors" then experience a 60 percent attrition

Table 17.2

COMPOUNDING OF GROWTH RATES

Annual Growth Rate (%)	Population after Specified Years as Percent of Initial Level					
	3	5	10	15	20	30
1.0	103.0	105.1	110.5	116.1	122.0	134.8
1.5	104.6	107.7	116.1	125.0	134.7	156.3
1.8	105.5	109.3	119.5	130.7	142.9	170.8
2.0	106.1	110.4	121.9	134.6	148.6	181.1
2.2	106.7	111.5	124.3	138.6	154.5	192.1
2.5	107.7	113.1	128.0	144.8	163.9	209.8
3.0	109.3	115.9	134.4	155.8	180.6	242.7

Table 17.3A

MODEL OF GAINS AND LOSSES IN NURSING PERSONNEL

Years Since Graduation	Permanent Attrition (%)	"Survival" Rates (%)	Temporary Dropout, Re-entry (%)	Hypothetical Experience-- Cohort of 1,000
under 5	30	70	-30	1,000
5 - 9	40	60	+30	700 - 300 = 400
10 - 14	50	50		240 + 300 = 540
15 - 19	60	40		270
20 - 24	70	30		108
25 - 29	100	0		32
				0

Table 17.3B

APPLICATION OF MODEL TO PRODUCE 20-YEAR PROJECTION

Years Since Graduation	Year				
	1980	1985	1990	1995	2000
under 5	482	530	583	642	706
5 - 9	307-131 = 176	337-145 = 192	371-159 = 212	408-175 = 233	257
10 - 14		106+131 = 237	115+145 = 260	127+159 = 286	140+175 = 315
15 - 19			118	130	143
20 - 24				47	52
25 and up					14
					1,487

rate, and so forth, until 100 percent retirement is reached thirty years after graduation.

The preceding calculations follow a cohort of graduates throughout their career.
The work force at a particular time to be projected is made up of a number of cohorts
who are at various stages in their careers. It is assumed that the attrition rates of Table
17.3A are applicable to each. If the rates are changing for each new cohort, separate
estimates must be made and applied uniquely to each group.

Let us suppose that, on the basis of 1980 data, we wish to estimate the number of
nursing personnel likely to be available in the year 2000. We need to know something
about the "birth rate," that is, expected trends regarding new graduates. Suppose that
the number of recent graduates in 1980, 482, is 10 percent above 1975 and that the
trend is expected to continue. This gives the first row of figures in Table 17.3B.

We must then "age" each cohort as far as necessary to determine the number of
"survivors" anticipated in 2000. From Table 17.3A we note that only 40 percent of
the 1995 cohort of 642 persons will be present in 2000. Similarly, the 1990 cohort of
583 will be reduced to 233 in 1995, but 175 of the dropouts will be temporary. By
2000 we expect 60 percent of the 233, or 140, to remain active and to be rejoined by
the 175 temporary dropouts. Comparable calculations are applied to data for earlier
years until we accumulate an expected total of 1,487 nurses to be available in 2000.

Such modeling can be useful for testing a series of alternatives. What if nursing
school enrollment were increased by 20 percent instead of 10 percent? How much
would attrition rates have to be reduced to achieve a similar effect? In general what
are the relative trade-offs between increased training capacity and improved retention
of those trained?

Changes in Other Population Characteristics

The way in which variables of importance other than age are to be taken into
consideration differs greatly according to individual conditions, all of which cannot
be detailed here. In general, however, projected changes in population composition
require assessment of shifts in average status and patterns of dispersion from that
average. The principle will be illustrated with respect to income changes.

Consider a population of 3 million with a present per capita income of $600.
National income is growing by 5 percent per year, while annual population growth is
2 percent. What per capita income can be expected in ten years?

Noting that national income is presently $1,800 million, we apply the concept of
compound interest to both income growth and population growth as follows:

$$\frac{1,800(1.05)^{10}}{3.0(1.02)^{10}} = \frac{2,932.010}{3.657} = \$802.$$

A simple approximation to this result can be obtained by assuming a 3 percent
annual increase in per capita income based upon the difference between income and
population growth rates. Then we obtain

$$600(1.03)^{10} = \$806.$$

Given a projected increase in real income by about one-third on the average, the
planner must consider how individual members of the population are likely to share

the increase. The simplest approach is to shift the present income distribution upward by approximately $200, leaving the overall shape of the distribution unchanged. On the other hand, if income disparities are expected to decrease or increase, the form of these changes must be quantified in some systematic way.

AGGREGATED EFFECTS OF CHANGING POPULATION CHARACTERISTICS

Projection of Population Detail from Marginal Totals

As suggested earlier, the presence of interactive effects makes it necessary to project jointly the population factors involved in the interaction. Consider the data in Table 17.4, for example. Marked differences in services utilization are seen between urban and rural areas and likewise among educational groups. Furthermore it is not possible to consider these factors independently. Virtually no difference exists between urban and rural poor, whereas the highly educated urban dwellers use more than half again as many services per capita as their rural counterparts. Depending upon the nature of future educational shifts, urban/rural differences in utilization could be either narrowed or increased. In either case it is necessary to obtain educational projections for urban and rural populations separately.

Frequently such detail is not available to the planner. The following scenario is typical. A 5 percent annual growth rate is likely in urban areas for the next decade, whereas rural growth will be 1 percent annually. In ten years one-fourth of the total population is expected to be "highly educated," while 40 percent will be in the middle education group. Educational projections in greater detail have not been made.

Applying this information to the population data of Table 17.4, we obtain the marginal totals of Table 17.5. To obtain the estimates needed in the individual cells of the table, the following statistically validated iterative procedure is recommended.

As a first approximation, apply the baseline urban/rural distribution by education group to the projected numbers. Since 109/1,147 of the baseline poorly educated were urban, a similar proportion is assigned to the 885 projected to be poorly educated ten years from now. Specifically,

$$\frac{109}{1,147} \times 885 = 84.$$

When the approximation procedure is applied to each column, it produces row totals that do not agree with the original projections. In order to bring the first row total from 589 to the desired 627, each entry in the row is multiplied by the adjustment factor 627/589. Similarly, each second-row entry is multiplied by 1,901/1,939. While the Step 2 procedure corrects the row discrepancies, it introduces errors in the column totals.

In the third step adjustments are made by column in the same way that row adjustments were made in Step 2. In particular each entry in the first column is adjusted by the factor 885/874. Not unexpectedly, row errors are reintroduced, and the back-and-forth process may seem to be endless. In fact, however, the row discrepancies at Step 3 are much smaller than at Step 1. The iterative process is therefore continued until Step 5, when agreement is found in both row totals and column totals.

Table 17.4

EVIDENCE OF INTERACTION IN SERVICES UTILIZATION RATES

Baseline Population (Thousands)

	Education			
	Low	Medium	High	
Urban	109	183	93	385
Rural	1,038	540	143	1,721
	1,147	723	236	2,106

Total Services (Thousands)

	Education			
	Low	Medium	High	
Urban	414	983	826	2,223
Rural	3,715	3,355	829	7,899
	4,129	4,338	1,655	10,122

Services Per Capita

	Education			
	Low	Medium	High	
Urban	3.8	5.4	8.9	5.8
Rural	3.6	6.2	5.8	4.6
	3.6	6.0	7.0	4.8

Summarization by Example

We began the chapter with the principle that detailed population forecasts are necessary only insofar as the population mix is expected to change with respect to factors associated with a resultant variable, such as services utilization, of importance in planning. We then introduced specific techniques for taking some of these factors into consideration. In this concluding section we illustrate how several population factors, assessed by any means deemed appropriate, are combined in the overall planning endeavor.

Table 17.5

ITERATIVE DERIVATION OF DETAILED POPULATION PROJECTIONS

Marginal Projections (Thousands)

	Education			
	Low	Medium	High	
Urban				627
Rural				1,901
	885	1,011	632	2,528

1. First Approximation

84	256	249	589
801	755	383	1,939

2. Row Adjustment

89	273	265
785	740	376
874	1,013	641

3. Column Adjustment

90	272	261	623
795	739	371	1,905

4. Row Adjustment

90	274	263
793	738	370
883	1,012	633

5. Final Adjustment

90	274	263	627
795	737	369	1,901
885	1,011	632	2,528

We suppose it has been determined that services utilization is a function of residence location, educational attainment, and health insurance eligibility. The first two factors interact as shown in Table 17.4, whereas the effect of insurance status is independent of the other factors. In particular, compared with a national average of 4.8 visits per capita, those covered by private health insurance schemes typically make 6.2 visits annually. The added 1.4 visits applies equally to insured residents of urban and rural areas across all educational levels. Controlling for the effects of education and residence location, persons eligible for standard government insurance coverage make 5.0 visits annually on the average, and those with no insurance whatsoever average 3.2 visits. In ten years the population size is expected to be as shown in Table 17.5, with private and public insurance covering 10 and 60 percent, respectively.

To estimate total utilization one decade hence, assuming no changes in rates within each subgroup, we begin with one factor or interacting set of factors, such

Table 17.6

ILLUSTRATIVE PROJECTION OF SERVICES UTILIZATION

Group	Population Size (M)	Per Capita Use	Number of Services (M)
Urban - Low Education	90	3.8	342.0
- Medium Education	274	5.4	1,479.6
- High Education	263	8.9	2,340.7
Rural - Low Education	795	3.6	2,862.0
- Medium Education	737	6.2	4,569.4
- High Education	369	5.8	2,140.2
Initial Estimate			13,733.9
Private Insurance	253	+1.4	+ 354.2
Public Insurance	1,517	+0.2	+ 303.4
No Insurance	758	-1.6	-1,212.8
Final Estimate			13,178.7

as education and residence location. Use rates from Table 17.4 are applied to the projected population levels derived in Table 17.5 to produce the initial projections of service levels in Table 17.6.

Adjustments are then made for other factors of concern, only insurance eligibility in the present case. After initial estimates have been made to reflect average conditions, only deviations from the average are of interest in accounting for the influence of additional factors. Thus, the use rates of 6.2, 5.0, and 3.2 for the three insurance groups are translated into deviations from the overall average of 4.8. The per capita differences, +1.4, +.2, and -1.6 are then applied to the projected populations in each category. This results in the final estimate of utilization in Table 17.6, 13.2 million visits. If other factors had been found to influence utilization, further adjustments for their effects would have been made in the same way.

REFERENCES

1. Carrier, Norman, and John Hobcraft, *Demographic Estimation for Developing Societies,* London: The Population Investigating Committee, London School of Economics, 1971.

PRIMARY READINGS

Barclay, George W., *Techniques of Population Analysis,* New York: John Wiley & Sons, 1958.
A clear exposition of basic demographic procedures. Although one of the earlier works, this is still a good basic reference.

Shryock, Henry S., and Jacob S. Siegel, *The Methods and Materials of Demography,* U.S.
    Bureau of the Census, Washington: U.S. Government Printing Office, 1973. A system-
    atic presentation of the methods used by technicians and research workers in demographic
    analysis. Data availability and analytical methods for statistically underdeveloped areas
    are emphasized.

SECONDARY READINGS

Carrier, Norman, and John Hobcraft, *Demographic Estimation for Developing Societies,* Lon-
    don: The Population Investigating Committee, London School of Economics, 1971.
Olurunfemi, J. F., "Population in Health Planning," *Social Science in Medicine,* 17, 9:597–
    600, 1983.

18

Measurement of Health Needs and Services Utilization

WILLIAM A. REINKE

The preceding chapter established the need for the planner to consider the projected size and characteristics of the client population. This information is of little consequence in its own right, but only as it helps to pinpoint services need in that population. We recall from the discussion of epidemiologic principles in Chapter 9 that such needs assessment includes consideration of the vulnerability of disease to service intervention and the propensity for those in need to make use of services, as well as the magnitude and distribution of the need itself. The measurement of service needs and utilization is the focus of attention in the present chapter.

CONSIDERATIONS AND CONSTRAINTS IN MEASUREMENT

While our aim is quantification of human need, we must recognize that impersonally objective priority setting may not be entirely realistic or appropriate in matters as emotionally charged as the valuation of human life. At a time when the United States had a president afflicted with poliomyelitis, public support for a foundation to combat that disease was ten times as high as that given to the Heart Association, even though morbidity and mortality from rheumatic fever were double those of polio. We also see evidence of an almost mystical "dread disease" factor at work in setting priorities. To illustrate, a city in the United States would be thrown into panic by several rabies deaths in one month, whereas much greater loss of life through motor vehicle injuries arouses relatively little concern. Similarly, a cholera epidemic resulting in fifty deaths would be considered newsworthy almost anywhere, whereas a much larger ongoing death toll from diarrhea among weaning-age children is hardly considered to be a departure from "normal."

How to enter age into the measurement is another matter on which consensus has not been reached. Some planners emphasize losses in productivity from disease and accordingly limit attention to affliction during economically active years. Others assign priority to childhood disease because of its magnitude, preventability, and long-term effects. Still others consider the lives of an infant, a forty-year-old family breadwinner, and an eighty-year-old retiree to be equally valuable.

Another issue of concern in measurement is the relative weights to be assigned to mortality, morbidity, and disability. Some health indices count one day of disability as equivalent to death one day prematurely. Thus a disease that causes twenty people to die at an age that averages five years less than life expectancy ($20 \times 5 = 100$ person-years lost) would be considered equally as serious as one that produced ten days of disability, but no deaths, among 3,650 individuals ($3,650 \times [10/365]$ days per year $= 100$ person-years). In contrast, some measurement procedures establish separate indicators of mortality, morbidity, and disability and combine them in a purely subjective manner or through application of the Delphi technique or another semiobjective means of appraisal.

Finally, the planner must be cognizant of the potential impact of preventable illness as well as the prevalence of overt disease. In assessing the importance of measles and measles immunization, for example, consideration must extend beyond existing cases to the disease load that would arise if vaccinations were curtailed. A corollary point is that measurement of a large part of service need is based upon demographic data and professional judgment rather than direct measures of disease prevalence. Thus, a population of 10,000 that averages 40 births per thousand population is considered to have a need for 400 deliveries annually by a trained birth attendant.

ECONOMIC COST OF ILLNESS

The preceding discussion has alerted us to the dangers of overly simplistic epidemiologic measures formed on narrow economic grounds. Nevertheless measures of productivity loss can provide a useful starting point in the determination of comparative importance among diseases, provided that we not lose sight of the caveats expressed regarding limitations in interpretation.[1,2] In this section we illustrate the basic computations involved by means of a hypothetical example. Various nuances and limitations in application of these measures to cost-benefit analysis are covered more fully in Chapter 20.

We suppose that hypertension in a specified population results in 4,000 deaths annually at an average age of sixty-two and in addition disables 15,000 persons for an average period of six months. The cost of medical care averages $300 for the former group and $1,400 for the latter. Each group has average earnings of $8,000 annually. What is the economic cost of hypertension in this population?

We first assume that the costs in lost productivity are applicable only to age sixty-five. We further assume that potential earnings in years prior to that age are to be discounted. The principle is that associated with any investment, for here we are dealing with an investment in human capital. If $1,000 is invested today to yield a 10 percent rate of return, it will be worth $1,100 in one year. The return during the second year is expected to be 10 percent of $1,100, or $110, increasing the value of the investment to $1,210. In general the value t years hence will be $(1,000)(1.10)^t$. It follows that $1,210 payable two years from now is equivalent to $1,000 today. In other words future earnings must be discounted back to present value. This conforms to human preferences in that individuals are willing to forego present benefits only in exchange for greater benefits in the future.

The discount rate to be used with regard to the value of future years of life is not as clear as that applicable to return on monetary investment. For purposes of illustration, however, we continue to assume a 10 percent rate of return and a corresponding discount factor. Considering the average individual who loses three years of productive life through death at age sixty-two, the current discounted value of those foregone earnings is calculated as follows:

$$\text{First year: } (8,000)/(1.10) = \$7,273$$
$$\text{Second year: } (8,000)/(1.10)^2 = 6,612$$
$$\text{Third year: } (8,000)/(1.10)^3 = \underline{6,011}$$
$$\$19,896$$

The disability loss of one-half year amounts to $4,000 each for the 15,000 disabled persons. Adding in the cost of medical care, we obtain total costs, direct and indirect, of

$$4,000(19,896 + 300) + 15,000(4,000 + 1,400) = \$161,784,000.$$

DECISIONS ON SCREENING

We have repeatedly stressed the fact that the health planner is interested in disease prevalence mainly in relation to the potential for service invention and prospects for the actual utilization of those services. The evaluation of screening strategies clearly conveys this merging of interests and represents a useful application of decision analysis.[3]

To illustrate the analytic approach, suppose that 20 percent of the members of a defined population have a certain health problem that will cost $100 per case to treat if it results in symptomatic disease. Early detection at the asymptomatic stage permits treatment at a cost of only $85. Early detection is possible through a screening test that can be performed for $1 per person. The test has a sensitivity of 80 percent, meaning that the screening test will fail to detect one-fifth of the cases (false-negative results). The specificity of 90 percent leads to 10 percent of well individuals' being falsely classified as having positive findings. Unnecessary follow-up of such individuals costs $10 per case. Identification as "positive" in screening does not guarantee that the individual will comply with the prescribed treatment; specifically a 60 percent compliance rate is assumed on the basis of past experience.

This scenario has all of the elements needed for making a rational decision: disease prevalence, cost and effectiveness of screening, likelihood of utilization of needed services, and cost of those services. We then ask whether potential cost savings are available from the screening program.

Figure 18.1 presents the two options schematically for a hypothetical population of 1,000 individuals. In the absence of screening, 200 cases would be treated eventually at a cost of $20,000. Branching at each stage of the screening program would lead to 6 subgroups with different characteristics and associated costs. Of the 200 true positive cases, for example, 160 would be identified in screening, and 96 of these would receive needed early treatment. The other 64, while screened correctly, would be no better off than the false-negative individuals because of noncompliance with treatment. Analogously among the 800 true negative results, there would be 80 false positive individuals, 48 of whom would receive unnecessary follow-up. This cost would be saved in the 32 noncompliant false-positive cases.

Summing up over the 6 subgroups, total costs associated with screening slightly exceed $20,000. Hence screening is not advised. The branching shows graphically why this conclusion is reached, apart from cost considerations regarding screening and the relative benefits of early detection. The results are affected by the prevalence rate, the effectiveness of screening, and the rates of compliance. Changes in any of these factors could make screening cost-effective. For example, identification of a high-risk group with higher prevalence of disease could make screening more attractive. Likewise, improvement in the sensitivity and/or specificity of the screening

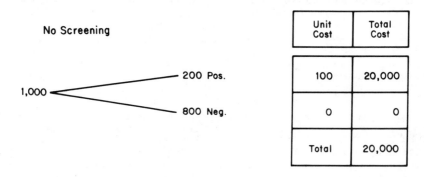

No Screening

	Unit Cost	Total Cost
200 Pos.	100	20,000
800 Neg.	0	0
Total		20,000

1,000

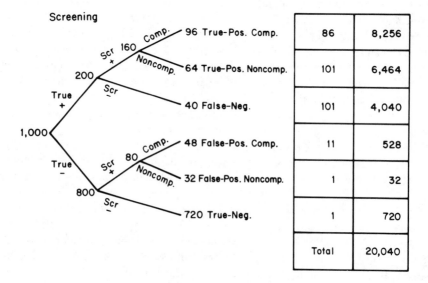

Screening

	Unit Cost	Total Cost
96 True-Pos. Comp.	86	8,256
64 True-Pos. Noncomp.	101	6,464
40 False-Neg.	101	4,040
48 False-Pos. Comp.	11	528
32 False-Pos. Noncomp.	1	32
720 True-Neg.	1	720
Total		20,040

Figure 18.1   Evaluation of screening strategies

test, thereby reducing unnecessary costs, would favor screening. Finally, it can be shown that if compliance among screened positive cases could be brought above 62.5 percent, the screening program would become worthwhile.

ANALYSIS OF SERVICES UTILIZATION

Service statistics are among the most widely available data for planning purposes. Information of utilization is routinely compiled at all service points, and additional data on service behavior are often available from special surveys. The quality of the information frequently fails to match the quantity, however, either because the client population is not clearly defined or because the data have not been transformed into meaningful indicators for decision making. As indicated earlier, the methodology of functional analysis attempts to overcome this problem through intensive analysis of the minimal body of information necessary.[4] Two examples of the organization and analysis of utilization statistics are presented in the following paragraphs.

Determinants of Services Utilization

Consider a survey of three health areas in which a total of 1,904 medical care visits were reported to the area health posts during a prior two-week period. Visits to the individual posts were as shown in Table 18.1. Although such service volume statistics are all that is sometimes reported, they are not very useful for comparative purposes because of area differences in population. The calculated utilization rates, also shown in the table, are therefore advised, and conversion to an annual basis is likely to be even more meaningful to planners and managers.

Comparison of rates suggests that Area A lags behind the others in service coverage, but the reason is not apparent from the data. Three possibilities exist: (1) Area A may have experienced less *morbidity* and consequent need for services; (2) perhaps a relatively small proportion of illnesses in Area A received care, that is, the *extent* of service coverage was low; (3) perhaps some individuals in Areas B and C were served repeatedly; that is, *intensity* of utilization was high. Each of these factors would be interpreted differently and lead to separate actions. In particular

Table 18.1

CURSORY ANALYSIS OF UTILIZATION

Measure	Area			
	A	B	C	Total
Patient Visits in 2 wks.	481	488	935	1,904
Individuals Surveyed	8,416	6,129	11,392	25,937
Util. Rate (%)	5.7	8.0	8.2	7.3
Util. Rate (Visits/Yr.)	1.49	2.07	2.13	1.91

it is helpful to know whether a service area has achieved broad coverage or whether a few individuals are being served to the point of overutilization whereas the majority remains without services.

Compilations as shown in Table 18.2 permit analysis of the three possibilities noted. Tests of statistical significance highlight the sources of real differences between areas, which can then be compared by means of appropriate indices. The data are organized to permit independent assessments of the three factors. To illustrate with respect to Area A, we first determine whether 946 persons with illness in a total of 8,416 individuals is exceptional, that is, statistically significant. Then we establish the significance of 359 service users among the 946 cases of morbidity. Because the 946 persons who provided the first-stage numerator become the denominator and sole basis for second-stage analysis, the latter is not influenced by the first-stage outcome.

From the findings in Table 18.2 we observe that the areas exhibit similar morbidity rates and differ mainly in their consultation rates. Nearly half of the illnesses in Area C receive attention, compared with 38 percent in Area A. Although Areas B and C show similar overall utilization rates in Table 18.1, they do differ regarding extent of coverage and intensity of use. The relatively high utilization rate in Area C occurs mainly because it achieves relatively broad services coverage, whereas the high rate in Area B is due to high intensity of use among fewer individuals.

Characteristics of Service Users

Because utilization is affected by the accessibility and acceptability of services, planners are interested in identifying physical, economic, and sociocultural factors

Table 18.2

DETAILED ANALYSIS OF UTILIZATION

Measure	Area			
	A	B	C	Total
Individuals Surveyed	8,416	6,129	11,392	25,937
Persons with Illness	946	707	1,374	3,027
Service Users	359	322	660	1,341
No. with Multiple Visits	105	126	223	454
Total Visits	481	488	935	1,904

Indicator	Basic Rates			Percent of Average			χ^2
	A	B	C	A	B	C	
Morbidity Rate (%)	11.2	11.5	12.1	96	99	103	3.24
Consultation Rate (%)	37.9	45.5	48.0	86	103	108	23.56***
Visits per Consulter	1.34	1.52	1.42	94	107	100	7.60*

* $- p < .05$
*** $- p < .001$

that inhibit use of services.[5] The already noted importance of basing analysis on a clearly defined population denominator becomes especially significant in the matter of physical access as pointed out in the following example.

Suppose that a health center finds that 70 percent of its patients reside within three kilometers of the center, and the remaining 30 percent travel three to six kilometers. The finding is a typical indication of the importance of travel time and distance in limiting service use. The situation is probably worse than this superficial appraisal suggests, however. The reason is that area is a function of the square of the distance, not the distance itself. Specifically, of the area encompassed within a circle of six kilometers' radius, only one-fourth, not one-half, lies within three kilometers. If population density were uniform, therefore, three-fourths of the target population, not one-half, would reside at a distance of three to six kilometers. When we recognize this, the fact that that ring contributes only 30 percent of the patients is especially striking. Population density is not uniform, of course, but population dispersion in many rural areas makes such an assumption reasonable as a first approximation.

To appraise the importance of selected population characteristics on utilization, construction of certain indicators and display according to the format of Table 18.3 are suggested. Economic status is used to illustrate the analytic procedure. As in the previous example the data are assumed to come from a survey of morbidity and utilization experience during a recent two-week period.

First, morbidity and consultation rates are calculated by economic status, and the significance of differences is noted. The presumed preventability of the complaints is also ascertained to guide determination of the extent and focus of preventive and promotive services to be offered. The illness episodes are then divided into two groups for further analysis. Those who sought medical attention are appraised regarding patterns of care-seeking behavior; those not seeking medical attention are classified according to reasons for that behavior.

Not all episodes of illness stand to benefit from medical care. The functional analysis methodology therefore includes provision for determination of need for professional attention and computation of a *need sensitivity index*. The factors determining need are category of illness, duration, and severity. An earache, for example, is considered worthy of medical attention regardless of duration, whereas certain other classes of illness are presumed to need attention only if they persist for at least seven days or result in more than three days' loss from work, school, or other normal activity.

All reported illnesses are separated into two categories, depending upon whether they are deemed to need medical attention. The proportion of those in each category who actually received care is then calculated. Suppose that 60 percent of those needing care actually received it, whereas 30 percent of the others also received care despite the lack of evidence of benefit. The need sensitivity index (NSI) is then

$$\text{NSI} = \frac{60}{30} = 2.$$

Ideally all those needing attention should get it; thus the numerator should be 100, whereas the denominator should be near zero. A large NSI, therefore, provides evidence of an efficient, discriminating system of care in which resources are used beneficially. On the other hand, if care is sought indiscriminately without regard to

Table 18.3

INFLUENCE OF ECONOMIC STATUS ON UTILIZATION

Economic Status	Persons		Those with Illness		
	Number	Percent Ill	Number	Percentage	
				Preventable	with Consultation
Low	11,336	13.1	1,482	35.8	41.6
High	14,601	10.6	1,545	35.1	46.9
χ^2		38.43***		0.14	9.01**

Economic Status	Consulters				Non-Consulters			
	No.	Percentage Use			No.	Percentage Reason		
		Pvt. Qual.	Govt.	Indig.		Economic	Access	No Need
Low	616	20.5	31.0	48.5	866	56.2	25.1	18.7
High	725	32.1	37.4	30.5	820	42.1	22.4	35.5
χ^2		48.78***				63.08***		

$** - p < .01$
$*** - p < .001$

real need, the numerator and denominator of the index will be similar and the index itself will be near one.

When the index has been applied in practice, it has been found to increase with education. When education is held constant, higher socioeconomic groups tend to be less discriminating than poor people in their use of services.

PROVIDER-INITIATED SERVICES

Underlying the preceding discussion was the attempt to understand and quantify client demand for services. Such assessment usually includes some preventive services, for instance, visits to under-fives clinics. In large part, however, these are likely to require provider initiated outreach services based upon professional determination of need rather than client-expressed demand. This requires a coupling of demographic information with the professional standards as illustrated in Table 18.4 for selected services.

The table assumes that the health unit of interest serves a population of 100,000 with a crude birth rate of 32. Of every 100 children born, 20 are expected to die before the age of five, 12 during infancy, 4 during the second year of life, 2 during the third year, and 1 each during years four and five. In the target population this translates into 3,200 births, 2,816 of whom reach the age of one, 2,688 who reach age two, 2,624 who reach age three, and 2,560 who survive to age five. On average

Table 18.4

PROFESSIONALLY-BASED LEVELS OF SELECTED SERVICES NEED

Demographic Calculations

3,200		Births		
	384	Deaths 1st Year	3,008	Avg. 0-1
2,816		1st Birthday		
	128	Deaths 2nd Year	2,752	Avg. 1-2
2,688		2nd Birthday		
	64	Deaths 3rd Year	2,656	Avg. 2-3
2,624		3rd Birthday		
	32	Deaths 4th Year	2,608	Avg. 3-4
2,592		4th Birthday		
	32	Deaths 5th Year	2,576	Avg. 4-5
2,560		5th Birthday		
	640	Total Deaths		

Service Type	No. Persons	Service Standard	Volume	
Well-child Visits 1st year 2nd and 3rd years 4th and 5th years	3,008 5,408 5,184	9 visits each 4 visits each 2 visits each	27,072 21,632 10,368	59,072
DPT Immunizations 1st year 3rd year booster	3,008 2,656	3 doses 1 dose	9,024 2,656	11,680
Nut. Supplement Ages 1-3	5,408	25% (based on spl. study) x 2 feedings/ day x 365 days/year		986,960

then we can assume there are 3,008 infants, 2,752 between the ages of one and two, an additional 2,656 less than three years old, and 5,184 between the ages of three and five. Applying these numbers to the desired service standards listed in Table 18.4, we derive the total volume of services needed.

The presentation of techniques for epidemiologic assessment has been illustrative but by no means exhaustive, though we have tried to cover the principal aspects of interest. Regardless of the type of analysis conducted, the purpose for planning is not simply to quantify the burden of disease but to guide decision making regarding the most feasible and appropriate ways to meet the defined need.

REFERENCES

1. Rice, Dorothy, "Estimating the Cost of Illness," *American Journal of Public Health*, 57, 3:424–440, 1967.

2. Cooper, Barbara, and Dorothy Rice, "The Economic Cost of Illness Revisited," *Social Security Bulletin*, 39, 2:21–36, 1976.

3. Reinke, William A., "Decisions About Screening Programs: Can We Develop a Rational Basis?" *Archives of Environmental Health*, 19:403–411, 1969.

4. Department of International Health, Johns Hopkins University, *The Functional Analysis of Health Needs and Services*, Ch. 2, pp. 35–152, New Delhi: Asia Publishing House, 1976.

5. Siegmann, Athilia, "Classification of Sociomedical Health Indicators: Perspectives for Health Administrators and Health Planners," *International Journal of Health Services*, 6, 3:521–538, 1976.

PRIMARY READINGS

Chen, Martin K., and Bertha E. Bryant, "The Measurement of Health: A Critical and Selective Overview," *International Journal of Epidemiology*, 4, 4:257–264, 1975. Various health status indices are classified, and strengths and weaknesses are discussed.

Department of International Health, Johns Hopkins University, *The Functional Analysis of Health Needs and Services*, Ch. 2, pp. 35–152, New Delhi: Asia Publishing House, 1976. Discusses design of data collection and sample selection, as well as analysis and presentation of results from a survey of community health needs and actions.

Hansluwka, H. E., "Measuring the Health of Populations: Indicators and Interpretations," *Social Science and Medicine*, 20, 12:1207–1224, 1985. A key paper that highlights the mainstream of recent developments in health measurement and lists main points of controversy in the search for health status indicators.

Morley D., and M. Woodland, *See How They Grow: Monitoring a Child's Growth for Appropriate Health Care in Developing Countries*, Hampshire, England: MacMillan Press, 1979. Demonstrates use of a simple chart to monitor growth and to observe effects of various diseases on nutritional status.

Murnaghan, J. H., "Health Indicators and Information Systems for the Year 2000," *Annual Review of Public Health*, 2:299–361, 1981. A review of problems, priorities, and guidelines for developing a health information system for promoting and monitoring health. One section is devoted specifically to situations in developing countries.

Rice, Dorothy, "Estimating the Cost of Illness," *American Journal of Public Health*, 57, 3:424–440, 1967. Presents the classic economic approach to assessment of the burden of disease.

Risk Approach for Maternal and Child Health Care, WHO Offset Publication No. 39, Geneva: World Health Organization, 1978. The approach described for screening priority health problems of mothers and children has gained wide use as a management tool.

SECONDARY READINGS

Fanshel, S., "A Meaningful Measure of Health for Epidemiology," *International Journal of Epidemiology,* 1, 4:319–337, 1972.

Hennes, James D., "The Measurement of Health," *Medical Care Review,* 29, 11:1268–1288, 1972.

Patrick, Donald L., "Constructing Social Metrics for Health Status Indexes," *International Journal of Health Services,* 6, 3:443–453, 1976.

Sommer, A., *A Field Guide to the Detection and Control of Xerophthalmia,* Geneva: World Health Organization, 1978.

19
Personnel Analysis

WILLIAM A. REINKE

In view of the long time frame associated with the training of many health professionals, it is not surprising that supply seldom matches personnel requirements at a specific point in time. In the absence of effective planning, the more severe the shortage of personnel, the more drastic and overreactive is the remedial action likely to be, and the more serious the consequent surplus that eventually emerges. Techniques for establishing and maintaining a balance between available personnel and requirements are therefore among the more useful planning tools.

In matching supply and demand, we have already observed that the supply of personnel must be related to the demand for services. Thus the supply of personnel must be translated into the supply of services through productivity assessments that define the volume of services each worker is able to provide.

These considerations lead to two categories of labor force analysis to be considered here. First, we examine at a macrolevel the long-term impact of various strategies of training and patterns of personnel retention. Second, we undertake a microanalysis of worker activity profiles. The *macroanalysis* deals quantitatively with the numbers of personnel to plan for, while the *microanalysis* relates more qualitatively to ways in which those personnel can and should be employed. These deployment decisions begin with an assessment of local service needs, as described in the previous chapter, and are therefore a continuation of the functional analysis methodology.

MACROANALYSIS

Projected Growth of Population and Service Requirements

In Chapter 17 we saw the value of disaggregated demand projections whenever service need or demand differs among population segments that also exhibit differential growth rates. As a point of departure for the present discussion we consider a population in which the rapidly growing urban segment utilizes more services per capita than the more stable rural segment.

In particular, we envisage a population of one million that is currently 80 percent rural. Urban areas are growing by 5 percent annually, whereas the rural population growth rate is 1 percent annually. Rural residents average two health center visits per capita each year, whereas the urban average is three per capita, 50 percent higher.

What is the current volume of services provided, and how is this likely to change over the next thirty years?

Separate calculations for the urban and rural segments yield populations of 864,388 and 1,078,279, respectively, thirty years hence. Thus, the projected population of 1,942,667 is expected to be 44 percent urban, compared to 20 percent at present. Assuming no change in utilization patterns, the number of services to be provided will reach 4,749,722 in all, compared to 2,200,000 currently. Whereas the population size is projected to increase by 94 percent, services growth is expected to total 116 percent.

One year from the present we can expect 808,000 rural residents and 210,000 urban residents. The total of 1,018,000 represents an overall growth rate of 1.8 percent. This can be stated more generally as

$$G_t = P_r G_r + P_u G_u, \tag{19.1}$$

where

G_t = overall annual growth rate
G_r = rural annual growth rate
G_u = urban annual growth rate
P_r = proportion of initial population that is rural
P_u = proportion of initial population that is urban

In the present case

$$G_t = (.8)(1) + (.2)(5)$$
$$= 1.8 \text{ percent per year.}$$

This initial growth rate will not remain constant, for over time the trend toward urbanization will cause the high urban growth rate to receive greater and greater weight in Equation 19.1. Assuming constant values of G_r and G_u, we observe from Table 19.1 that in ten years the overall population growth rate will reach

Table 19.1

POPULATION PROJECTIONS
with and without Disaggregation

Projected Years Ahead	Disaggregated Population (Thousands)					Approximation	
	1% Inc. Rural	5% Inc. Urban	Total	Percent Urban	Composite Increase	Assumed 1.8% Inc.	% Error
0	800	200	1,000	20.0	1.80	1,000	0
10	884	326	1,210	26.9	2.08	1,195	1.2
20	976	531	1,507	35.2	2.41	1,429	5.2
30	1,078	864	1,942	44.5	2.78	1,708	12.0

$$G_t = (.731)(1) + (.269)(5)$$
$$= 2.08 \text{ percent.}$$

Thus, the table shows that projection of a constant 1.8 percent increase in population produces underestimates of population growth. For moderate time horizons the discrepancy is slight; however, a thirty-year projection of constant rate of population increase would result in a 12 percent underestimate of the total population, again assuming that the segmented growth rates are, in fact, sustained over such a period of time. In such circumstances the improved precision from disaggregated projections is apparent.

Services utilization per capita, S_t, is a weighted average of rural and urban utilization, S_r and S_u, respectively. Initially the overall rate is

$$S_t = P_r S_r + P_u S_u \qquad (19.2)$$
$$= (.8)(2) + (.2)(3)$$
$$= 2.20.$$

This is also subject to continual change because of the increasing weight of urbanization. In particular, after ten years

$$S_t = (.731)(2) + (.269)(3)$$
$$= 2.27.$$

The rate of growth in overall service volume is weighted by both the differential rates of rural and urban population growth and by differentials in services utilization. At any point in time the rate of increase in services volume, V_t, is

$$V_t = \frac{P_r G_r S_r + P_u G_u S_u}{P_r S_r + P_u S_u} \qquad (19.3)$$
$$= \frac{P_r G_r S_r + P_u G_u S_u}{S_t}$$

In the present case this is calculated initially as

$$V_t = \frac{(.8)(1)(2) + (.2)(5)(3)}{(.8)(2) + (.2)(3)}$$
$$= \frac{(.8)(2) + (.2)(15)}{(.8)(2) + (.2)(3)}$$
$$= 2.09 \text{ percent per year.}$$

This rate of services increase exceeds the rate of population growth because the rapidly expanding number of high-use urban residents exerts a double-barreled influence on the right-hand component of the numerator in Equation 19.3. In particular, after ten years

$$V_t = \frac{(.731)(2) + (.269)(15)}{(.731)(2) + (.269)(3)}$$
$$= 2.42 \text{ percent}$$

Table 19.2 shows that thirty-year service projections based upon current population growth rate (Eq. 19.1) and constant overall per capita utilization levels contain two

Table 19.2

SERVICES PROJECTIONS
Based upon Varied Degrees of DISAGGREGATION

Projected Yrs. Ahead	Projected Services (Thousands)				Percent Error		
	(1)	(2)	(3)	(4)	(1)	(2)	(3)
0	2,200	2,200	2,200	2,200			
10	2,630	2,706	2,661	2,745	4.2	1.4	3.1
20	3,143	3,327	3,315	3,544	11.3	6.1	6.5
30	3,757	4,092	4,274	4,750	20.9	13.9	10.0

Assumptions:

(1) 1.80% Annual Population Growth; Constant per capita utilization 2.2 visits annually

(2) 2.09% Annual Services Growth

(3) Disaggregated Population Growth; Constant per capita utilization 2.2 visits annually

(4) Disaggregated Population Growth; Disaggregated per capita utilization

faulty assumptions that produce estimates that are in error by more than 20 percent. Estimates that include provision for changing per capita utilization levels (Eq. 19.3) but fail to update the changes are somewhat more accurate but are still in error by nearly 14 percent after thirty years. Estimates that recognize the dynamics of population growth but incorrectly assume a constant composite level of per capita services utilization are not much better, showing a 10 percent error after thirty years.

In summary, fully disaggregated projections are desirable where differential rates of population growth and levels of services utilization exist. In many cases, however, relatively short-term approximations based upon Equation 19.3, or even 19.1, may be adequate. The dynamics of individual circumstances vary, of course, along with the effects of approximation methods.

Supply Projections: Accounting for Attrition

Personnel projections are based upon two factors: (1) the rate of entry into the work force and (2) the rate of retention.[1] The simplest case is that in which a constant number of individuals is recruited or trained each year, and a fixed percentage of trained workers leave the field each year, regardless of length of employment. The assumption of a constant rate of attrition is unlikely to be entirely realistic, but it can be useful in making rapid, "order of magnitude" supply projections.

Assuming a 10 percent annual attrition rate, for example, how many personnel in a present work force of 500 will still be employed three years from now? After fifteen years? Ninety percent of the 500, or 450, can be expected to remain after one year. A similar percentage of the 450, or 405, are expected after two years, and 365 should be present after three years. More directly we find that

$$500(.9)^3 = 365.$$

More generally,

$$W_i = W_0 R^y,$$ (19.4)

where

W_0 = current number of workers
W_i = number of initial workers remaining after y years
R = annual retention rate

Thus after fifteen years we expect

$$W_i = 500(.9)^{15}$$
$$= 103.$$

Equation 19.4 has been applied to selected attrition rates and periods of time to provide Table 19.3. With a 10 percent attrition rate, for example, we observe that 79.4 percent of the original work force would depart within fifteen years. If that work force totaled 500, the remaining 20.6 percent would amount to 103 individuals, as calculated previously.

Work Force Augmentation

We now consider augmentation, as well as attrition. Suppose that each year a training program graduates 100 recruits who are then subject to a 10 percent annual attrition rate. What will be the net addition to the work force after three years? After fifteen years?

One hundred personnel will be added during the first year. Ten of these will be lost during the second year, but 100 others will be added, resulting in a net gain of 90. Of the 190 workers present at the end of the second year, 19 will leave during the third year and 100 will be added. The net gain of 81 will yield 271 workers at the end of the third year.

Table 19.3

GROWTH/ATTRITION FACTORS
According to Time Covered and Attrition Rate

Years of Effect (y)	Cumulative Effect $100(1-R^y)$ by Annual Attrition Rate $100(1-R)$		
	5%	10%	20%
5	22.6	41.0	67.2
10	40.1	65.1	89.3
15	53.7	79.4	96.5
20	64.2	87.8	98.8
25	72.3	92.8	99.6
30	78.5	95.8	99.9

To continue the iterative process for long-term projections could become tedious. An adaptation of Equation 19.4 can be used instead. Specifically, assuming that T new workers are trained or recruited per year, W_0 in the the earlier equation is replaced by $T/(1 - R)$, and R^y is replaced by $(1 - R^y)$ to reflect augmentation rather than attrition. Then the net gain, (W_g), after y years is calculated as

$$W_g = \frac{T(1 - R^y)}{1 - R}. \tag{19.5}$$

For the preceding example after three years

$$W_g = \frac{100(1 - .9^3)}{1 - .9}$$
$$= 271.$$

After fifteen years (referring to Table 19.3)

$$W_g = \frac{100(.794)}{1 - .9}$$
$$= 794.$$

Composite Effects and Implications for Training

Combining Equations 19.4 and 19.5, we determine the total supply of workers (S) after y years to be

$$S = W_0 R^y + \frac{T(1 - R^y)}{1 - R}. \tag{19.6}$$

In the present example, after fifteen years

$$S = 103 + 794$$
$$= 897.$$

Equation 19.6 is based upon a predetermined annual addition of new workers. Frequently the key planning question is, How many new workers must be added each year in order to reach a predetermined supply level within a defined time frame? The variable to be determined is now T, and Equation 19.6 becomes

$$T = \frac{(1 - R)(S - W_0 R^y)}{1 - R^y} \tag{19.7}$$

To illustrate, how many workers must be trained annually to reach a total work force of 800 within five years? As before we assume an initial work force of 500 and a 90 percent retention rate. Again with the aid of Table 19.3 we find

$$T = \frac{[1 - .9][800 - (500)(.590)]}{.410}$$
$$= 123.$$

More detailed analysis reveals that the initial work force of 500 will be reduced to 295 after five years, but the addition of 123 new recruits each year will yield a net gain of 505 over that time period, bringing the total to 800.

Quick Approximations

Although the preceding equations are not especially unwieldy, quick approximations in using them would be desirable. The approximations are obtained by considering the maximum augmentation (M) obtained from the annual addition of T workers with a nominal work life (N). If annual attrition is $(1 - R)$, the nominal work life is

$$N = \frac{1}{1 - R} \qquad (19.8)$$

and maximum augmentation is

$$
\begin{aligned}
M &= TN \\
&= \frac{T}{1 - R}.
\end{aligned} \qquad (19.9)
$$

Consider the earlier case in which 100 workers are added each year and they suffer a 10 percent annual attrition rate. Then

$$
\begin{aligned}
N &= \frac{1}{1 - .9}, \\
&= 10
\end{aligned}
$$

and

$$
\begin{aligned}
M &= \frac{100}{1 - .9} \\
&= 1,000.
\end{aligned}
$$

The simplistic view that emerges is one in which 100 workers are trained each year and employed for ten years. At the end of that time there are 1,000 workers, but thereafter each 100 new workers simply replace a similar number hired ten years earlier. In reality the process is much more gradual, of course, but the simplistic view is useful as a starting point, as a closer look at Table 19.3 shows.

With a 5 percent attrition rate the nominal work life is twenty years, and the table indicates that attrition at that time, in fact, reaches 64.2 percent. With 10 percent attrition N is ten years, at which time cumulative attrition is 65.1 percent. A 20 percent annual attrition rate gives a nominal work life of five years and cumulative attrition of 67.2 percent at that time. Thus, the cumulative effect of attrition after nominal work life is within a narrow range for various attrition rates. A useful rule of thumb states that by the end of the nominal work life cumulative attrition reaches about 65 percent regardless of annual rate of decline.

The relationship holds for percentages of nominal work life other than 100. For example, after 150 percent of nominal work life (fifteen years in the case of a 10 percent attrition rate), cumulative attrition amounts to about 79 percent, regardless of attrition rate. This leads to the tabulation of general factors (Table 19.4) for rapid approximations of relationships of interest.

Consider the initiation of training for a new cadre of community health workers with the expectation that 20 percent of the workers present at the end of a particular year are no longer active a year later. How many must be trained each year in order to have 1,000 in the work force after nine years? The answer is found in Equation 19.7

Table 19.4

GROWTH/ATTRITION FACTORS (APPROXIMATE)
According to Percent of Nominal Career Length

Yrs. Effect as % Nominal $[100y(1-R)]$	Cumulative Effect $[100(1-R^y)]$	Yrs. Effect as % Nominal $[100y(1-R)]$	Cumulative Effect $[100y(1-R^y)]$
10	10.0	120	71.8
20	19.0	150	79.4
30	27.1	180	85.0
40	34.4	220	90.2
50	41.0	260	93.5
60	46.9	300	95.8
80	57.0	350	97.5
100	65.1	400	98.5

with the number of workers initially (W_0) equal to zero. The 20 percent attrition rate means that the nominal work life is five years, and nine years is 180 percent of this. According to Table 19.4 the corresponding value of

$$1 - R^y = 85.0 \text{ percent.}$$

Equation 19.7 then becomes

$$T = \frac{(1 - .8)(1,000 - 0)}{.850}$$
$$= 235.$$

If 235 workers were trained each year as suggested, how many would be functioning after four years? The nominal work life of five years indicates that the maximum work force will be 5×235, or 1,175. Table 19.4 shows that after four years, that is, 80 percent of nominal, 57 percent of the maximum is reached. This works out to 670 workers.

Finally the effect of high attrition rates can be determined quickly by using the approximation technique. If annual attrition were 10 percent instead of 20 percent, for example, how many must be trained annually to reach 1,000 in nine years? Equation 19.7 now becomes

$$T = \frac{(1 - .9)(1,000 - 0)}{.850}$$
$$= 118.$$

As might be expected, if annual losses could be cut in half, the number added each year could be cut in half. If the incentives needed to produce such an effect on attrition were less costly than the savings from training 117 fewer individuals each year, then the incentive scheme should be implemented.

Incongruities Between Supply and Demand

Normally projections of designated supply levels are intended to conform to expected needs (demand) at a specified time in the future. Suppose, for example, that 1,000 personnel of a given type are needed currently and demand is growing by 3 percent annually, whereas current supply is only 500. Assuming 10 percent annual attrition rates, how many personnel must be trained annually in order for supply to match needs within ten years?

In ten years demand will be

$$1,000(1.03)^{10} = 1,344,$$

and this is also the required supply (S) in Equation 19.7. Thus

$$T = \frac{[1 - .9][1,344 - (500)(.9)^{10}]}{[1 - (.9)^{10}]}$$

$$= \frac{(.1)(1,344 - 174)}{.651}$$

$$= 180.$$

Although a training program that graduates 180 persons annually will succeed in bringing supply into line with demand within ten years, the program will become inadequate soon thereafter because of differences in the character of the demand and supply curves, as shown in Figure 19.1. Demand continues to accelerate over time, whereas supply levels off through attrition. Because of these dynamic differences, supply and demand are equalized at only a single point in time. This suggests the initiation of a program that gradually increases the number of trainees over time in accordance with the changing effects of both attrition and demand. Labor force planning must cope dynamically with an adequately broad time horizon in order that the supply curve may be shaped to conform to the demand curve.

Another feature of the preceding illustration is that it gradually reduces the personnel deficit over a ten-year period. In practice, the policymakers and planners do

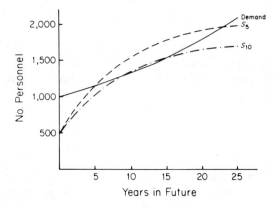

Figure 19.1   Illustration of dynamic relationship between personnel supply and demand

not always exhibit such patience. What if it were required to erase the deficit within five years?

In five years, demand is expected to be

$$1,000(1.03)^5 = 1,159.$$

Application of Equation 19.7 to these conditions raises the number of trainees annually to 211. As shown in Figure 19.1, supply will overshoot the mark, creating a surplus for more than fifteen years after compensation for the initial deficit. Again, the supply curve must be manipulated to conform with the demand curve over a reasonable time frame.

MICROANALYSIS

Macroplanning of labor force requirements well into the future is clearly essential but should be accompanied by microanalysis. Only at the point of health services delivery is it possible to ascertain service needs, convert these to specific activities and skills required, and determine the appropriate mix of personnel needed to provide the requisite services.[2] Aggregation of resulting personnel mixes over the various service units then becomes the basis for macroplanning and establishment of relevant training programs.

Distribution of Effort by Personnel Category

Documentation of specific worker activities can be accomplished through maintenance of detailed diaries or work logs. More simply, estimates of past performance or contemplated activity patterns might be made. For example, a standard of six patients per hour per physician might be set.

Better yet, work sampling has been found to be a simple, yet realistically objective and quantifiable, means of portraying worker activity. Tasks conducted within facilities employing several workers are recorded through randomized intermittent instantaneous observations. The observations, made at two-minute intervals, are distributed among workers in a chance sequence that takes account of the desired frequency of observation. Presumably physicians and others performing more complex and varied tasks would be observed more frequently in order to ensure inclusion of relatively rare events in the recorded observations. The probability of selection for observation at any instant would be adjusted accordingly.

Observation of community activity precludes the tracking of more than one worker at a time by a single observer. Conversely, it does permit the maintenance of a continuous log of activity, but in this setting, too, we have found the instantaneous intermittent observation approach to be simpler and virtually as definitive as the continuous log approach. We do, however, maintain a continuous count of service contacts, compiled by type of contact, category of service recipient, and location of the service.

The recording of activities is accomplished with the aid of a prestructured form that contains a simple checklist of functions and activity categories within functions. The recommended functional breakdown includes such service categories as medical relief

(curative), personal preventive services (e.g., well-child care), community-level preventive services (e.g., mass immunization), and family planning. Activity categories
are associated with direct service (e.g., history taking or giving an injection), supportive services (e.g., supervision or record keeping), travel, and nonproductive personal
time. Table 19.5 illustrates a simplified tally of findings that might be obtained from
a health unit with three types of workers performing four basic functions.

Overview of Service Unit Activity

Although work sampling only yields counts of observations, these can be readily
translated into estimated hours devoted to the activity of interest. Table 19.5 shows,
for example, that 63 of 500 observations of the professional, that is, 12.6 percent,
were associated with direct curative care. If the health unit operates 30 hours per week
and sampling is conducted randomly over the period of operation, we can estimate
that the professional devotes 12.6 percent of the 30 hours, or 3.8 hours per week, to
curative care.

We see from the table that the relative frequency of observation did not correspond
with the size of the work force. Whereas the 500 observations of the professional are
representative of 30 hours of effort per week, the 300 paraprofessional observations
reflect 60 worker-hours of effort. Conversion of observations to hours in Table 19.6
must be performed separately for each personnel category. In particular the conversion
factor for the professional is 30/500, whereas that for the paraprofessional is 60/300.
Thus the 15 curative service observations for the latter are converted to

$$\left(\frac{60}{300}\right)(15) = 3.0 \text{ hours.}$$

After observations have been transformed into work hours for each category of
worker, the hours can be summed to obtain a profile of the proportional distribution of
effort for the health unit as a whole. We find overall, for example, that 38.5 percent
of the available time in the health unit is spent nonproductively.

Data from Table 19.6 might also be organized to show the relative contribution
each type of worker makes to the total effort in specified functional areas. To illustrate,
of the 5.4 hours per week devoted to communicable disease control (CDC),

Table 19.5

ILLUSTRATIVE TALLY OF WORK-SAMPLING OBSERVATIONS

Worker Category	Direct Service				Support. Act.	Travel	Non- Prod.	Total Obs.	No. Workers
	Cur.	MCH	CDC	FP					
Professional	63	17	0	5	197	72	146	500	1
Para-prof.	15	18	9	16	75	83	84	. 300	2
Auxiliary	8	8	6	5	38	43	92	200	4

Table 19.6

A HYPOTHETICAL WORKWEEK
(Activity-Hours)

Worker Category	Direct Service				Support. Act.	Travel	Non- Prod.	Total Hrs.
	Cur.	MCH	CDC	FP				
Professional	3.8	1.0	0.0	0.3	11.8	4.3	8.8	30.0
Para-prof.	3.0	3.6	1.8	3.2	15.0	16.6	16.8	60.0
Auxiliary	4.8	4.8	3.6	3.0	22.8	25.8	55.2	120.0
All	11.6	9.4	5.4	6.5	49.6	46.7	80.8	210.0
Percent	5.5	4.5	2.6	3.1	23.6	22.2	38.5	100.0
Serv. Units	243	84	29	112				

auxiliaries contribute two-thirds, that is, 3.6 hours. Is this appropriate? Are they adequately trained to perform this function?

By associating time distribution with units of service provided, one can measure time per unit of service and ultimately cost per service for considerations of efficiency.

All of the foregoing indicators of current status become a basis for future planning. In view of the relative inattention currently given to CDC activities, for example, a doubling of CDC effort might be proposed. The additional burden would presumably fall mainly on auxiliary staff. There seems to be plenty of idle time, however, to accommodate the possible 3.6 hours of additional direct service time required, along with corresponding increases in supportive activities and travel. In other circumstances the data may suggest the need to reassign tasks or to alter the personnel mix.

MACRO- AND MICROANALYSIS IN PERSPECTIVE

The health planner must determine the extent to which professionally determined needs are to be addressed, along with the felt needs that are already being satisfied through effective demand. The resulting projections of services utilization must be associated with requisite skills and activities that translate into personnel requirements. At times these considerations take place at the macrolevel of policy analysis regarding the balance in numbers of personnel of various types and the consequent adequacy of training capacity. Other planners operate at the services interface where the principal issue is the efficient and effective utilization of personnel to satisfy the objectives of a local community project. Microanalyses of the latter type are hardly divorced from macroanalysis, however, for realistic macropolicy decisions must consider the aggregation of jobs to be done and the optimal organization of tasks to perform them. To ask how many nurses are needed is an idle question until service loads have been

established, along with determination of the extent to which nurses have, or should
be provided, the skills associated with the requisite services.

REFERENCES

1. Hornby, P., et al., *Guidelines for Health Manpower Planning: A Coursebook*, Geneva:
World Health Organization, 1980.
2. Department of International Health, Johns Hopkins University, *The Functional Analysis
of Health Needs and Services*, Ch. 3, pp. 153–238, New Delhi: Asia Publishing House, 1976.

PRIMARY READINGS

Department of International Health, Johns Hopkins University, *The Functional Analysis of
Health Needs and Services*, Ch. 3, pp. 153–238, New Delhi: Asia Publishing House,
1976. Detailed description of methods of job analysis for realigning tasks and determin-
ing training needs.
Hall, T., and A. Mejia (eds.), *Health Manpower Planning: Principles, Methods, Issues*,
Geneva: World Health Organization, 1978. Comprehensive overview of national health
personnel planning.
Hornby, P., et al., *Guidelines for Health Manpower Planning: A Coursebook*, Geneva: World
Health Organization, 1980. This practical follow-up to the Hall-Mejia volume employs
a self-instruction format for implementation.

SECONDARY READINGS

Golladay, F. L., et al., *Health Manpower Planning and Efficient Health Manpower Utilization*,
Health Economics Research Center, Madison: University of Wisconsin, 1972.
Golladay, F. L., et al., "Policy Planning for Mid-level Health Workers: Economic Potentials
and Barriers to Change," *Inquiry*, 13:80–89, 1976.
Smith, K. R., et al., "Analytic Framework and Measurement Strategies for Investigating
Optimal Staff in Medical Practice," *Operations Research*, 24:5,1976.
Verderese, M. L., and L. M. Turnbull, *The Traditional Birth Attendant in Maternal and Child
Health and Family Planning: A Guide to Her Training and Utilization*, WHO Offset
Publication No. 18, Geneva: World Health Organization, 1975.

20

Cost-Benefit and Cost-Effectiveness Analysis of Health Programs

ALAN L. SORKIN

Where several candidate programs must compete for limited resources, comparison of the costs of each in relation to potential benefits gives a rational basis for priority setting. Programs with diverse objectives are compared by means of cost-benefit analysis, whereas cost-effectiveness analysis is used to evaluate alternative ways of reaching the same objective.

Comparisons involving different objectives require use of a common measure of benefit. Most often benefits are specified in monetary terms[1] and each program is then evaluated in terms of the dollars of benefits produced per dollar of expenditure.[2] All programs with such benefit-cost ratios exceeding one are worthy of consideration, and those with the highest ratios are assigned priority in the use of limited funds. This approach is useful in determining, for example, whether an area would be more profitably employed in growing pineapples or in providing a tourist resort. Comparison of the benefits of health programs in relation to educational endeavors is more problematic. Even within the health field programs yielding different results in different target populations are difficult to evaluate in cost-benefit terms.

Cost-effectiveness analysis is most often the technique of choice in the health field. Sometimes it is conducted to establish the least costly means of achieving a defined objective, for example, protecting a target population of ten thousand infants against measles. In other instances cost-effectiveness calculations are made to derive the maximum benefit that can be achieved from a fixed budget. Thus the question may be, How many children can be immunized for twenty thousand dollars?

GENERAL FEATURES OF THE ANALYSIS

To illustrate the cost-benefit approach, assume one had to make a choice as to which of the six programs outlined on page 262 is to be funded.

If the total budget available for these programs is $50,000 and the sole criterion for project selection is to maximize benefit per dollar of expenditure (the benefit/cost ratio), then only the measles vaccination program, irrigation project, and port dredging activities should be funded. However if $100,000 were available, all the projects except the crime prevention program could be funded.

Program	Expected Benefits	Expected Costs	Benefit/Cost Ratio
Measles Vaccination	$110,000	$10,000	11/1
Irrigation Project	250,000	28,000	9/1
Dredging of Port	70,000	9,000	8/1
Maternal and Child Health Program	210,000	35,000	6/1
Primary Schooling	50,000	12,000	4/1
Crime Prevention	120,000	60,000	2/1

Present Value

While planners and administrators must decide whether or not to initiate a project in the present, the project itself often yields benefits for many years in the future. In order to determine the *present value* of these benefits one must discount them using an appropriate formula. For example, suppose a planner is considering the implementation of an irrigation project. The project is expected to result in an increase of farm income in a particular region (the measure of benefits) for a period of twenty years. Let us assume that this annual benefit is $100,000. Thus, the present value of total expected benefits (ΣB) is equal to:

$$\Sigma B = \frac{100,000}{(1+r)} + \frac{100,000}{(1+r)^2} + \frac{100,000}{(1+r)^3} + \frac{100,000}{(1+r)^4} \cdots\cdots + \frac{100,000}{(1+r)^{20}}$$

Similarly, if the construction of the irrigation facilities is expected to take five years at a cost of $50,000 per year, the present value of total expected costs (ΣC) is equal to:

$$\Sigma C = \frac{50,000}{(1+r)} + \frac{50,000}{(1+r)^2} + \cdots\cdots + \frac{50,000}{(1+r)^5}$$

The present value of total benefits is divided by the present value of total costs to obtain the *benefit/cost ratio*. The result depends, of course, upon the discount rate *(r)* that is used. The *discounting procedure*, which recognizes that benefits or costs which accrue in the future have a lower present value than an equivalent dollar amount today, provides a link between the present value of benefit and costs and expected future values.

Microanalysis

One theoretic problem with cost-benefit analysis is that it operates from a partial framework and is basically a tool for microanalysis. Thus, it is assumed that the programs being analyzed will only have a marginal impact on the economic, social, or demographic fabric of society.[3] This assumption may be called into question where the incidence and prevalence of certain infectious and parasitic diseases is very high. Thus, if malaria were to be completely eradicated, there would be major demographic impacts on society, particularly fifteen to thirty years after the health intervention. Without a more sophisticated analytic framework capable of considering such macroeconomic impacts, the public policy decisions based on the results of a microeconomic cost-benefit analysis may be misleading.[4]

SPECIAL CONSIDERATIONS

There are a number of other factors that must be considered when undertaking a cost-benefit analysis. These include (1) effect of inflation, (2) risk and uncertainty, (3) distribution of benefits, and (4) intangibles. Moreover health program analyses have their own peculiar difficulties.

Inflation

Inflation can be appropriately handled by either of two methods: estimate all future benefits and costs in constant prices (that is, simply assume no inflation); or estimate all future costs and benefits in current (that is, inflated) prices, and use as the discount rate an estimate of the prevailing rate of interest.

Risk and Uncertainty

One approach to dealing with uncertainty in a benefit-cost framework is to treat estimated benefits and costs as random variables that can be described by some probability distribution. Suppose, for instance, that an analysis of historic flood patterns suggests that the discounted benefits from a flood control project will range from 0 (if there is no flood) to $100 million (if the worst possible flood occurs). In addition the same analysis would also reveal the probability that floods of intermediate severity would be experienced. Suppose for illustrative purposes that we can identify only four possible outcomes, as well as the probability of their occurrence:

Value of Discounted Benefits	Probability of Occurrence
0	0.3
$ 30 million	0.4
$ 50 million	0.2
$100 million	0.1

The method of determining the expected value of benefits when this type of information is available is as follows:

$$\text{Expected Value of Benefits} = (0 \times .3) + (30 \text{ million} \times .4) + (50 \text{ million} \times .2) + (100 \text{ million} \times .1) = \$32 \text{ million.}$$

The primary difficulty with this method of dealing with uncertainty is the lack of data necessary to determine the probability distribution.

Distribution of Benefits

A third issue which the decision maker must consider is the distribution of benefits. Suppose a planner or administrator is faced with the following situation:

Project	B/C Ratio	Gains to Poverty Population
A	8/1	20,000
B	7/1	25,000
C	5/1	29,000
D	2.5/1	32,000
E	1.5/1	34,000

In this hypothetical example, the most efficient project, using cost-benefit criteria and assuming a fixed budget, is Project A with a benefit/cost ratio (B/C ratio) of 8/1, but the project with the greatest gain to the poverty population is Project E—a project that has the lowest benefit/cost ratio of any of the five projects considered. Given this situation, the analyst must subjectively weigh efficiency and distributional considerations. However, an explicit formulation of the information available will make the alternatives as clear as possible.

Intangibles

A further consideration is the allowance for intangibles. For example, in a Ford Foundation labor force program the primary objective was to reduce the number of dropouts from the St. Louis public schools. The expected direct benefit of such a program was an increase in the expected lifetime income of high school graduates in comparison with high school dropouts. Included among the intangible benefits were improved self-esteem of students, increased social and political consciousness, and reduction in the incidence of crime and delinquency. Intangible factors are difficult, if not impossible, to quantify, particularly in dollar terms. One of the primary problems with the inclusion or consideration of intangibles is that they are sometimes used to justify inefficient projects.

Health Applications: Direct and Indirect Costs

In cost-benefit analysis of particular health or disease control programs the total cost of the disease serves as a measure of the potential benefits derived if that disease or condition could be prevented or eliminated.[5] Total cost comprises three elements: (1) loss of production, (2) expenditures for medical treatment, and (3) pain, discomfort, and suffering that accompany illness. Because economists concentrate on measuring the first two components, the third is generally neglected as a result of lack of data and appropriate methodology. However, pain and suffering are important intangible costs of illness.

Expenditures for medical care to treat a disease (or injury) are not the total costs of that disease. The economic costs of illness comprise at least two components: direct costs and indirect costs. *Direct costs* are the expenditures for health services attributable to the disease, such as costs for in-patient care, physicians' fees, and drugs. These expenditures reflect the use of resources. Indirect costs are associated with the loss of output attributable to the disease as a result of premature death or disability.

Thus, the total (direct plus indirect) costs of a disease serve as a measure of the benefits derived from a program that would achieve eradication or control of the disease. In a cost-benefit calculation the comparison is between the contemplated additional expenditures for health services and the anticipated reduction in existing costs. This is the essential conceptual framework.

Two categories of costs are omitted—transfer payments and taxes. When income loss is used as a measure of indirect costs, adding pension or relief payments would be double-counting. As for tax payments, it would be double-counting to add income tax losses to losses of earnings, and triple-counting if the tax receipts were used for public payments for health care.

Utilizing information on the direct and indirect costs of illness in the United States in 1972, Barbara Cooper and Dorothy Rice computed the total costs of illness for sixteen disease categories or conditions.[6] For example, the total cost of diseases of the digestive system in 1972 was $17 billion. Of this total, $11 billion was accounted for by treatment costs, $2.6 billion was due to morbidity, and $3.2 billion resulted from premature mortality. The total cost of a number of diseases or conditions is presented in Table 20.1.

In 1975 the direct cost of ill health in the United States was approximately $119 billion. The cost of morbidity was estimated at $58 billion, and the cost of mortality at about $88 billion.[7] Thus, in 1975 the total cost of illness was more than $265 billion, about 17 percent of the gross national product (GNP). Of that total, 55.2 percent was indirect costs and 44.8 percent was direct costs. If recent trends continue, it has been estimated that by the year 2000 direct costs will be $416.4 billion (1975 dollars), and indirect costs will be $176.7 billion.[8]

To calculate the economic loss of premature mortality, one multiplies the number of deaths by the expected value of an individual's discounted future earnings.[5] This method of calculation must consider the changing pattern of earnings at successive ages, varying the labor force participation rates, the work-life expectancy for different age and sex groups, and the appropriate discount rate to convert a stream of costs or benefits into its present worth.

In order to accurately estimate the present value of future losses resulting from morbidity, longitudinal data on the patterns of illness by diagnosis are required. A certain illness that affects an individual in youth may affect future productivity and earnings. Some illnesses leave a person partially or totally disabled; others have a minimal effect on subsequent health status. If one can obtain longitudinal data relating to morbidity patterns by diagnosis, the analyst can assess the total economic impact of morbidity from specific illnesses. Since longitudinal data are not generally available, estimates are usually made by multiplying individuals' annual earnings by the fraction of the year they are unavailable for employment. This procedure assumes no loss in future earning power due to the illness.

Table 20.1

TOTAL COST OF ILLNESS IN THE UNITED STATES, BY DIAGNOSIS, 1972[a]

Diagnosis	Amount (in Millions)	Percentage Distribution
Infective and Parasitic Diseases	$ 3,443	1.8
Neoplasms	17,367	9.2
Endocrine, Nutritional and Metabolic Diseases	5,939	3.1
Diseases of the Blood and Blood Forming Organs	921	0.5
Mental Disorders	13,917	7.4
Diseases of the Nervous System and Sense Organs	10,931	5.8
Diseases of the Circulatory System	40,060	21.2
Diseases of the Respiratory System	16,454	8.7
Diseases of the Digestive System	17,487	9.3
Diseases of the Genito-Urinary System	6,456	3.4
Complications of Pregnancy, Childbirth and the Puerperium	2,932	1.6
Diseases of the Skin and Subcutaneous Tissue	2,052	1.1
Diseases of the Musculo-Skeletal System and Connective Tissue	8,948	4.7
Congenital Anomalies	1,903	1.0
Accidents, Poisoning and Violence	26,678	14.1
Other	13,924	7.0
Total	188,789	100.0

[a]Present value of future earnings is calculated at a 4 percent discount rate.

Source: Barbara Cooper and Dorothy Rice, "The Economic Cost of Illness Revisited," Social Security Bulletin, February 1976, p. 31.

METHODOLOGIC ISSUES

The Discount Rate

As indicated previously, a given amount of money has different values when it is realized or spent at alternative periods in the future. The process of discounting converts a stream of benefits or costs into its present value. The higher the rate of discount the lower the present value of costs or benefits. Discounting is particularly important when evaluating programs in which benefits or costs will accrue for a long period of time such as thirty to fifty years after the initial outlay.

What rate of discount should be utilized in benefit-cost studies? The discount rate should represent the value of the funds in alternative uses (opportunity cost). If one is considering a public program, it can be maintained that the appropriate discount rate is the long-term bond rate. This is because the long-term bond rate represents the cost of long-term borrowing for the government. A different view is that government projects should not be undertaken unless they are as efficient or productive as those operating in the private sector; as such, the proper rate should be that charged by commercial banks for business loans. In 1983 the long-term bond rate in the United States was 8 percent, while the prime interest rate was 11 percent. Thus a moderate range of possible choices of discount rates exists. Moreover one could argue that neither rate is appropriate. The discount rate should balance the productivity of an investment and the reluctance of society to sacrifice current for future consumption.[9] Given the uncertainty in the literature, it is sensible to use a range of discount rates so that the planner can determine the sensitivity of the benefit-cost ratio to the choice of discount rate.

Rate of Employment

Even if the entire working age population were in a perfect state of health, some persons would be unemployed or absent from the labor force. A portion of the population is unwilling or unable to find jobs as a result of such factors as lack of demand for labor or structural imbalances in the labor market. Estimates of losses in output due to death or illness assume that the persons affected have the same employment and labor force experience as those in the same age and sex categories who are physically or mentally healthy. For example, assume that the average earnings of males aged thirty-five to forty-four is $12,000 with a labor force participation rate of 96 percent and an unemployment rate of 5 percent. Thus, the expected earnings of a thirty-five to forty-four-year-old male is $12,000 (.96) (.95), or $10,920. This assumes that the employment potential of persons cured of illness is the same as those who were never ill. In a severely depressed economy in which unemployment rates are 15 to 25 percent, the indirect costs of illness would be far less than under conditions of nearly full employment.

Homemakers' Services

Earnings and labor force participation rates of women are generally lower than those of males. Thus the cost of illnesses primarily affecting women would be greatly underestimated if only market earnings were used in the calculation of indirect costs. As a result the economic value of homemakers' services must also be included in the computation of indirect costs.

In an early study by Rice,[10] the value of homemakers' services was based on the earnings of a domestic servant. Most observers considered this method of valuation resulted in an underestimate of the value of those services. More recently other approaches to the problem have been developed, including the opportunity-cost and market-cost methods of valuation.[11] Briefly, the opportunity-cost approach assumes the economic value of unpaid work to be at least as much as the wage rate the same person would obtain in the marketplace. The wage rate would be a function of age, education, and on-the-job training. In essence if a woman chooses homemaking over employment, the value of homemaking must be equal to or greater than that of foregone employment.[12] One criticism of this method of valuing homemakers' services is that it would not be consistent with the approach used for the employed population. In the latter case one's present activity is valued as opposed to what one could be doing. A physician in research or academic medicine, for example, could earn much more in private practice, yet only the earnings as a researcher or teacher are counted.

The market value approach values each duty a homemaker performs. Based on a time-motion study of homemakers, the relevant market wages for various services performed are multiplied by the number of hours reported for performing that service.[13] That figure represents an estimate of the cost of replacing the homemaker with employed individuals who would do the same work. It takes into consideration the homemaker's age, number of children, and age of youngest child. The psychic value of a homemaker to her family or society is not considered in this calculation. An estimate of the latter would be highly subjective.

Expected Earnings or Willingness to Pay

There have been objections to the "human capital" approach to cost-benefit analysis that values one's life in terms of expected earnings. This is partly because it assumes that changes in earnings streams bear a direct relationship to what society values in terms of health program outputs. Because of income differences men are valued more highly than women and those in the prime working ages more highly than the very young and very old.[6]

Economists have begun to reflect upon difficulties with this approach to benefit measurement. In particular, they are troubled by the lack of a direct relation between the "costs" of illness (as defined previously) and the preferences of individuals as quantified in their willingness to pay. This has led to the view that program benefits must be defined as reductions in the *risk* of mortality or morbidity, since the identity of the program beneficiaries is usually not known in advance and many, if not all, persons are potential beneficiaries.[14] Then the most appropriate benefit measure is assumed to be based upon individual willingness to pay for the reductions in the risk of morbidity and/or mortality provided by a program. As a practical matter, though, it is very difficult to develop such a benefit measure. Direct surveying of individuals to determine their willingness to pay is a costly process and requires respondents who are well informed about the nature of the benefits and able to understand probabilistic concepts. While surveys have indicated fairly reasonable results in uncomplicated situations, such as those in which benefits can be described simply as a reduced probability of death, their usefulness in cases in which the benefits are more complex is questionable.

An alternative to surveys is to use observed market behavior, such as the amount of additional wages that must be paid to attract workers to risky occupations.[15] This, too, has only been applied to the simple case of reduced mortality risk.

Developing Country Circumstances

The data requirements to undertake a sophisticated benefit-cost study are severe. One requires information on earnings by age and sex; labor force participation and unemployment rates by age and sex; life tables, which are used to calculate the probability of living to retirement age; information on direct expenditures for health services; as well as data on the distribution of deaths and morbidity for the disease or diseases under consideration. Much of this information has never been collected in developing countries, forcing planners to make approximations or even guesses at the magnitudes of the parameters involved.

Moreover, agricultural and other subsistence level workers in many developing countries are often not a part of the cash economy, although they may occasionally undertake some market transactions. Nevertheless, they do engage in production and consumption of commodities, and their premature mortality and morbidity have economic consequences. With a significant amount of the labor force in developing countries engaged in subsistence agriculture, the measurement of the economic cost of disease for this group is a major and important challenge.

Finally, there is considerable evidence that chronic unemployment exists in many developing countries, especially in the agricultural regions. This may amount to as much as one-fourth of the labor force.[16] To determine the value of lost production due to premature mortality and morbidity given unemployment of this magnitude is an extremely difficult task, especially if it is seasonal. An epidemic during the harvest season could be devastating, whereas occurrence during a relatively slack period might have only minor economic repercussions.

COST-BENEFIT ANALYSIS OF FAMILY PLANNING PROGRAMS: A CASE STUDY

Cost-benefit analysis has been applied to determine the efficiency of family planning programs in a number of developing countries. Besides the present value of the unborn child's consumption, this takes into account government savings on educational expenses for that child, plus the fact that workers in the existing population would produce more per dollar paid to them because, with fewer people being born, more public funds will have been available to invest in the health or education of each of them prior to their joining the labor force. (See Figure 20.1.)

One example of a cost-benefit analysis using the preceding approach is presented in Table 20.2. In this example discounted benefits exceed discounted costs by a considerable margin, indicating that the program is probably a good investment, although funding priorities depend on the benefits and costs of other worthy programs. Notice that the choice of discount rate does affect the magnitude of benefits and costs.

One serious problem with the application of cost-benefit analysis to a reduction in births is the exclusion of psychic income which parents receive from child rearing.[17]

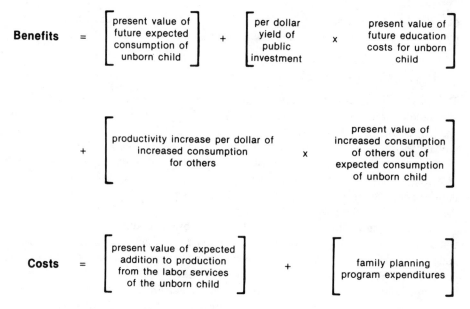

Figure 20.1   Human investment approach to cost-benefit analysis to family planning programs

Moreover, particularly in agrarian societies, parents may have a relatively large number of children to assure themselves of adequate support in their old age. Since these countries lack social security systems, older persons must rely on their children for financial assistance.

COST-EFFECTIVENESS ANALYSIS

Special Features

Most of the techniques and difficulties of cost analysis raised in connection with cost-benefit considerations are equally applicable to cost-effectiveness analysis. The unique feature of the latter is that costs are calculated and alternative ways are compared for achieving a specific set of objectives. The aim is not just to use funds efficiently; a defined outcome must be realized as well.

The result is not generally expressed in dollars but in terms of a particular health objective, such as years of life saved, number of cases of blindness prevented, number of births averted, or number of addicts successfully treated. Such indicators can be at least as meaningful in the health sector as monetary measures, are more readily determined, and avoid the questionable assumptions that must be made in translating benefits into dollar terms. As in the case of cost-benefit analysis program costs are summarized into a single number, benefits are stated in another number (though not necessarily in the same units), ratios of the two are formed, and simple decision rules for comparison are applied.[18] Several disease control programs might be compared, for example, to determine which one incurs the lowest cost per death averted. The

Table 20.2

COST-BENEFIT ANALYSIS OF FAMILY PLANNING
IN EGYPT DURING THE 1960s*

Benefits	Using 10 Percent Discount Rate	Using 15 Percent Discount Rate
1. Consumption	222-351	109-206
2. Wage productivity effect	16-21	9-14
3. Public savings effect	37	24
4. Total	275-409	142-244
Costs		
5. Productivity	79-91	24-31
6. Family planning services	4-20	
7. Total	83-111	28-51
8. Differences between benefits and costs	164-326	91-216
9. Benefit/cost ratios	2.5-4.9	2.8-8.7

*Numbers are Egyptian pounds per prevented birth.

Source: George Zaidan, "The Costs and Benefits of Family Planning Programs,"
World Bank Occasional Paper No. 12 (Washington, D.C.:   World Bank,
1971).

method is particularly useful, therefore, in the analysis of preventive health programs
addressing different problems, and perhaps different target populations.[19]

Example of a Cost-Effectiveness Study

In rural Punjab State in India, three experimental groups of villages were identified on
the basis of the type of service provided.[20] Persons in the first group of villages were
provided with both nutrition and health care services (NUTHC). Those in the second
group of villages received nutrition services only (NUT), and those in the third group
received health care only (HC). Table 20.3 summarizes the cost-effectiveness ratios
obtained with respect to four outcomes of interest in the three experimental groups.

The lowest cost per perinatal death averted was found to be $7.75 in the NUT
experimental group, whereas the HC package of services was most cost-effective in
averting infant ($25.35) and older child ($30.65) deaths. NUT services were more

Table 20.3

COST-EFFECTIVENESS RATIOS FOR THE THREE EXPERIMENTAL GROUPS
(Indices Created by Equating Lowest Cost in Any Category to 1)

I (a)   Cost[1] per death averted

	Perinatal		Infant		1-3 Year Old	
NUTHC	1.3	($9.85)	1.5	($37.35)	3.3	($101.45)
NUT	1.0	($7.75)	1.4	($36.40)	2.3	($71.75)
HC	1.8	($14.15)	1.0	($25.35)	1.0	($30.65)

   (b)   Cost[2] per day of illness averted

NUTHC			1.4	($0.56)	1.1	($0.39)
NUT			*		*	
HC			1.0	($0.40)	1.0	($0.35)

II (a)   Cost[3] per additional cm growth
                       at 36 months

NUTHC	1.0	($26.25)
NUT	1.2	($30.40)
HC	*	

   (b)   Cost[3] per additional percentage
              point increase in psychomotor
              development scores over the first
                    three years of life

NUTHC	1.0	($5.05)
NUT	2.7	($13.60)
HC	*	

[1] using a proportion of total program costs equal to the age specific mortality rate

[2] using all health care costs minus costs counted under mortality

[3] using all nutrition costs minus costs counted under mortality

*small or no effects produced large or infinite cost-effectiveness ratios.

Source: Parker, Robert L., et al., "Evaluation of Program Utilization and Cost
         Effectiveness," in Arnfried Kielmann, et al., Child and Maternal Health
         Services in Rural India, The Narangwal Experiment; Vol. 1: Integrated
         Nutrition and Health Care, Baltimore: The Johns Hopkins Press, 1983, p.
         254.

than twice as costly per one- to three-year-old death averted ($72), while NUTHC
services were at least three times as costly ($101).

    The number of days of illness due to nine selected symptoms was used as the
morbidity indicator. The table indicates that only villages with health care services
produced any reduction in days of morbidity. In infants the cost per day of illness

averted was $0.40 in HC villages and $0.56 in NUTHC villages. For children one to three years of age the costs were $0.35 and $0.39, respectively.

The NUTHC experimental group of villages had the best cost-effectiveness ratios for both growth indicators. Nutritional costs per additional centimeter of growth attained by three years of age in comparison to control were $26 in NUTHC and $30 in NUT villages. Costs per percentage point of gain in psychomotor scores was $5 for NUTHC villages and $14 for NUT villages.

In summary, the analysis shows that infant and one- to three-year-old mortality are decreased with least cost by health care alone, but perinatal mortality is prevented for the least cost through nutrition services. To decrease morbidity, health care alone is the most cost-effective approach, but increases in growth and development are obtained for the least cost through the combined program. Which combination of services is to be preferred overall depends upon subjective judgments regarding the relative importance of each of the outcome indicators. Unless one- to three-year-old mortality is of overriding importance, however, it appears that comprehensive care (NUTHC) is most attractive in producing multiple benefits at little more than the minimum cost required to achieve a single benefit.

SUMMARY

The cost of ill health comprises three elements—direct costs, indirect costs (premature mortality and morbidity), and pain and suffering. In a cost-benefit exercise, a comparison is made between expected program expenditures and anticipated reduction in the cost of illness (the measure of benefits).

A number of methodologic issues must be considered when carrying out a cost-benefit study of a health program. These include the choice of discount rate, determination of rates of employment, and valuation of homemakers' services.

Cost-benefit analysis has been criticized for assuming that variations in expected lifetime income are directly related to what society values in terms of the output of health programs. This results in lower values being assigned, for example, to females and members of minority groups because their incomes are relatively low.

The "willingness to pay" approach to valuing the output of health services does not suffer from the previously mentioned weakness, but requires a highly sophisticated populace in order to obtain even minimally useful results.

Cost-effectiveness analysis is a less demanding alternative for evaluating health programs. This method examines cost differences among several potential programs for achieving a specified outcome. It has the advantage that output is not expressed in dollars. Thus, the analyst does not have to deal with the thorny problem of determining the money value of human life.

REFERENCES

1. Crystal, Royal, and Agnes Brewster, "Cost-Benefit and Cost-Effectiveness in the Health Field: An Introduction," *Inquiry*, 3,4:3–13, December 1966.

2. Smith, Warren, "Cost-Effectiveness and Cost-Benefit Analyses for Public Health Programs," *Public Health Reports*, 83,11:899–906, November 1968.

3. Dunlop, David, "Benefit-Cost Analysis: A Review of Its Applicability in Policy Analysis for Delivering Health Services," *Social Science and Medicine*, 9,3:133–139, March 1975.

4. Barlow, Robin, *The Economic Effects of Malaria Eradication*, Research Series No. 15, Ann Arbor: University of Michigan, School of Public Health, 1968.

5. Weisbrod, Burton, *Economics of Public Health*, Philadelphia: University of Pennsylvania Press, 1961.

6. Cooper, Barbara, and Dorothy Rice, "The Economic Cost of Illness Revisited," *Social Security Bulletin*, 39,2:21–36, February 1976.

7. Berk, A., L. C. Paringer and S. J. Mushkin, *The Economic Cost of Illness, 1975*, Washington: Georgetown University Public Services Laboratory, 1977, p. 37.

8. Mushkin, S. J., et al., "Cost of Disease and Illness in the United States in the Year 2000," *Public Health Reports*, Supplement, 93,5:494–588, September–October 1978.

9. Hufschmidt, Maynard, *Standards and Criteria for Formulating and Evaluating Federal Water Resources Developments*, Washington: U.S. Bureau of the Budget, 1961, p. 11; and Morglin, Stephen, "Economic Factors Affecting System Design," in Arthur Maass, et al., *Design of Water Resources Systems* Cambridge, MA: Harvard University Press, 1962, p. 194.

10. Rice, Dorothy, "Estimating the Cost of Illness," *American Journal of Public Health*, 57,3:424–440, March 1967.

11. Broady, Wendyce, *Economic Value of a Housewife*, Research and Statistics Note No. 9, Washington: Social Security Administration, Office of Research and Statistics, 1975.

12. Gronau, Reuben, "The Measurement of Output of the Nonmarket Sector: The Evaluation of Housewives' Time," in Milton Moss (ed.), *The Measurement of Economic and Social Performance*, New York: National Bureau of Economic Research, 1973, pp. 168 and 171.

13. Walker, Katherine, and William Gauger, "The Dollar Value of Household Work," *Information Bulletin*, 60:16, 1973.

14. Schelling, Thomas, "The Life You Save May Be Your Own," in S. B. Chase (ed.), *Problems in Public Expenditure*, Washington: The Brookings Institution, 1968.

15. Thaler, R., and S. Rosen, "The Value of Saving a Life: Evidence from the Labor Market," in N. Terleckyj (ed.), *Household Production and Consumption*, New York: Columbia University Press, 1976.

16. Buchanan, N. S., and H. S. Ellis, *Approaches to Economic Development*, New York: Twentieth Century Fund, 1955, p. 45.

17. Blandy, R., "The Welfare Analysis of Fertility Reduction," *The Economic Journal*, 84,333:109–129, March 1974.

18. Shepard, Donald, and Mark Thompson, "First Principles of Cost-Effectiveness Analysis in Health," *Public Health Reports*, 94,6:535–543, November–December 1979.

19. Lane, J. R., et al., "Economic Impact of Preventive Medicine," in *Preventive Medicine, U.S.A.*, New York: Prodist, 1976, pp. 675–714.

20. Parker, Robert L., et al., "Evaluation of Program Utilization and Cost Effectiveness," in Arnfried A. Kielmann, et al., *Child and Maternal Health Services in Rural India, The Narangwal Experiment; Vol. 1: Integrated Nutrition and Health Care*, Baltimore: The Johns Hopkins University Press, 1983.

PRIMARY READINGS

Mills, A., and M. Thomas, *Economic Evaluation of Health Programmes in Developing Countries*, Evaluation and Planning Centre for Health Care, London: London School of

Hygiene and Tropical Medicine, 1984. A thorough exposition of both cost-benefit and cost-effectiveness analysis with special attention to the health and methodologic problems of developing countries.

Reynolds, Jack, and K. Celeste Gaspari, *Cost-Effectiveness Analysis*, Pricor Monograph Series: Methods Paper 2, Chevy Chase, MD: Center for Human Services, 1985. A nontechnical presentation of the fundamentals of cost-effectiveness analysis with simplified examples from the health field.

SECONDARY READINGS

Barlow, Robin, *The Economic Effects of Malaria Eradication*, Research Series No. 15, Ann Arbor: University of Michigan School of Public Health, 1968.

Creese, A. L., and R. H. Henderson, "Cost-Benefit Analysis and Immunization Programmes in Developing Countries," *WHO Bulletin*, 58,3:491–497, 1980.

Dunlop, David, "Benefit-Cost Analysis: A Review of Its Applicability in Policy Analysis for Delivering Health Services," *Social Science and Medicine*, 9,3:133–139, 1975.

Feingold, Alan, "Cost-Effectiveness of Screening for Tuberculosis in a General Medical Clinic," *Public Health Reports*, 90, 6:544–547, 1975.

Isaac, M. K., and R. L. Kapur, "A Cost-Effectiveness Analysis of Three Different Methods of Psychiatric Case Finding in the General Population," *British Journal of Psychiatry*, 137:540–546, 1980.

McNeil, B. J., M. Thompson and S. J. Adelstein, "Cost- Effectiveness Calculations for the Diagnosis and Treatment of Tuberculosis Meningitis," *European Journal of Nuclear Medicine*, 5,3:271–276, 1980.

Shepard, Donald, and Mark Thompson, "First Principles of Cost-Effectiveness Analysis in Health," *Public Health Reports*, 94,6:535–543, 1979.

21

Synthesis of Health Needs and Resources

WILLIAM A. REINKE

The planning approach we have advocated begins with the identification of major health problems and determination of their magnitude in relation to various population groups to be served. This permits establishment of priorities for allocating limited resources to defined service functions. Resource allocation involves decisions about personnel, facilities, and finances, as well as their organization into an adequately efficient, effective, and equitable health services delivery system. Each of these aspects of planning has been covered separately. In practice, of course, the dynamics of planning does not permit the piecemeal approach we have found useful for purposes of exposition. Enumeration of service needs is little more than an academic exercise apart from concern for access to bases for service delivery. Provision of facilities is in turn meaningless unless they can be adequately staffed. Then decisions about staffing and associated support have obvious budgeting implications.

Moreover, no neat formulas have been derived for bringing the various considerations together into an assuredly optimal services mix.[1] No one can say for sure (and be believed) that in a specified population with $5 per capita to spend on health services, the way to maximize the health status of the population is to spend $1.29 on maternity care, $0.83 on immunizations, $1.16 on potable water, and so on.

This is not to denigrate the importance of documentation of need and objective analysis of alternative means of satisfying it. The point being made is that even under the most favorable circumstances the setting of priorities and objectives, as well as the choice of programs for fulfilling them, is bound in the end to be somewhat arbitrary. Furthermore, when objectives are established arbitrarily, there is no guarantee that they will be mutually compatible.

This concluding chapter addresses these two points. First, after gathering as much hard data as is feasible and organizing it in the most intelligible form, we consider ways of making the remaining arbitrariness as rational and analytic as possible. The seemingly reasonable conclusions are then examined for internal consistency to ensure their mutual compatibility.

TRANSLATING FACTS INTO PRIORITIES

The health needs in various functional areas can be quantified for a defined population by means of community surveys, knowledge of the demographic characteristics of the population, and application of professional standards as described in Chapter 18. Likewise, methods of functional analysis, including sampling of work patterns presented in Chapter 19, can determine the extent to which services are being provided to meet the specified needs. Actual results from such an exercise carried out in Punjab State, India,[2] have been reproduced in part in Table 21.1 in terms of a base population of 100,000.

The analytic approach makes evident the varying shortfalls in service delivery among functional categories, but the evidence serves to highlight questions rather than to provide immediate answers regarding program priorities. For example, is the 52 percent shortfall in meeting patient needs for medical care of similar importance for the government health center as the 51 percent deficit in malaria surveillance visits? On the one hand it could be argued that the medical relief deficiency is more significant because it involves a larger absolute number of service contacts, while on the other hand it might be contended that the inadequacy of the malaria services should be of greater concern because the health center alone has the capacity for remedial action, whereas numerous providers exist in the private sector to meet curative needs.

Obviously, any comparison must also consider the cost and difficulty of providing additional services as well as their likely effectiveness and the amount of benefit to be expected if they are effective. Would the vast increase in visits apparently needed

Table 21.1

ILLUSTRATIVE PARTIAL COMPARISON OF ANNUAL HEALTH NEEDS AND SERVICES
PER 100,000 POPULATION--
BASED UPON DATA FROM PUNJAB STATE, INDIA

Function	Service Category	Service Quantity		Service Deficit	
		Need	Received	Quantity	Percent
Medical Care	Patient Visits	733,000	351,000	382,000	52
Maternal and Child Health	Maternity Care School Health Contacts	32,800 12,500	15,000 1,000	17,800 11,500	54 92
Family Planning	Motivation Visits Acceptors	40,400 1,010	45,000 800	+4,600 210	+11 21
Communicable Diseases Control	Malaria Surveillance Visits Malaria Blood Smears	401,000 24,060	195,000 14,000	206,000 10,060	51 19
Environmental Sanitation	Visits for Water, Drainage	54,100	1,200	52,900	98

Source: Adapted from The Functional Analysis of Health Needs and Services, Table 4.4, page 266.

for advice on water and drainage, for example, be effective in inducing real changes in community conditions, and by how much would such changes improve the health status of the population affected?

Finally, we must recall that the calculated needs are based upon assumptions regarding appropriate standards that are in many respects arbitrary. As a case in point, the achieved level of family planning motivation visits appears adequate according to the standards employed, but their quality or quantity was evidently still insufficient to yield the targeted number of acceptors. A general review of the figures suggests that for most of the functions involved there is need for simply increasing the input of services. Concerning family planning, however, the indication that a service input somewhat in excess of the standard is falling short of the acceptor target gives evidence that a qualitative change in methods might be introduced.

While the data sharpen the issues, a means for seeking agreement on their resolution is still needed. The nominal group and Delphi techniques (Chapter 15) have each proved useful for obtaining group consensus through systematic organization of informed judgment. Either approach would be reasonable in the present situation. For purposes of discussion we illustrate the possibility of using both together.

Let us suppose that a panel of five individuals is assembled to grapple with the questions of priority. To begin with, it is easier to place the service gaps of Table 21.1 in rank order, rather than trying to score each on, say, a scale from 0 to 100. The nominal group technique first permits the listing of additional items for priority attention, even if relevant data are limited or absent, and then calls for the ranking of the items as we have suggested. We suppose that the process adds four items to the eight listed in Table 21.1, producing twelve in all, as shown in Table 21.2. We further suppose that all members of the panel are asked to choose what they consider to be the top eight, giving eight points to the first priority, seven to the second, and so on. Illustrative results are given in Table 21.2.

Maternity care, family planning, and medical care are uniformly considered to be of high priority. Nutrition and malaria surveillance, along with measles immunization, receive strong, but not universal, support. Not more than one or two individuals stress the importance of other items, and they are dropped from the next stage of appraisal.

Focusing attention on the six items about which members have indicated they feel most strongly, the panel should be able to translate those views into more refined priority scores. The Delphi technique is used to assemble and compare their ratings. It is to be hoped that the results indicate consensus regarding not only the order of priorities but the relative distance between them.

COMPATIBILITY AMONG PRIORITIES AND OBJECTIVES

No matter how systematically the matter of priority setting may be pursued, the element of human judgment remains. Objectives growing out of the priorities are likewise somewhat arbitrary. As indicated earlier, individually reasonable intentions may not make sense when taken together. To put this assertion into concrete terms we consider one priority function, maternity care, and certain simple program objectives that emerge from it.

Table 21.2

ILLUSTRATIVE RANKING OF SERVICE PRIORITIES
USING NOMINAL GROUP TECHNIQUE

Service Category	Group Member Vote					Total Points	Priority
	A	B	C	D	E		
Documented List							
Patient Visits	4	8	4	6	5	27	III
Maternity Care	8	7	3	4	8	30	I
School Health Contacts		1		3	1	5	
Family Planning Motivation Visits	7			1		8	
Family Planning Acceptors	6	6	8	2	7	29	II
Malaria Surveillance Visits	3	4	6	7		20	V
Malaria Blood Smears			5			5	
Visits for Water, Drainage	2		2		3	7	
Other Items							
BCG Vaccination		2		5		7	
Measles Immunization	1	5		8	4	18	VI
Well Chlorination			1		2	3	
Nutrition Surveillance	5	3	7		6	21	IV

Source: Adapted from The Functional Analysis of Health Needs and Services, Table 4.5, page 269.

The Setting and Objectives

Assume that we are planning for a region of 250,000 population fairly evenly distributed over an area of 3,000 square kilometers. For simplicity, furthermore, we suppose that our plan is limited to maternity care, noting that the region's crude birth rate is 40 per 1,000 population, and approximately 30 percent of pregnancies are high-risk according to defined criteria.

The basic goal is to provide 80 percent of pregnant women access to maternity care of acceptable quantity and quality. The hierarchy of services contemplated include clinics (CL) with doctor (DR) to serve 25,000 population each, health posts (HP) with midwife (MW) for each 2,500 population, and one community health volunteer (CHV) per 1,000 population.

Being well-versed in planning techniques, we recognize the importance of stating objectives in measurable terms. Accordingly, acceptable care has been defined to include one physician visit and four midwife visits in case of normal pregnancy and twice as many contacts of each type in high-risk cases. Regardless of risk eight contacts with the CHV are planned.

A survey of provider availability and productivity has led to the following annual performance standards: 1,000 maternity contacts per DR, 600 service contacts per MW, and 400 contacts per CHV.

Services are considered *accessible* if there is a health post within five kilometers of the patient and a clinic within ten kilometers.

Implications

Individually the preceding definitions, standards, and targets seem quite reasonable; indeed similar ones in actual use could easily be cited. But what are the implications, and are they mutually compatible?

These questions need to be addressed in relation to three types of indicators that emerge from the preceding scenario: (1) numbers of facilities required, (2) personnel required and their organization by facility type, and (3) maximum travel distances to facilities. The scenario also includes three categories of targets to be considered in sequence in the following three sections. Data from the resulting analyses are summarized in Table 21.3.

Resources/Population Ratios

The specification that a population of 250,000 is to be served by one clinic per 25,000 staffed by a doctor suggests a need for ten clinics and a comparable number of physicians. Similarly, the specified population per health post dictates the requirement for 100 health posts and midwives. It might be assumed that additional midwives would be employed at the clinics, but such staffing standards have not been made explicit. Finally, the stated target for coverage by CHVs carries with it the need for 250 community workers.

Designation of the number of facilities to be operated in an area of 3,000 square kilometers connotes travel distances, regardless of whether these are made explicit. In particular if ten clinics are uniformly distributed over the region, each will cover 300 square kilometers. The service area might be considered to be in the form of a circle, but circles arranged tangentially to one another leave slight gaps between

Table 21.3

REVIEW OF RESOURCES INDICATORS

Basis for Targets	Facilities		Personnel			Max. Travel	
	CL	HP	DR	MW	CHV	M_{CL}	M_{HP}
Resources/Population	10	100	10	100	250	10.7	3.4
Acceptability	11	70	11	70	160	10.2	4.1
Accessibility	12	47	12	47	-	10.0	5.0

Targets Enclosed are Implied from Others.

them. Instead, we consider service areas in the form of hexagons nested together in honeycomb fashion. Using M to symbolize the distance from the center of the hexagon to each vertex; that is, the maximum distance from the centered facility to the most peripheral area, the area (A) of the hexagon, can be calculated as

$$A = 1.5\sqrt{3}M^2 \qquad (21.1)$$
$$= 2.6M^2.$$

For specified A, then,

$$M^2 = \frac{A}{1.5\sqrt{3}},$$

or

$$M = 0.62\sqrt{A}. \qquad (21.2)$$

Thus with $A = 300$,

$$M_{CL} = 0.62\sqrt{300}$$
$$= 10.7 \text{ kilometers.}$$

Comparably the 100 health posts would each serve 30 square kilometers and

$$M_{HP} = 0.62\sqrt{30}$$
$$= 3.4 \text{ kilometers.}$$

Note that M_{CL} and M_{HP} differ in the terms $\sqrt{300}$ and $\sqrt{30}$, respectively. That is, M_{CL} is $\sqrt{10}$ times as large as M_{HP}. The relationship arises from the fact that there are to be ten times as many health posts as clinics.

Acceptability Considerations

The acceptability criteria have direct implications for personnel requirements, as determined in Table 21.4. First, a crude birth rate of 40 in a population of 250,000 leads to 10,000 deliveries annually, 30 percent of which are expected to be high-risk cases. Eighty percent coverage means services in 5,600 normal pregnancies and 2,400 high-risk cases (apart from further assumptions regarding more complete coverage of the latter).

The tally of individual services provided for this caseload on the basis of defined service standards is shown to the right in Table 21.4. To illustrate, the 5,600 normal pregnancies receiving one physician contact each, coupled with two visits for each of the 2,400 high-risk cases, yields 10,400 doctor contacts in all. Since each physician can handle 1,000 antenatal visits per year, 10.4 physicians are needed. This has been rounded upward in Table 21.3 to the next highest integer. Similarly, the need for 70 midwives and 160 community workers has been transferred to Table 21.3.

The personnel requirements translate into a need for 11 health centers and 70 health posts, or fewer, considering the possibility that some of the midwives might be assigned to clinics, which would serve, in effect, as health posts for the nearby population. In any case, considerations of service need and productivity, that is, acceptability criteria, suggest that 100 health posts and 250 CHVs would be excessive.

Table 21.4

CALCULATION OF SERVICE LOADS

Measure	Cases		Services		
	Total	80% Cov.	DR	MW	CHV
Normal Preg.	7,000	5,600	5,600	22,400	44,800
High-Risk	3,000	2,400	4,800	19,200	19,200
Total	10,000	8,000	10,400	41,600	64,000
Productivity			1,000	600	400
Personnel			10.4	69.3	160.0

Would as few as 70 health posts provide satisfactory access, however? Seventy posts distributed over three thousand square kilometers implies service areas

$$A_{HP} = \frac{3,000}{70}$$
$$= 43 \text{ square kilometers.}$$

Application of Equation 21.1 yields, in turn,

$$M_{HP} = 0.62\sqrt{43}$$
$$= 4.1 \text{ kilometers,}$$

which is still well below the five kilometer limit considered tolerable.

By the same token

$$A_{CL} = \frac{3,000}{11}$$
$$= 273 \text{ square kilometers,}$$

and

$$M_{CL} = .62\sqrt{273}$$
$$= 10.2 \text{ kilometers.}$$

Accessibility Criteria

Considering the requirement that all members of the population be within ten kilometers of a clinic, we find (Eq. 21.1) that the resulting service area would be

$$A = (2.6)(10)^2$$
$$= 260 \text{ square kilometers.}$$

Over the total area of three thousand square kilometers, then,

$$\frac{3,000}{260} = 11.5,$$

or 12 clinics would be needed. Similar calculations for health posts shows a need for 46.2, or 47, facilities. The staffing implications of these results suggest a need for at least 12 doctors and 47 midwives, shown in Table 21.3.

We see in Equation 21.1 that the service area, and consequently the number of facilities required for coverage, is a function of the square of the maximum travel distance. Thus if maximum travel to a health post is to be half that to a clinic, then health posts must be four times as numerous as clinics. This is a much different ratio from that associated with the arbitrary stipulation that the population served by a clinic should be ten times that served by a health post.

Attainment of Compatibility

The three approaches to target-setting summarized in Table 21.3 produce widely different resources indicators. The need for health posts and midwives is especially ambiguous, depending upon the basis for determining need.

Ambiguities arise when resources planning proceeds arbitrarily apart from considerations of the magnitude of health problems and consequent service requirements. Population/resource ratios are commonly specified, but their realism is by no means assured. Nor is any one ratio uniformly valid in all settings.

More appropriately one begins the planning process with identification of the principal health problems of the community, translates these into service requirements, and then derives resource needs and their configuration. The first iteration of this process is likely to produce derived resource requirements that cannot feasibly be met. Following this approach, however, the further iterations in the process made necessary by the need for compromise will lead to rational priority setting based upon factual information rather than seemingly reasonable, but arbitrary and possibly unrealistic, targets.

In the illustrative case, we proceed from a service program that dictates the need for at least 11 physicians, 70 MWs, and 160 CHVs. Assignment of the doctors to eleven clinics would provide adequate accessibility in that virtually everyone would reside within ten kilometers of a facility. Each clinic might also be staffed by a midwife and serve, in effect, as a health post for the adjacent population. Fifty-nine separate health posts would be needed in addition.

More detailed job analysis might lead to the staffing of each clinic by 1 doctor and 2 midwives. The remaining midwives employed in forty-eight health posts would be within the requisite five kilometers of all residents.

For service purposes, 160 CHVs would be adequate, but this would mean one worker per 1,600 population rather than 1,000. This distribution may or may not be satisfactory, depending upon the size and configuration of communities. If, for accessibility reasons, 250 workers are required, consideration might be given to the assignment of additional tasks. Indeed decisions regarding all aspects of the organization of care flow from the initial assumptions regarding service standards, work assignments, and productivity levels. These assumptions might be questioned and the ramifications of other assumptions investigated.

While relatively simplistic, the illustration we have followed in detail conveys the fundamentally important message that planning should focus first and foremost on the realistic satisfaction of priority human needs, taking care that the planning efforts result in mutually compatible and achievable measures of input (resources indicators) and output (accessible services of acceptable quantity, quality, and efficacy).

REFERENCES

1. Correa, Hector, and Wafik A. Hassouna, "Model for the Integration of Health and Nutrition Planning", *Development and Change*, 3,4:51–61, 1975.
2. Department of International Health, Johns Hopkins University, *The Functional Analysis of Health Needs and Services*, Ch. 4, pp. 239–281, New Delhi: Asia Publishing House, 1976.

PRIMARY READINGS

Department of International Health, Johns Hopkins University, *The Functional Analysis of Health Needs and Services*, Ch. 4, pp. 239–281, New Delhi: Asia Publishing House, 1976. A comprehensive description of the streamlined application of functional analysis to the routine appraisal of services delivery.
Feldstein, Martin S., M. A. Piot and T. K. Sundaresan, *Resource Allocation Model for Public Health Planning: A Case Study of Tuberculosis Control*, Department of Economics, Cambridge, MA: Harvard University, 1973. Analysis of resource allocation in a situation in which derivation of a mathematically optimum solution is possible.
Stiffman, Lawrence H., *Some Health Sector Analysis Methods for Developing Nations*, School of Public Health, Ann Arbor: University of Michigan, 1974. Describes highly structured computer models that can be useful in teaching health planning.

SECONDARY READINGS

Correa, Hector, and Wafik A. Hassouna, "Model for the Integration of Health and Nutrition Planning," *Development and Change*, 3,4:51–61, 1975.
Dietz, K., L. Molineaux and A. Thomas, "A Malaria Model Tested in the African Savannah," *WHO Bulletin*, 50:347–357, 1974.
Hansen, James V., "Computer-Assisted Planning for Regional Health Care Programs," *Socioeconomic Planning Science*, 9,5:239–245, 1975.

Index

Acceptable care, 279, 281–82
Accessibility, 282–83
Accountability, 27, 158
Accounting of program operations, 51
Action research, 33. *See also* Operations research
Additive law of probability, 194
Adjusted rates, 124
Advisory groups, 79–80
Age-specific fertility rates, 228. *See also* Birth rates
Age structure, 103–6
Alma Ata Conference, 172, 174
Annual plan and budget, 5
Associations of causality, 34, 123
Attrition, 229–31, 251–52. *See also* Personnel losses
Availability of services, 114

Banfield, Edward C., 82
Baseline estimates, 227–28
Benefit-cost ratio. *See* Cost-benefit analysis
Birth rates, 103–6. *See also* Age-specific fertility rates
Births averted, 270
Blum, Henrik L., 79
Budgeting, 157–69
    capital budgets, 165
    development budgets, 165
    line-item budgets, 166
    performance budgets, 167–69
    program budgets, 166–67
    recurrent cost budgets, 165
    routine budgets, 165
Bureau of the Census, 114

Capitation, 164
Categories, health personnel, 132–33
Centralized responsibilities, 8–9
Chain of command, 188–89
Chile, 81, 83

Committee approach to planning, 6
Communicable disease reports, 126
Communications, 179, 191–94. *See also* Management information systems
Community action model, 82
Community financing, 160, 180–81
Community health workers, 177
Community laboratories, 40
Community organization, 176–77
Community surveys. *See* Sample surveys
Comparative analysis, 32, 222–23
Comparative method of supply analysis, 139
Component method, 114–15
Composition, population, 229–35
Comprehensive planning, 6
Conscientization, 175
Constituencies, 77
Constraints, 67–68, 75, 152–53
Construction costs, 149–51
Consultants, use of, 153–54
Consumer participation, 10, 23, 34, 77, 80, 172–84
Continuing education, 26
Cooper, Barbara, 265
Cost analysis, 90–92, 157
Cost-benefit analysis, 261–70
Cost centers, 159
Cost control, 158
Cost-effectiveness, 49, 157, 261, 270–73
Cost recovery, 34
Cost of uncertainty, 196
Current Population Survey, 107

Deaths averted, 270–72
Debt servicing, 151
Decentralization, 7–8, 9–10, 16, 22, 27, 34, 159
Decision analysis, 43–44, 194–98, 239–41
Deficit financing, 95, 163
Delbecq, Andre, 204
Delphi technique, 205–6, 278